Principles and Practice of

TRAUMA CARE

Principles and Practice of TRAUMA CARE

SECOND EDITION

SK Kochar MS (Gen Surg)
Formerly Senior Adviser and Head
Department of Surgery
Army Base Hospital
New Delhi, India

Past President
Indian Association of Traumatology and Critical Care

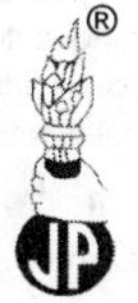

JAYPEE BROTHERS MEDICAL PUBLISHERS (P) LTD

New Delhi • London • Philadelphia • Panama

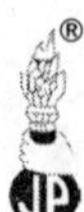

Jaypee Brothers Medical Publishers (P) Ltd

Headquarters

Jaypee Brothers Medical Publishers (P) Ltd
4838/24, Ansari Road, Daryaganj
New Delhi 110 002, India
Phone: +91-11-43574357
Fax: +91-11-43574314
Email: jaypee@jaypeebrothers.com

Overseas Offices

J.P. Medical Ltd
83 Victoria Street, London
SW1H 0HW (UK)
Phone: +44-2031708910
Fax: +02-03-0086180
Email: info@jpmedpub.com

Jaypee-Highlights Medical Publishers Inc.
City of Knowledge, Bld. 237, Clayton
Panama City, Panama
Phone: +507-301-0496
Fax: +507-301-0499
Email: cservice@jphmedical.com

Jaypee Brothers Medical Publishers Ltd
The Bourse
111 South Independence Mall East
Suite 835, Philadelphia, PA 19106, USA
Phone: + 267-519-9789
Email: joe.rusko@jaypeebrothers.com

Jaypee Brothers Medical Publishers (P) Ltd
17/1-B Babar Road, Block-B, Shaymali
Mohammadpur, Dhaka-1207
Bangladesh
Mobile: +08801912003485
Email: jaypeedhaka@gmail.com

Jaypee Brothers Medical Publishers (P) Ltd
Shorakhute, Kathmandu
Nepal
Phone: +00977-9841528578
Email: jaypee.nepal@gmail.com

Website: www.jaypeebrothers.com
Website: www.jaypeedigital.com

Inquiries for bulk sales may be solicited at: jaypee@jaypeebrothers.com

Principles and Practice of Trauma Care

First Edition: 1998

Second Edition: **2013**

ISBN 978-93-5025-717-3

Printed at Rajkamal Electric Press, Plot No. 2, Phase-IV, Kundli, Haryana.

Contributors

Alok Kumar Jha
MS MCh
Consultant Urologist
Sitaram Bhartia Hospital
New Delhi, India

B Easwaran
MS
Senior Associate Professor
Department of Surgery
School of Medicine
The Asian Institute of Medicine, Science and Technology (AIMST) University
Bedong, Kedah, Malaysia

(Brig) Gurjit Singh
MS FACS FAIS
Professor and Head
Department of General Surgery
Padmashree DY Patil Medical College
Pune, Maharashtra, India

(Brig) PK Sahoo
MS (Gen Surg) MCh (Neuro Surg)
Chief Neurosurgeon
Tata Hospital
Jamshedpur, Jharkhand, India

(Brig) VK Sinha
MS (Gen Surg) DNB (Ortho)
Professor
Department of Orthopedics
Armed Forces Medical College
Pune, Maharashtra, India

(Col) Kumud Rai
MS FICS FIACS
Director Vascular Surgery
Max Hospital
New Delhi, India

(Col) M Arora
MS MCh
Senior Adviser and Professor
Department of Pediatric Surgery
Army Base Hospital
New Delhi, India

(Col) SK Kochar
MS (Gen Surg)
Formerly Senior Adviser and Head
Department of Surgery
Army Base Hospital
New Delhi, India

(Col) Subhash Kotwal
MS MCh (Urology)
Chief Urologist
Sitaram Bhartia Hospital
New Delhi, India

DK Sarma
MS
Professor
Department of Surgery
Guwahati Medical College
Guwahati, Assam, India

PM Deka
MS MCh
Professor and Head
Department of Urology
Guwahati Medical College
Guwahati, Assam, India

Siddharth Pramod Dubhashi
MS
Associate Professor
Padmashree DY Patil Medical College
Pune, Maharashtra, India

Preface to the Second Edition

Till recently, trauma was limited to military precincts and trauma care evolved under constraints of military operations. Slow and difficult evacuation, poor lighting and operative conditions, nonavailability of diagnostic aids, inadequate and irregular supply of blood, paucity of potent antibiotics, primitive intensive care facility, transient patient and surgeon population were some of the controlling factors for safe and staged procedures to evolve. Stress was to save the life and limb, and the morbidity took the back seat. Principles of trauma surgery learned and practiced during war became the Bible for surgeons in civil practice, who, as such, had sporadic exposure to trauma care.

However, the scene has changed. Wars have become far and few, industrialization, increased road traffic accidents, upsurge of violence and terrorism have brought trauma at the doorsteps of the surgeon whether he is at subdistrict hospital or in a university hospital. Simultaneously, with it has evolved, rapid evacuation, energetic resuscitation, easy availability of blood, good paraoperative care, ideal operative conditions, potent antibiotics, widespread use of diagnostic peritoneal lavage and ready availability of ultrasonography (USG) and computed tomography (CT) scan. These developments are responsible for the current trends in trauma care. Older concepts have been challenged and new methods of treatment have been advocated, leaving the poor surgeon in a dilemma. The aim of this book is to steer clear of controversies and present a balanced view. It was intended to be a single author effort; but, I soon realized that in this era of superspecialization, multidisciplinary approach is the order of the day. My colleagues in the Armed Forces Medical College and trauma experts in the civil services soon joined hands and we produced the first edition in 1998.

Since the first edition, there have been increasing understanding the need of organizing and providing trauma care. Prehospital and inhospital trauma care is finding its way into planning of health care, diagnostics had a quantum jump. Computed tomography (CT) scan and magnetic resonance imaging (MRI) are easily available and affordable. Ambulances have improved. Noninvasive investigations and nonoperative management is making headway; endoscopy and laparoscopy are being added to the trauma surgeon's armamentarium. All these changes have necessitated the need of second edition. Few chapters have been written by new authors and few new chapters have been added.

I am grateful to Professor (Brig) Gurjit Singh, Professor Siddharth Pramod Dubhashi, Dr (Col) SV Kotwal, Dr Alok Kumar Jha, Dr (Col) Kumud Rai, Dr (Brig) PK Sahoo, Dr (Brig) VK Sinha, Professor PM Deka, Professor DK Sarma, and (Col) M Arora, for contributing specialized chapters. Illustrations by nursing colleagues Swapna Basu and Tara Rajan have been retained. You may write a book but it cannot see the light of the day till it is not published. M/s Jaypee Brothers Medical Publishers (P) Ltd, New Delhi, India, extended their golden hand no sooner than I approached them. Their constant inspiration and support boosted my morale.

Well, the person who suffers most when you spend your leisure hours sitting in front of computer and burn midnight electricity is none other than your better half. My sincere gratitude to Dr (Mrs) Shalini Kochar for bearing with me. I am indebted to Professor GC Sharma, Maj Gen P Subhas, Air Marshal NB Amaresh, my "Gurus"and mentors in surgery, who have greatly influenced my surgical practice.

SK Kochar

Preface to the First Edition

Till recently trauma was limited to military precincts and trauma care evolved under constraints of military operations. Slow and difficult evacuation, poor lighting and operative conditions, nonavailability of diagnostic aids, inadequate and irregular supply of blood, paucity of potent antibiotics, primitive intensive care facility, transient patient and surgeon population were some of the controlling factors for safe and staged procedures to evolve. Stress was to save the life and limb, and the morbidity took the back seat. Principles of trauma surgery learned and practiced during war became the Bible for surgeons in civil practice, who as such had sporadic exposure to trauma care. However, the scene has changed. Wars have become far and few, industrialization, increased road traffic accidents, upsurge of violence and terrorism have brought trauma at the doorsteps of the surgeon whether he is at subdistrict hospital or in a university hospital. Simultaneously, it has evolved, rapid evacuation, energetic resuscitation, easy availability of blood, good paraoperative care, ideal operative conditions, potent antibiotics, widespread use of diagnostic peritoneal lavage and ready availability of ultrasonography (USG) and computed tomography (CT) scan. These developments are responsible for the current trends in trauma care. Older concepts have been challenged and new methods of treatment have been advocated, leaving the poor surgeon in a dilemma. The aim of this book is to steer clear of controversies and present a balanced view. It was intended to be a single author effort; but, I soon realized that in this era of superspecialization, multidisciplinary approach is the order of the day. My colleagues in the Armed Forces Medical College and trauma experts in the civil services soon joined hands and here we are with our efforts. I am grateful to Col SK Kotwal, Lt Col Kumud Rai, Lt Col PK Sahoo, Lt Col VK Sinha, Professor A Indrayan, Professor PS Ramani, Professor AK Mahapatra, Professor PM Deka, Professor DK Sarma and Professor DP Sanan, for contributing specialized chapters. Illustrations became a necessity and my nursing colleagues Swapna Basu and Tara Rajan chipped in with excellent diagrams. You may write a book but it cannot see the light of the day till it is not published. M/s Jaypee Brothers Medical Publishers (P) Ltd, New Delhi, India, extended their golden hand no sooner than I approached them. Their constant inspiration and support boosted my morale. Well, the person who suffers most when you spend your leisure hours sitting in front of computer and burn midnight electricity is none other than your better half. My sincere gratitude to Dr (Mrs) Shalini Kochar for bearing with me. I am grateful to Brig YD Sharma, Commandant, 151 Base Hospital, for encouraging me from time-to-time and granting me permission to publish the work. I am indebted to Professor GC Sharma, Formerly Professor and Head, Department of Surgery, Sawai Man Singh (SMS) Medical College, Jaipur, Rajasthan, India, and Brig (Dr) P Subhas, my teachers and Guru in surgery, who have greatly influenced my surgical practice.

SK Kochar

Contents

PLATE 1

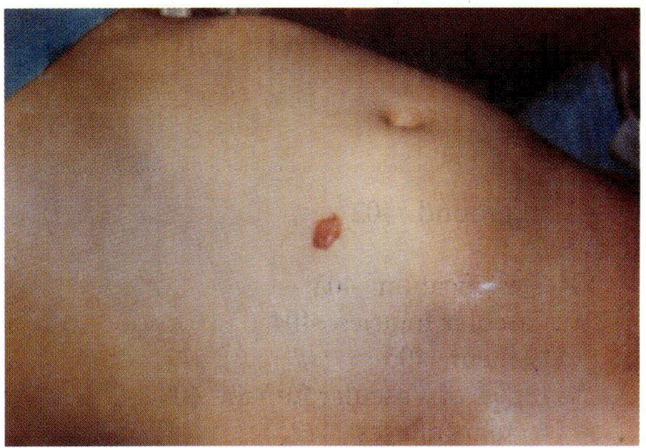

Fig. 4.2: Point of exit of bullet in Figure 4.1 case

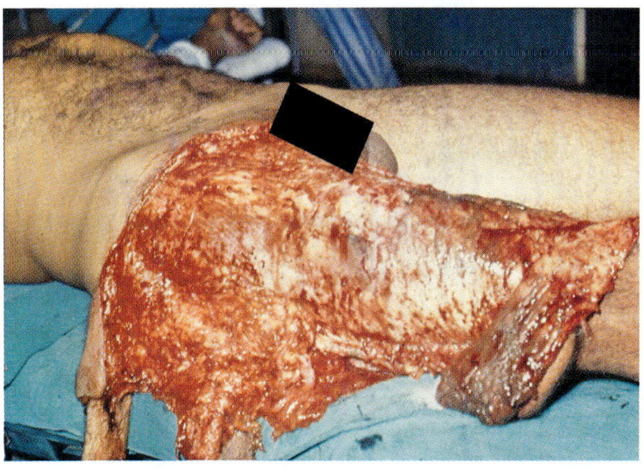

Fig. 6.1: Extensive degloving injury in RTA

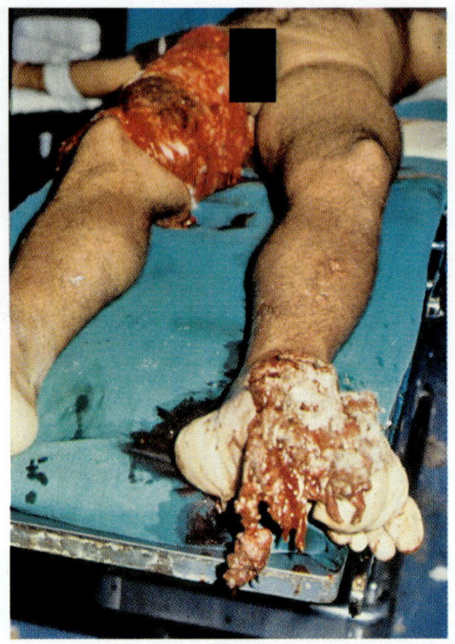

Fig. 6.2: Extensive injury in a rail accident victim

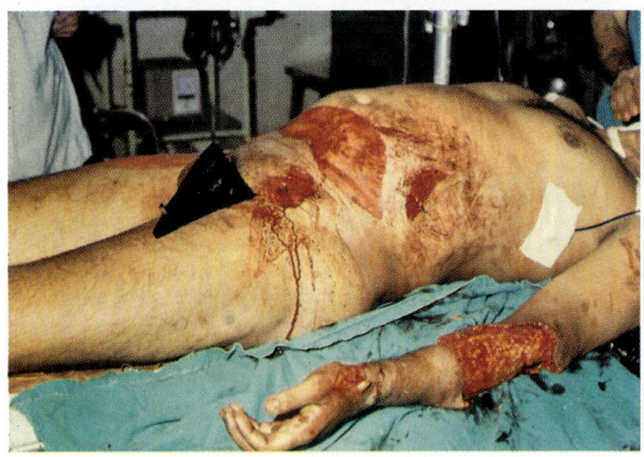

Fig. 6.3: Polytrauma in road traffic accident

PLATE 3

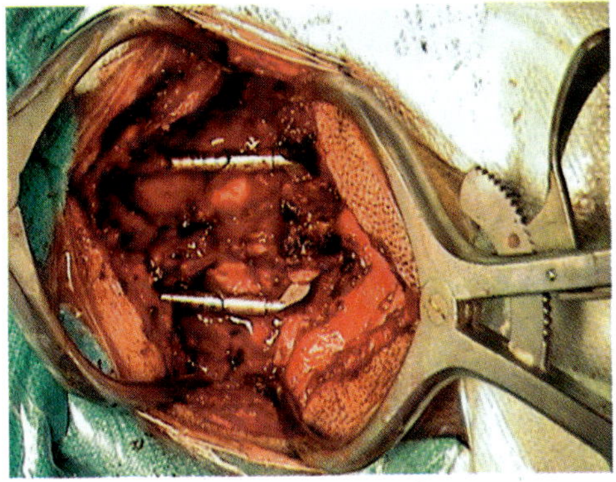

Fig. 10.14: Posterior cervical fusion by Apofix

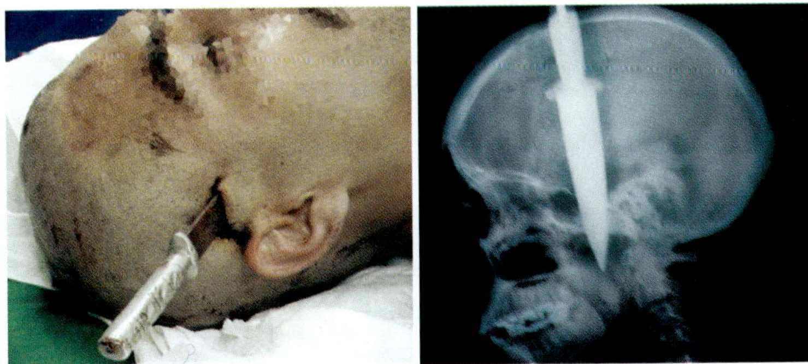

Fig. 11.7: Penetrating injury head with knife

PLATE 4

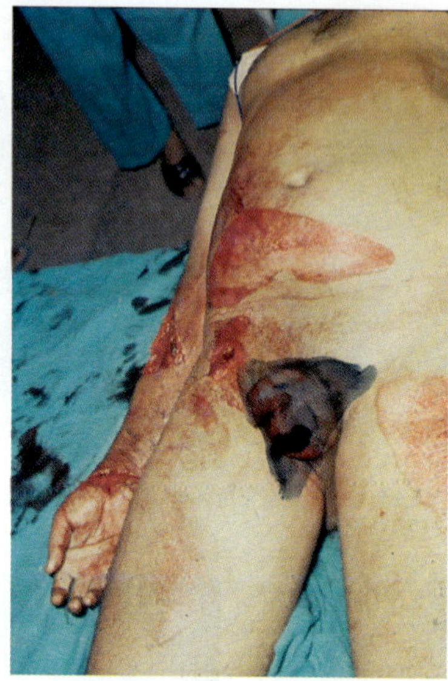

Fig. 16.7: Road traffic accident. Tell tale abrasions on the abdominal wall

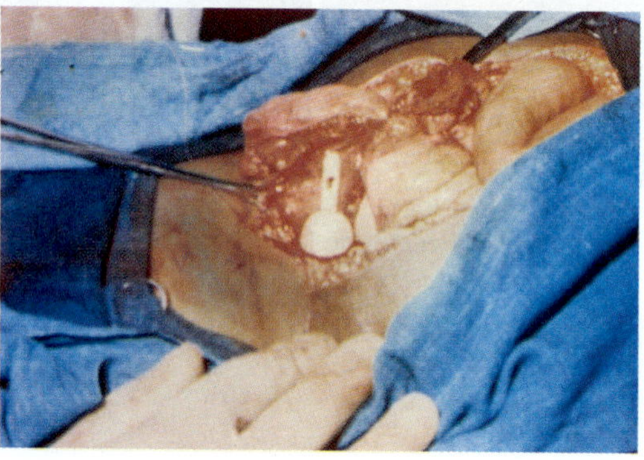

Fig. 16.8: Blunt injury abdomen, transection of sigmoid colon and bladder rupture

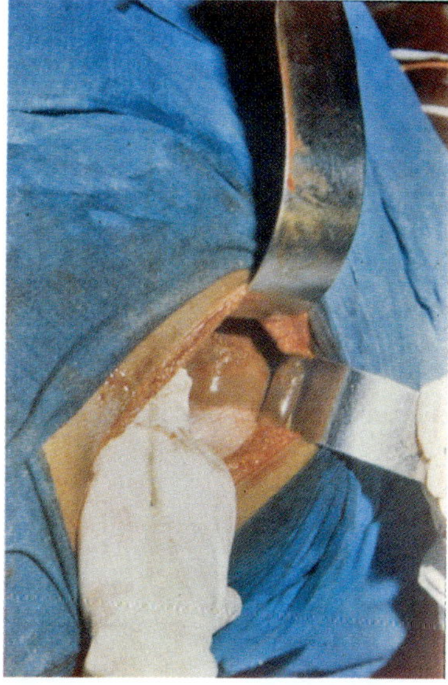

Fig. 16.9: Gunshot wound abdomen grazing the liver which could have been treated conservatively

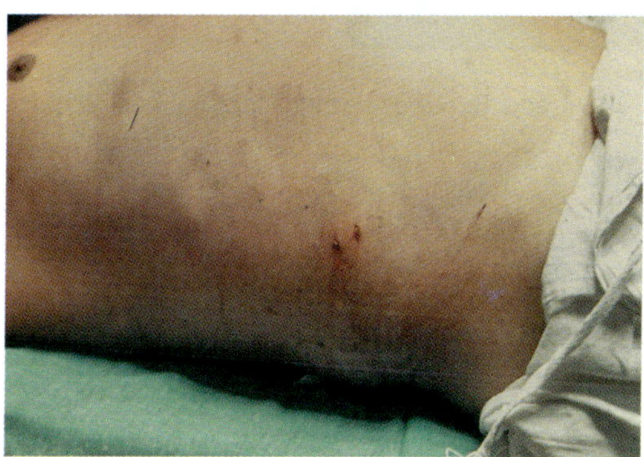

Fig. 16.10: Penetrating injury abdomen

PLATE 6

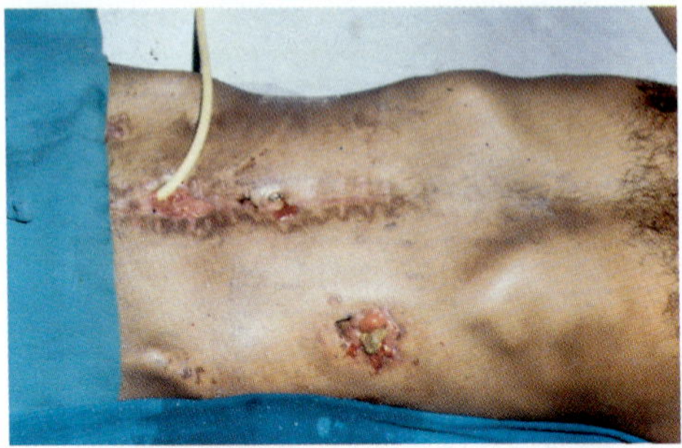

Fig. 23.3: Gunshot wound abdomen. Colonic injury treated with proximal colostomy

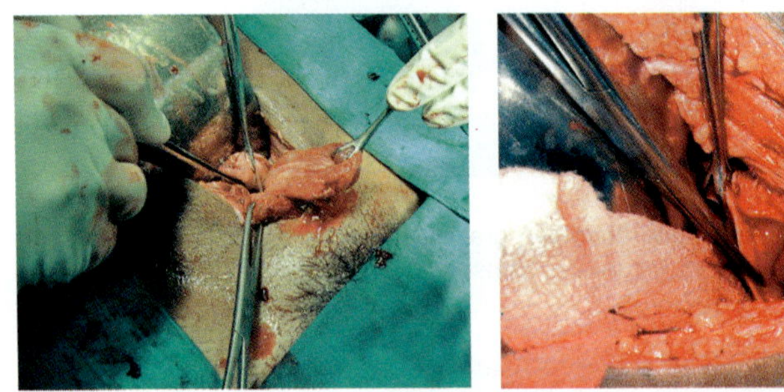

Figs. 24.9A and B: Repair of intraperitoneal rupture of bladder

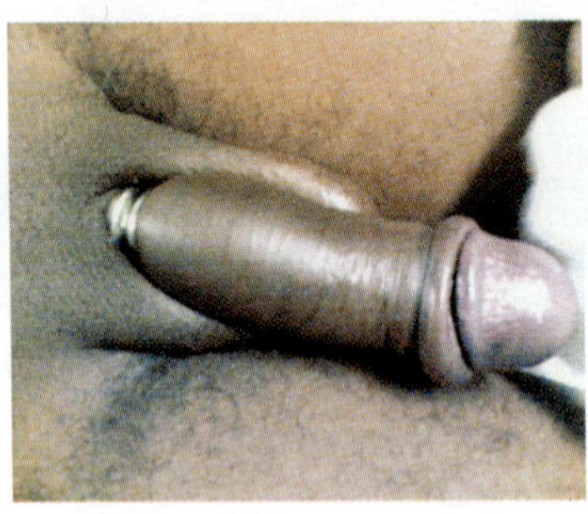

Fig. 25.1: Metal ring around root of penis (strangulation injury of penis)

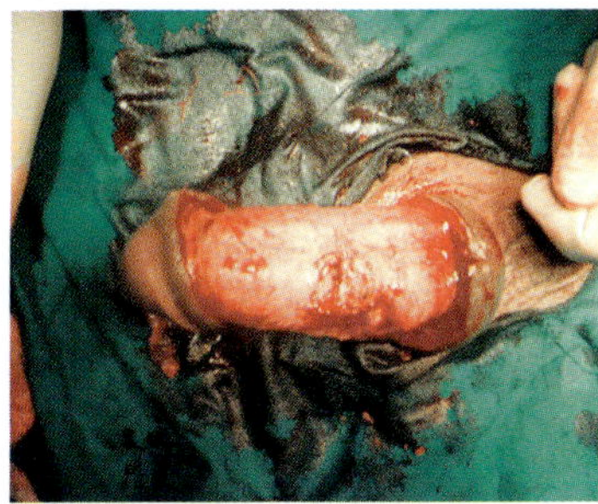

Fig. 25.2: Degloving injury of penis

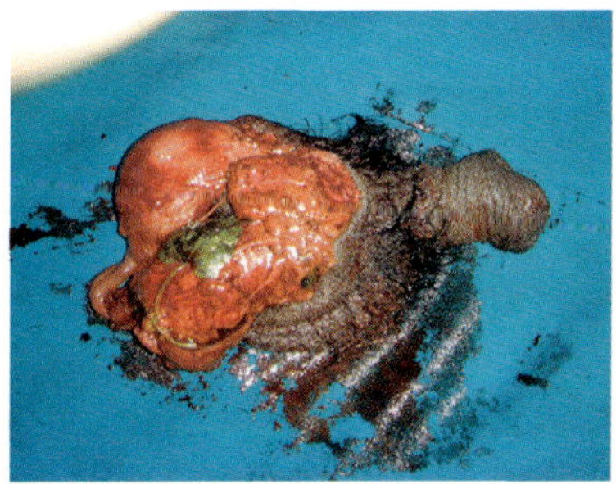

Fig. 25.3: Machine tool injury of penis

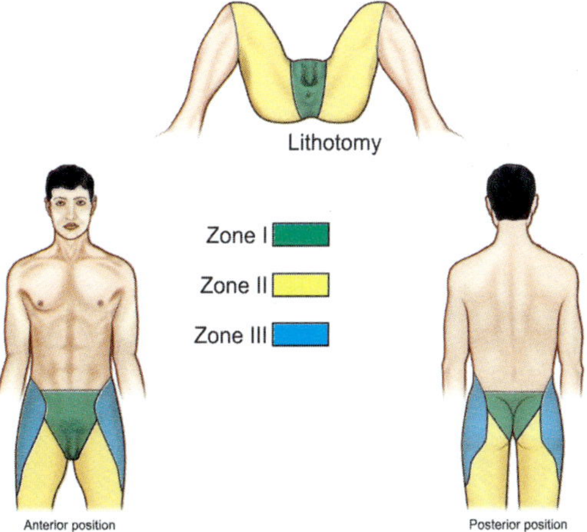

Fig. 27.10: Faringer's classification of wounds in different zones. Zone I injuries often require colostomy, zone II injuries are diverted selectively, with wounds into subcutaneous fat of anterior groin or medial thigh possibly requiring colostomy. Diversion is rarely required for zone III wounds

Essential Trauma Care

SK Kochar

Over 1.2 million people die each year on the world's roads, and between 20 and 50 million suffer non-fatal injuries (Table 1.1). Research from Bangalore, India found that mortality from road traffic injuries was 13.1 and 48.1 per 100000 in the poorer socioeconomic groups of urban and rural populations respectively, compared to 7.8 and 26.1 per 100000 among their more affluent urban and rural counterparts.[1] Poor families are less likely to have finance resources to pay the direct and indirect costs related to a road crash. Road traffic injuries account for 20-50% of emergency room registrations and, 60-70 of people hospitalized with traumatic brain injuries.[2]

In most regions of the world this epidemic of road traffic injuries is still increasing. In the past five years most countries have endorsed the recommendations of the World report on road traffic injury prevention which give guidance on how countries can implement a comprehensive approach to improving road safety and reducing the death toll on their roads. To date, however, there has been no global assessment of road safety that indicates the extent to which this approach is being implemented.

The Global status report[3] presents a number of key findings: low-income countries have higher road traffic fatality rates (21.5 and 19.5 per 100,000 populations, respectively) than high-income countries (10.3 per 100,000). Over 90% of the world's fatalities on the roads occur in low-income and middle-income countries, which have only 48% of the world's registered vehicles. Almost half of those who die on the road traffic crashes are pedestrians, cyclist or users of motorized two wheelers-collectively known as vulnerable road users"-and this proportion is higher in poor

Table 1.1: Leading causes of death, 2004 and 2030 compared

Year 2004 *Rank leading cause%*	*Year 2030* *Rank leading cause%*
• Ischemic heart disease 12.2	• Ischemic heart disease 12.2
• Cerebrovascular disease 9.7	• Cerebrovascular disease 9.7
• Lower respiratory infections 7.0	• Chronic obstructive pulmonary disease 7.0
• Chronic obstructive pulmonary disease 5.1	• Lower respiratory infections 5.1
• Diarrheal diseases 3.6	• Road traffic injuries 3.6
• HIV/AIDS 3.5	• Trachea, bronchus, lung cancers 3.5
• Tuberculosis 2.5	• Diabetes mellitus 2.5
• Trachea, bronchus, lung cancers 2.3	• Hypertensive heart disease 2.3
• Road traffic injuries 2.2	• Stomach cancer 2.2
• Prematurity and low birth weight 2.0	• HIV/AIDS 2.0
• Neonatal infections and other 1.9	• Nephritis and nephrosis 1.9
• Diabetes mellitus 1.9	• Self-inflicted injuries 1.9
• Malaria 1.7	• Liver cancer 1.7
• Hypertensive heart diseases 1.7	• Colon and rectum cancer 1.7
• Birth asphyxia and birth trauma 1.5	• Esophagus cancers 1.5
• Self-inflicted injuries 1.4	• Violence 1.4
• Stomach cancer 1.4	• Alzheimer and other dementias 1.4
• Cirrhosis of the liver 1.3	• Cirrhosis of the liver 1.3
• Nephritis and nephrosis 1.3	• Breast cancer 1.3
• Colon and rectum cancers 1.1	• Tuberculosis 1.1

(***Source:*** World health statistics 2008 www.who.int/whosis/whostat/2008/en/index.html)

economies of the world. The adoption and enforcement of traffic laws appears inadequate in many countries. The development and effective enforcement of legislation is critical in reducing drink-driving and excessive speed and in increasing the use of helmets and child restraints. The report shows that huge gaps remain in the quality and coverage of the data that countries collect and report on road traffic injuries. Reliable data on fatalities and nonfatal injuries are needed by countries to assess the scope of the road traffic injury problem, to target responses to it and to monitor and evaluate the effectiveness of intervention measures.

Key Recommendation of Global Status Report Are

Government need to take into consideration the need of all road users when making policy decisions that impact on road safety. To date the needs of vulnerable road users have been neglected in many countries and should be given renewed emphasis, particularly when decisions are made about road in infrastructure, land use planning and transport services.

Government need to enact comprehensive laws that require all road users to be protected through enforcement of speed limits that are appropriate to the type and function of the road, through the stipulation of blood alcohol concentration limits to reduce drink-driving, and through the use of appropriate occupant protection measures.

The enforcement of comprehensive and clear legislation with appropriate penalties and accompanied by public awareness campaigns is a critical factor in reducing road traffic injuries and deaths. Government needs to ensure that the institutions nominated as responsible for action on road safety are fostering multisectorial collaboration and the necessary human and financial resources to act effectively.

Systems Approach to Road Safety

A. Admission to the system, Licensing of vehicle and people
B. Enforcement of road rules
C. Understanding of crashes and risks
D. Education and information
E. Safe vehicle
F. Safe speed safe roads and road sides
G. Working to prevent crashes that result in serious injury or death.
H. Human tolerance to physical force, crash helmet, seat belt, air bag, child restraints.

Evaluation of road traffic safety program from India as done by global safety report is shown in Table 1.2.

Table 1.2: Traffic safety program India (Global safety report)

INDIA	
Population	1,169,015,509
Income group	Low
Gross national income per capita	45000INR
POST-CRASH CARE	
Formal, publicly available pre-hospital care system	Yes
National universal access number DATA	Yes
Reported road traffic fatalities	(2006)
105725 (84% males, 16% females)	
Reported non-fatal road traffic injuries 452922	(2006)
Costing study availableYes (deaths and injuries)	
Police data, defined as died within 30 days of the crash	
INSTITUTIONAL FRAMEWORK	
Lead agency department of road transport and highways	
Funded in national budget	Yes
National road safety strategy	
Measurable targets funded	Yes
Not formally endorsed by government	
REGISTERED VEHICLES	
72,718,000 total (2004)	
Trucks and Lorries	3%
Light motor vehicles (goods and passengers)	5%
Buses	1%
Two wheelers	71%
Cars, jeeps and taxis	13%
Tractors and trailers	6%
Other	15
TRENDS IN ROAD TRAFFIC DEATHS	
Number of road traffic deaths	
Year 2002	80,000
Year 2006	100,000
Source: National Crime Records Bureau	
NATIONAL LEGISLATION	
Speed limits set nationally No (subnationally)	
Local authorities can set lower limits yes	
Maximum limit urban roads yes/no	
Enforcement yes/no	
Drink–driving law	Yes
BAC limit—general population 0.03 g/dl	

Contd...

Contd...

BAC limit—young or novice drivers	0.03 g/dl
Random breath testing and/or police checkpoints	yes
Road traffic deaths involving alcohol	
Enforcement 3/10	
Motorcycle helmet law	Yes
Applies to all riders	Yes
Helmet standards mandated	Yes
Helmet wearing rate	-
Enforcement	2/10
Seat-belt law	Yes
Applies to all occupants	Yes
Seat-belt wearing rate	--
Enforcement	2/10
Child restraints law	No
Enforcement	NA
Enforcement score represents consensus based on professional opinion of respondents, on a scale of 0 to 10 where 0 is not effective and 10 is highly effective.	
VEHICLE STANDARDS	
Car manufacturers required to adhere to standards on	
Fuel	No
Seat-belt installation for all seats	No
ROAD SAFETY AUDITS	
Formal audits required for major new road construction projects	No
Regular audits of existing road infrastructure	No
PROMOTING ALTERNATIVE TRANSPORT	
National policies to promote walking or cycling	Yes
National policies to promote public transportation	Yes
(Data cleared by the Ministry of Health and Family Welfare)	
DEATHS BY ROAD USER CATEGORY	
Source: ("Road Accidents in India 2006." Ministry of Shipping, Road Transport and Highways)	
Passenger cars and taxis	(15%)
Unspecified	(11%)
Riders motorized 2- or 3-wheelers	(27%)
Cyclists	(4%)
Pedestrians	(13%)
Other	(29%)
Driver's 4-wheelers	(3%)
Other	(4%)

Essential trauma treatment services should realistically be made available to almost every injured person worldwide. By reinforcing inputs of: (1) human resources (training and staffing); and (2) physical resources (supplies and equipment). There are notable disparities in mortality rates for injured patients around the World. For example, one study looked at the mortality rates for all seriously injured adults (injury severity score of 9 or more) in three cities, in countries at different economic levels. The mortality rate (including both pre-hospital and in-hospital deaths) rose from 35% in a high-income setting to 55% in a middle- income setting, to 63% in a low-income setting.[4] Considering only patients who survive to reach the hospital, a similar study demonstrated a six-fold increase in mortality for patients with injuries of moderate severity (injury severity score of 15–24). Such mortality increased from 6% in a hospital in a high-income country to 36% in a rural area of a low-income country,[5] there is a tremendous burden of disability from extremity injuries in many developing countries.[5,6] By comparison, head and spinal cord injuries contribute a greater percentage of disability in high-income countries.[7] Much of the disability from extremity injuries in developing countries should be eminently preventable through inexpensive improvements in orthopedic care and rehabilitation.

Improved survival and functional outcome among injured patients in developed countries comes from high-cost equipment and technology. Unfortunatly, much of this may be unaffordable to the average injured person in the world for the foreseeable future. However, much of the improvement in patient outcome in higher-income countries has come from improvements in the organization of trauma care services.[8,9] Improvement in the organization of trauma services should be achievable in almost every setting and may represent a cost- effective way of improving patient outcomes.

Human Resources: Staffing and Training

It is important that the trauma center is adequately staffed with trained doctors, nurses and paramedics who had not only training in trauma care but in any area is likely to vary from 1 to 30 patients per day and it has a very serious effects on the revenues of the trauma center and staff and resources cannot be varied every other day and the idle staff and the facility drain the funds even in the developed countries. This one of the main criticism for having trauma centers. To offset this wastage of resources it will be very economical to couple up the trauma centers with emergencies of the hospital. A and E services record far better than the trauma centers. In fact there is growing trend to couple up trauma, emergencies and or acute care at these centers. Training of acute acre specialist, nurses and paramedics will encompass trauma, surgical emergencies Obs and medical emergencies at the present moments needs to be addressed separately.

Physical Resources Infrastructure, Equipment and Supplies

Many hospitals lack important equipment, some of which is inexpensive. The main reason for the absence of such vital equipment is a lack of organization and planning, rather than resource restrictions. Programs to assure the supply and maintenance of trauma-related equipment, appropriate to the specific circumstances of the given country, could help to address deficiencies of inexpensive but high-yield resources.

Process: Organization and Administration

In addition to assuring adequate supplies, improved administration could also assist in appropriate utilization. Delay at the casualty, delay in the X-ray and delay in activation of the operation theater are some of the week areas. These can be addressed by the medical audit and these are curable defects.

Efforts to Improve Trauma Care in Individual Countries

As an example of this, the American College of Surgeons (ACS) Committee on Trauma has significantly advanced the care of the injured in the United States and Canada by creating and promulgating the Advanced Trauma Life Support course (ATLS) and by the publication of Resources for optimal care of the injured patient.

In addition to efforts to improve care at individual hospitals, progress has been made by addressing the entire spectrum of the development of systems for trauma management. This involves political jurisdictions designating hospitals to fill the roles of trauma centers at varying levels of complexity, ranging from large urban centers to small rural hospitals. It also implies planning of emergency medical services, pre-hospital triage, transfer criteria and transfer arrangements between hospitals.

The planning of systems for trauma management implies several integrated functions, including political jurisdictions designating which hospitals are to fill the roles of trauma centers at varying levels of complexity, ranging from large urban trauma centers to small rural hospitals and clinics. It also implies the planning of mobile emergency medical services, pre-hospital triage (to determine which patients should go to which types of designated facilities), transfer criteria and transfer arrangements between hospitals.

When considering the relevance of these findings to the potential tility of similar organizational efforts in developing countries, it is important to note that the above improvements were mostly witnessed in comparison with environments with the same levels of resources. The enactment of an organized system for trauma management usually required inputs of resources that were fairly small in comparison with the overall cost of the existing system of care itself.

Rural clinics whose staff are not doctors are often the first source of care for injured patients in their communities. These are intermediate between pre-hospital and hospital-based in character, as regards trauma care. These can be categorized into three broad sets of needs:

1. Life-threatening injuries are appropriately treated, promptly and in accordance with appropriate priorities, so as to maximize the likelihood of survival.
2. Potentially disabling injuries are treated appropriately, so as to minimize functional impairment and to maximize the return to independence and to participation in community life.
3. Pain and psychological suffering are minimized.

Within these three broad categories, there are several specific medical goals that are eminently achievable within the resources available in most countries.

- Obstructed airways are opened and maintained before hypoxia leads to death or permanent disability.
- Impaired breathing is supported until the injured person is able to breathe adequately without assistance.

- Pneumothorax and hemothorax are promptly recognized and relieved.
- Bleeding (external or internal) is promptly stopped.
- Shock is recognized and treated with intravenous (IV) fluid replacement before irreversible consequences occur.
- The consequences of traumatic brain injury are lessened by timely decompression of space-occupying lesions and by prevention of secondary brain injury.
- Intestinal and other abdominal injuries are promptly recognized and repaired.
- Potentially disabling extremity injuries are corrected.
- Potentially unstable spinal cord injuries are recognized and managed appropriately, including early immobilization.
- The consequences to the individual of injuries that result in physical impairment are minimized by appropriate rehabilitative services.
- Medications for the above services and for the minimization of pain are readily available when needed.

The precise procedures that can optimally be applied to achieve these goals, as well as the human and physical resources needed to optimally carry out these procedures, will vary across the spectrum of economic resources of the nations of the world and the geographic location of the facilities concerned. However, these goals should be achievable for most injured patients in most locations. The provision of these services should not be dependent on ability to pay. Hence, cost recovery schemes, necessary though they may ultimately be, should not preclude the provision of initial emergency care nor of critical elements of definitive care. The provision of specific items of physical examination, diagnostic tests, medications and therapeutic procedures. Likewise, the ability of the health system to provide these items depends on the inputs of human resources (training and staffing) and physical resources (infrastructure, equipment and supplies).

Basic Facilities (Outpatient Clinics and/or Non-medical Providers)

Primary health care (PHC) clinics that are the mainstay of health care throughout many of the rural areas of low-income countries. These are almost exclusively staffed by non-doctor providers, such as village health workers, nurses and medical assistants. This category also includes outpatient clinics run by doctors, whether in urban or rural settings. In many cases, such facilities represent the first access for injured patients to the health care system. This is especially true in low-income countries where there are no formal emergency medical services (EMS).

Hospitals Staffed by General Practitioners

This includes hospitals without full-time specialist doctors, particularly those without a fully trained general surgeon. Such hospitals may or may not have operating theater capabilities. These facilities are usually referred to as district hospitals in Africa and primary health centers in India. In some areas, particularly in East Africa, certain medical assistants have been highly trained to act in the capacity of general practitioners, even performing operations such as cesarean section. The facilities in which they work are more likely to fall into this category, rather than the basic designation above.

Hospitals Staffed by Specialists

This includes hospitals whose personnel includes at least a general surgeon. Staff at such facilities may also include orthopedic surgeons and members of other subspecialties (i.e. specialists with responsibility for more narrowly defined fields within each specialty). Such facilities have operating theaters. These facilities are usually referred to as regional hospitals in Africa, community health centers or district hospitals in India, or general hospitals in Latin America.

Tertiary Care Hospitals

This includes hospitals with a broad range of subspecialties. Such facilities are usually, but not exclusively, teaching or university hospitals. They usually represent the highest level of care in a country or large political division within a country. There are notable differences in the capabilities of tertiary care hospitals worldwide. In some countries, surgical staff may be quite extensive in their range of subspecialties, and in others, more limited.

However, this is of great relevance to the accessibility of trauma care by the population of a country. These issues are addressed by broader planning activities and should be considered by those planning trauma services for their country or area. Likewise, it is recognized that the different levels of facility will play differing roles within overall trauma treatment in different countries. For example, facilities staffed by non-doctors and hospitals staffed by general practitioners are likely to care for a greater percentage of all injured patients in low-income countries, whereas specialist-staffed hospitals and tertiary care hospitals are likely to care for a greater percentage of all injured patients in middle-income countries.

TRAUMA SYSTEMS

There is considerable evidence that political jurisdictions that improve the organization of trauma services benefit from reduced trauma mortality, in comparison with similarly resourced jurisdictions that do not. Such evidence comes from panel reviews of preventable deaths, hospital trauma registry studies and population-based studies. Most studies confirm a reduction in mortality with the improved organization provided by a system for trauma management. For example, panel reviews show an average reduction in medically preventable deaths of 50% after the implementation of a system for trauma management.

To have trauma systems in place following are accepted criteria's.[10]

- Legislative authority for designation
- Formal designation process.
- American college of surgeons standard or equivalent.
- Use of nonbiased survey teams (out of town)
- Population or volume based trauma center designation.
- Triage criteria that require direct transport to trauma center
- Quality improvement systems
- Full geographical coverage.

Components of trauma systems are:

a. Access to care
   - Prehospital care
   - Hospital care
   - Rehabilitation

b. Prevention
   - Disaster medical planning
   - Patient education
   - Research
c. Prehospital communication
   - Transport system
   - Trained personnel
   - Qualified trauma care personnel
d. Peer review
   - Verification

Quality Improvement Systems

Trauma Center Facilities

Level I: Trauma centers are tertiary care hospitals that demonstrate a leadership role. The faculty has trauma surgeon, ortho- surgeon, neurosurgeon, vascular surgeon, reconstructive surgeon around the clock and facility has dedicated. Causality, operation theater, ward, radiological investigations and it takes on trauma research and training program. It addresses public education and preventive issues. They lead research efforts to advance care, which may extend from prehospital to rehabilitation. It is university level hospital.

Level II: Trauma centers provide definitive care to those who are injured and may be the principle provider in the community. Here approach to trauma is comprehensive and an attending trauma surgeon's availability is equivalent to a level I trauma center in the early care of patient. Graduate education and research are not required.

Level III: Trauma centers generally are large community hospitals that serve a community and lacks level I or level II facilities. Commitment is required to assess, resuscitate, and, when necessary, provide definitive operative therapy. When capabilities for definitive care are exceeded, transfer agreements and protocols are essential for level III trauma centers.

Level IV: Trauma centers usually are hospitals located in rural areas and expected to provide initial evaluation of patients who are acutely injured, with transfer to higher level of care anticipated. Transfer agreements and protocols must be in place, because of these hospitals have no definitive surgical capabilities on a regular basis.

Beside these designated centers facilities my be available at large general hospitals and specialist hospitals like, pediatric trauma, burn, spinal cord injury and hand injury centers.

Rehabilitation is as important as prehospital and hospital care. It is often the longest and most difficult phase of trauma care continuum for patient and families.

ANNEXURE

Resource Matrix

These are the guidelines as enumerated in "Guidelines for essential trauma care, Geneva, World Health Organization, 2004" Editors; Mock C, Lormand JD, Goosen J, Joshipura M, Peden M.

In this and subsequent resource matrices, the following key is used to indicate different levels of facilities:

Level IV, Level III, Level II, Level I

E: essential; D: desirable; PR: possibly required; I: irrelevant (not usually to be considered at the level in question, even with full resource availability).

Airway Management				
Airway: knowledge and skills LEVEL	IV	III	II	I
Assessment of airway compromise	E	E	E	E
Manual maneuvers (chin lift, jaw thrust, recovery position, etc.)	E	E	E	E
Insertion of oral or nasal airway	D	E	E	E
Use of suction	D	E	E	E
Assisted ventilation using bag–valve–mask	D	E	E	E
Endotracheal intubation	D	D	E	E
Cricothyroidotomy (with or without tracheotomy)	D	E		E
Airway: Equipment and Supplies				
Oral or nasal airway	D	E	E	E
Suction device: at least manual (bulb) or foot pump	D	E	E	E
Suction device: powered: electric/pneumatic	D	D	D	D
Suction tubing	D	E	E	E
Yankauer or other stiff suction tip	D	E	E	E

Contd...

Contd...

Laryngoscope	D	D	E	E
Endotracheal tube	D	D	E	E
Esophageal detector device	D	D	E	E
Bag–valve–mask	D	E	E	E
Basic trauma pack	D	E	E	E
Magill forceps	D	D	E	E
Capnography	I	D	D	D
Breathing: Knowledge and Skills				
Assessment of respiratory distress and adequacy of ventilation	E	E	E	E
Administration of oxygen	D	E	E	E
Needle thoracostomy	D	E	E	E
Chest tube insertion	I	E	E	E
Three-way dressing	E	E	E	E
Breathing: equipment and supplies stethoscope	E	E	E	E
Oxygen supply (cylinder, concentrator or other source)	D	E	E	E
Nasal prongs, face mask, associated tubing	D	E	E	E
Needle and syringe	D	E	E	E
Chest tubes	I	E	E	E
Underwater seal bottle (or equivalent)	I	E	E	E
Pulse oximetry	I	D	D	D
Arterial blood gas measurements	I	D	D	D
Bag–valve–mask	D	E	E	E
Mechanical ventilator	I	I	D	D
Circulation and Shock				
Circulation: knowledge and skills facility level				
Assessment and external control of hemorrhage				
Assessment of shock	E	E	E	E
Compression for control of hemorrhage	E	E	E	E
Arterial tourniquet in extreme situations	E	E	E	E
Splinting of fractures for hemorrhage control	E	E	E	E
Deep interfascial packing for severe wounds (e.g. landmine)	D	E	E	E
Pelvic wrap for hemorrhage control	D	E	E	E
Fluid Resuscitation				
Knowledge of fluid resuscitation	D	E	E	E
Peripheral percutaneous intravenous access	D	E	E	E
Peripheral cut down access	D	E	E	E

Contd...

Contd...

Central venous access for fluid administration	I	D	E	E
Intraosseous access for children under 5 years	D	D	E	E
Transfusion knowledge and skills	I	E	E	E
Monitoring				
Knowledge of resuscitation parameters	D	E	E	E
More advanced monitoring (central venous pressure)	I	D	D	D
More advanced monitoring (right heart)	I	I	D	D
Other				
Differential diagnosis of causes of shock	D	E	E	E
Use of pressors in neurogenic (spinal) shock	I	D	D	D
Use of fluids and antibiotics for septic shock	I	E	E	E
Recognition of hypothermia	E	E	E	E
External rewarming in hypothermia	E	E	E	E
Use of warmed fluids	I	D	E	E
Knowledge of core rewarming	I	D	E	E
Circulation: Equipment and Supplies				
Assessment and external control of hemorrhage				
Clock or watch with second hand	E	E	E	E
Stethoscope	E	E	E	E
Blood pressure (BP) cuff	E	E	E	E
Gauze and bandages	E	E	E	E
Arterial tourniquet in extreme situations	E	E	E	E
Fluid Resuscitation				
Crystalloid	D	E	E	E
Colloids	D	D	D	D
Blood transfusion capabilities	I	E	E	E
Intravenous infusion set (lines and cannulas)	D	E	E	E
Intraosseous needle or equivalent	D	D	E	E
Central venous lines	I	D	E	E
Monitoring				
Stethoscope	E	E	E	E
Blood pressure (BP) cuff	E	E	E	E
Urinary catheter	D	E	E	E
Electronic cardiac monitoring	I	D	D	D
Monitoring of central venous pressure	I	D	D	D
Right-heart catheterization	I	I	D	D
Laboratory facilities for hemoglobin or hematocrit	D	E	E	E

Contd...

Contd...

Laboratory facilities for electrolytes, lactate and arterial blood gases	I	D	D	D
Pressors (for neurogenic/spinal shock)	I	D	D	D
Nasogastric (NG) tube	D	E	E	E
Thermometer	E	E	E	E
Fluid warmers	I	D	D	D
Weighing scale for children	D	E	E	E
Head Injury				
Recognize altered consciousness; lateralizing signs, pupils	E	E	E	E
Full compliance with AANS1 guidelines for head injury	I	I	D	D
Maintain normotension and oxygenation to prevent secondary brain injury	D	E	E	E
Avoid over hydration in the presence of raised ICP2 (with normal BP)	D	E	E	E
Monitoring and treatment of raised ICP	I	I	D	D
CT scans	I	D	D	D
Burr holes (skill plus drill or other suitable equipment)	I	PR	D	E
More advanced neurosurgical procedures	I	I	PR	D
Surgical treatment of open depressed skull fractures	I	PR	D	E
Surgical treatment of closed depressed skull fractures	I	I	PR	D
Maintenance of requirements for protein and calories	I	E	E	E
Neck Injury				
Recognize platysmal penetration	D	E	E	E
External pressure for bleeding	E	E	E	E
Packing, balloon tamponade for bleeding	D	D	D	D
Contrast radiography, endoscopy	I	I	D	E
Angiography	I	I	D	D
Chest Injury				
Autotransfusion from chest tubes	I	D	D	D
Adequate pain control for chest injuries/rib fractures	D	E	E	E
Respiratory therapy for chest injuries/rib fractures	I	E	E	E
Rib block or intrapleural block	I	PR	E	E
Epidural analgesia	I	I	D	D
Skills and equipment for intermediate thoracotomy	I	I	D	E
Skills and equipment for advanced thoracotomy	I	I	I	D
Abdominal Injury				
Clinical assessment	E	E	E	E
Diagnostic peritoneal lavage (DPL)	I	D	E	E

Contd...

Contd...

Ultrasonography	I	D	D	D
CT scan	I	I	D	D
Skills and equipment for intermediate laparotomy	I	PR	E	E
Skills and equipment for advanced laparotomy	I	I	E	E
Extremity Injury				
Recognition of neurovascular compromise; disability-prone injuries	E	E	E	E
Basic immobilization (sling, splint)	E	E	E	E
Spine board	D	E	E	E
Wrapping of pelvic fractures for hemorrhage control	E	E	E	E
Skin traction	I	PR	E	E
Closed reduction	PR	PR	E	E
Skeletal traction	I	PR	E	E
Operative wound management	I	PR	E	E
External fixation (or its functional equivalent: pins and plaster)	I	PR	E	E
Internal fixation	I	I	E	E
Tendon repair	I	PR	E	E
Hand Injury: Assessment				
Basic splinting	E	E	E	E
Hands: debride, fix	I	PR	E	E
Measurement of compartment pressures	I	D	D	E
Fasciotomy for compartment syndrome	I	PR	D	E
Amputation	I	PR	E	E
X-ray	D	D	E	E
Portable X-ray	I	D	D	E
Image intensification	I	I	D	D
Proper management of immobilized patient to prevent complications	D	E	E	E
Spinal Injury				
Assessment—recognition of presence or risk of spinal injury	E	E	E	E
Immobilization: C-collar, backboard	D	E	E	E
Monitoring of neurological function	E	E	E	E
Assessment by International Classification System	I	I	D	E
Maintain normotension and oxygenation to prevent secondary neurological injury	D	E	E	E
Holistic approach to prevention of complications especially pressure sores and urinary retention/infection —	D	E	E	E

Contd...

Contd...

CT scan	I	D	D	D
MRI	I	I	D	D
Full compliance with AANS guidelines	I	I	D	D
Non-surgical management of spinal injury (as indicated)	I	PR	E	E
Surgical treatment of spinal injury	I	I	PR	E
Surgical treatment of neurological deterioration in the presence of spinal cord compression	I	I	PR	E
Burns and Wounds				
Assessment of depth and extent	E	E	E	E
Sterile dressings	D	E	E	E
Clean dressings	E	I	I	I
Topical antibiotic dressings	D	E	E	E
Debridement	I	PR	E	E
Escharotomy	I	PR	E	E
Skin graft	I	PR	E	E
Early excision and grafting	I	I	D	D
Physiotherapy and splints to prevent contractures in burn wounds	I	E	E	E
Reconstructive surgery	I	I	D	E
Wounds				
Assess wounds for potential mortality and disability	E	E	E	E
Non-surgical management: clean and dress	E	E	E	E
Minor surgical: clean, suture	PR	E	E	E
Major surgical debridement and repair	I	PR	E	E
Tetanus prophylaxis (toxoid, antiserum)	D	E	E	E
Rehabilitation				
PT/OT1 for recovery of extremity injuries	D	E	E	E
Full spectrum of physiotherapy	I	I	D	D
Full spectrum of occupational therapy	I	I	D	D
Prosthetics	I	I	D	E
Psychological counseling	D	E	E	E
Neuropsychology for cognitive dysfunction	I	I	D	D
Speech pathology	I	I	D	D
Physical medicine and rehabilitation specialist -level care	I	I	D	D
Electromyography	I	I	D	D
Specialized rehabilitative nursing	I	I	D	D
Discharge planning	I	E	E	E

REFERENCES

1. Aeron Thomas A, et al. The involvement and impact of road crashes on the poor: Bangladesh and India case studies Project PPRO 10. Crown Home, UK Transport Reasearch Lab 2004.
2. Gururaj G. Road traffic deaths, injuries and disabilities in India: current scenario. The National Medical Journal of India 2008;21:14-20.
3. Global status report on road safety: time for action. Geneva, World Health Organization, 2009.
4. Mock CN, et al. Trauma mortality patterns in three nations at different economic levels: implications for global trauma system development. The Journal of Trauma 1998;44:804-14.
5. Mock CN, et al. Trauma outcomes in the rural developing world: comparison with an urban level I trauma center. The Journal of Trauma 1993;35:518-23.
6. Mock CN, Denno D, Adzotor ES. Paediatric trauma in the rural developing world: low cost measures to improve outcome. Injury 1993;24:291-6.
7. MacKenzie EJ, et al. Functional recovery and medical costs of trauma: an analysis by type and severity of injury. The Journal of Trauma 1988;28:281-97.
8. Nathens A, et al. The effect of organized systems of trauma care on motor vehicle crash mortality. The Journal of the American Medical Association 2000;283:1990-4.
9. Nathens A, et al. Effectiveness of state trauma systems in reducing injury-related mortality: a national evaluation. The Journal of Trauma 2000;48:25-30.
10. Hoyat DB, Coimbra R.Trauma systems. Surg Clin N Amer 2007;87: 21-35.

Chapter 2

Prehospital Trauma Care

SK Kochar

According to Edwin Smith Papyrus by 1500 BC distinct triage and surgical protocol had been developed in Babylonia under the rule of Hammerabi.[1] Greeks required physicians to be present during the battle and Romans established the hospitals close to the battle field but truly speaking Dominique Larry (1776-1842) can be called the father of prehospital care. During the Campaign he organized a system of prehospital transportation to carry out the wounded from the scene of battle to a centralized location by a horse drawn wagon called the "Flying ambulance".[2] Surprisingly, it took almost 200 years before the army experience of prehospital care has been translated into organized trauma care in civil set up.

Compulsion of prehospital trauma care are dictated by the fact that every year in India over 3 lakhs people die of trauma and out of these 50,000 dies on the road. A three fold increase in mortality has been reported for every 30 minutes elapsed without care.[3] Time is a critical factor in the treatment of trauma. Retrospective review of trauma deaths, however postulates that up to 18% of patients died unnecessary during prehospital transportation.[4] These patients either exsanguate, had airway obstruction or ventilatory compromise, which could have been rapidly treated in the field before or during transportation.

Trimodal Distribution of Trauma Deaths

Death from trauma has trimodal distribution,[5] i.e. immediate, early and late. Immediate death, the first peak is the death occurring within seconds or minutes of injury. Invariably these deaths are due to laceration of:

i. Brain,
ii. Brainstem,
iii. Upper spinal cord,
iv. Heart aorta large veins.

Early deaths occurs within 2-3 hours and are due to:

i. Sub/extradural hematoma,
ii. Hemothorax,
iii. Ruptured spleen,
iv. Liver laceration
v. Multiple injuries with hypovolemic shock.

Late deaths are due to sepsis, infection and multiple organ failure.

Immediate deaths (50%) cannot be salvaged by any treatment but these can be prevented by improved crash worthiness of motor vehicle, compulsory use of crash helmet and safety belt. One fifth of the immediate accidents deaths could be saved by changes in the road environment, for example, by improving the junction design and traffic management, and another quarter by changes in driver behavior including enforcement of alcohol limits and safer speed. Late deaths (20%) occurs in the hospital late in the course of management and this number may decrease with intensive organ support and with better understanding of septicemia.

Aim of Prehospital Care

The aim of prehospital care is to prevent early deaths (30%) and sustain life till the patient reaches hospital where definite treatment can be provided. Time is an important factor as mortality is directly related to the time spent in shock. That is why this first hour has been called golden hour and platinum half hour. In fact every minute is important in a case of polytrauma who may have airway obstruction, ventilatory problem or circulatory collapse. To achieve this one has to cut down on the transport time between the accident and hospital but it may not be possible due to:

- Narrow roads,
- Rough weather/tough terrain,
- Lack of communication,
- Poorly maintained ambulances,
- Nonavailability of helicopters,
- General apathy of public (to be associated with accident victim).

Types/Systems of Prehospital Care

There is growing body of thought that claims that it is important to initiate resuscitation as soon as possible and to perform a limited number of definitive interventions to stabilize a trauma patient before transportation to a trauma care facility. Such procedures may include definitive protection of the airway by endotracheal intubation and initial resuscitation from hypovolemic shock by the establishment of peripheral venous access and fluid administration (Stabilize and Go). The rationale is that these components of definitive care are possible in the prehospital environment and that they contribute towards improving the outcome following severe trauma. A second school of thought claims that advance life support has no place in the prehospital management of trauma victims. The rationale is that the hospital is the definitive place for surgical attention and that a patient's clinical condition is unlikely to deteriorate during the short time needed for rapid transportation. Time to definitive operative treatment is felt to be the single most vital factor in influencing the outcome following injury (Scoop and Go).

Features of Prehospital Phase

- Extrication of casualty and protection of cervical spine
- Airway control
- Control of hemorrhage
- Venous access and intravenous fluids
- Treatment of:
  - Cardiac arrest
  - Sucking chest wound
  - Cardiac tamponade
  - Tension pneumothorax
  - Evisceration of viscera
- Splinting of fractures
- Administration of:
  - Analgesics
  - Antibiotics
  - Tetanus prophylaxis

All the features enumerated above forms what has been termed advance life support when airway is supported by endotracheal intubation and circulation is supported by venous access and intravenous fluid administration. Basic life support does not include these two features.

The value of field stabilization depends on time dependent patient categories; patient with long transport times; those with extremely time urgent, life-threatening problems, regardless of expected transport time, and finally those who fall into vast middle group of severity, stability and transport time. For all categories virtually all surgeons agree that spine immobilization, airway precautions, oxygen supplementations, pressure control of massive bleeding and ABC's of resuscitation should be performed as soon as possible, since these are all quick procedures the omission of which would have disastrous consequences. Even proponents of scoop and run would agree that in an area in which transport times are measured in hours some stabilization must be attempted.[6] Many patients will be stable enough to survive several hours without treatment although an increase in morbidity would be expected.

There is a set of circumstances in which field stabilization is obviously logical and that is in those trauma emergencies that must be resolved in a period shorter than even the shortest transportation: Complete airway obstruction, cardiac arrest and full blown tension pneumothorax (cyanosis, hypotension and moribund). None of these syndrome can be allowed to persist for more than a few minutes, which is less than virtually any transport time to any hospital anywhere. However, patient with slow internal hemorrhage, a tension pneumothorax, progressive airway obstruction, impending cerebral herniation or perhaps even cardiac tamponade, who cannot reach a hospital within 1-2 hours, will be doomed unless something is done in the interim. A short interval of time at the scene spent establishing the intravenous fluid administration is probably worthwhile. It is in this group of patients that contradictory reports/studies are coming and here is the value of, initial assessment and different factors like type of injury, distance involved, availability of facilities locally and trauma center.[6]

Prehospital Protocols

Extrication of Casualties and Protection of Spine

Extrication problems are acute in railway accidents, house collapse, and air disaster while it does not pose much problem in road traffic accidents. What is more important in a case of polytrauma while extricating is to avoid further injury to spine? Helmet is to be carefully removed. Cervical spine should be protected by a rigid collar at the earliest and patient be extricated and loaded on the stretcher in single piece.

Airway

With this begins the ABC of resuscitation. Airway must be cleared of blood, mucous, vomit, any foreign body or dentures. Tongue is pulled out and jaw braced forward and oropharyngeal airway placed *in situ*. Methods of airway control such as, esophageal obturator airway, endotracheal/nasotracheal tube, laryngeal airway or combi tube can consume a great deal of time if multiple attempts are necessary and it also entails presence of trained individuals. Their use is therefore reserved for the unconscious patients whose airway is immediately threatened by bleeding or facial or airway trauma and whose ventilation is inadequate. cricothyroidotomy, percutaneous transtracheal ventilation (PTTV) are beyond the scope of paramedics and needs expertise which does not justify its use in field conditions.[6] In desperate situation a 16-gauge needle pushed in the cricothyroid space and connected to oxygen cylinder with oxygen flowing at the rate of 10-12 liter/min will probably see the patient reach hospital alive. A portable suction apparatus is an essential adjuvant for a clear airway. Nasal catheter is preferred over face mask for oxygen delivery, as suction if required is not interfered with. There are several clinical scenarios that require the need for urgent airway intervention:

- Impending airway obstruction resulting from severe upper airway burns
- Expanding neck hematoma
- Direct trauma to the upper airway
- Inability to protect the airway because of altered level of consciousness
- Severe traumatic brain injury
- Severe respiratory compromise with the need for assisted ventilation.
- Endotracheal intubation (ETI) facilitated by neuromuscular blockade can be performed safely in prehospital settings with improved success at achieving appropriate endotracheal

placement and reduction in the need for surgical airway access. The question remains however whether or not prehospital ETI improves outcome for patients who are severely injured.[6a]

Breathing

Once the airway is cleared the patient's respiratory effort would be observed. Although the sucking chest wound is obvious, paramedics may not be able to diagnose tension pneumothorax or massive hemothorax. Sucking chest wound is closed by sterile vaseline gauge dressing with plenty of gauge and adhesive dressing. Rarely if the closer is watertight these patients may go into tension pneumothorax. Safer will be to close three sides while applying adhesive plaster. It may be very difficult to diagnose tension pneumothorax/massive hemothorax in the field settings and even when accompanied by emergency physician and diagnosed, chest tube is not advisable in field setting. In tension pneumothorax 16-gauge needle with a finger stall at the other end with a small hole in it (thus forming a nonreturn valve), pushed into 2nd space can see the patient through the journey. If not contraindicated due to other injuries, patient with chest trauma should travel propped up.

Appropriate ventilation has emerged as a critical factor that may have impact on outcome. Hyperventilation may be detrimental for patients who have severe TBI and those in hypovolemic shock. Hypoventilation in patients who have severe chest injury may be just as detrimental. Ventilation using a standard ambu bag is difficult to regulate, especially in often chaotic prehospital settings. Studies are required to evaluate the use of end tidal CO_2 monitoring; the use of transport ventilators; the use of a SMART BAG which resist excessive ventilation; and the addition of timing lights to prompt ventilatory rate.

Circulation

Most trauma patients have bleeding either external or internal. Pressure dressings are adequate for external bleeding. No attempt should be made in the field settings to apply hemostat. In case external bleeding cannot be arrested by pressure dressing, pneumatic tourniquet should be used. Indiscriminate use of tourniquet earned it a bad reputation and it resulted in more loss of limbs than it saved. It must be released intermittently and be mentioned either on the fore head or by a tag on the forearm that patient has been given a tourniquet. For internal hemorrhage pneumatic antishock garment (PASG) and administration of intravenous fluid had been advocated. Both these modalities have fallen in to controversy.

A universally accepted axiom for resuscitation of the hypovolemic/hypotensive patient has always been that improvement in blood pressure is a good sign.[7] However improving blood pressure and blood flow in a hypotensive patient will increase blood loss from injured major and minor vessels. The patient's hypotension acts to reduce blood loss from these vessels. Any treatment that restores blood pressure and blood flow to within normal limits will increase blood loss. Lewis[8] using a computer model, found that giving a patient intravenous fluids in the prehospital setting was a detrimental since the blood loss would be greater over the time than the fluid replaced at flow rates of less than 500 ml/min. However, a more detailed computer model by Wear and Winton showed a much improved survival rates when intravenous infusions were begun in the prehospital period.[9] Other studies[10,11] also support this view.

In a patient who will probably exsanguate in 15-40 min, the bleeding must be 60-200 ml/min as it requires a loss of 40-50 percent of blood volume to cause hypovolemic arrest. The patient threatened with exsanguation in less than 40 min therefore, loses more blood volume during the intravenous attempts (time taken 11 min) than can be given subsequently (maximum rate 1000 ml in 10 min) by the paramedics to make up for it. If the failure rate involved in starting field intravenous is considered it only tips the balance further against starting the intravenous. Obviously if total field time in excess of 40-60 min are encountered; the above analysis does not apply and the benefit of an intravenous might outweigh its disadvantages. This would occur in prolong extrication or long transport distances.[12] This situation is encountered in our country in majority of patient as the average transport time varies anywhere between 2-6 hours.[13,14] Ringer's lactate/isotonic saline is the fluid of choice although it is the rate of administration what is more important than the type of fluid.

- Control of hemorrhage and intravenous fluid has been the standards so far. There are several products which may aid in the control of external hge.
- Microporous polysaccharide hemispheres (Trauma DEX)
- Mineral zeolite (quick clot)
- Poly-N-acetylglucosamine (HemCon).
- Microporous hydrogel forming polyacrylamide (Bio-Hemostat).
- Fibrin impregnated bandages
- All these are still in trial phase and for now direct pressure and rapid transport seems to be the mainstay.
- Patients with long transport time will definitely need fluid resuscitation.
- Intravenous access is usually achieved in adults by using upper extremity peripheral veins. Although in some patients particularly in combat locations sternal intraosseous access has been preferred because of the simplicity of its use.
- The issue of what should be the ideal fluid for resuscitation has not been settled.

Fluids under investigations are:

- 7.5% saline with or without Dextran 70
- Polymerized hemoglobin blood substitutes, polyheme, hemolink, hemopure.
- The results of ongoing clinical trials are awaited and till then crystalloids solution remains the fluid of choice.

Indications for PASG in the mid 1990s were patients with severe intra-abdominal hge with blood pressure of less than 50 mm Hg. Major contraindications were hge outside the confines of the garment and diaphragmatic hernia.[15] Cardiac arrest in trauma patient occurs secondarily to exsanguinations, airway ventilation compromise and central nervous system injury. It is extremely difficult for the paramedics to diagnose the cause of cardiac arrest. Prehospital treatment of cardiac arrest consists of:

- Immediate establishment of an airway,
- Ventilation with 100 percent oxygen, if feasible with an endotracheal tube, and
- Initiation of external cardiac message. All the paramedics are trained in external cardiac message and recently pneumatic powered pistons to be placed over the sternum have been developed for proper compression. CPR with a mechanical

device such as the thumper provides better CPR than can be done manually in a moving vehicle.[16]

Cardiac Tamponade

It is difficult to diagnose in field setting and even if it is diagnosed, pericardiocentesis is not a feasible proposition in the field setting. Intravenous fluid loading and inotropic agents can tied over the crisis.

Immobilization

Splintage of the fractured limbs done at the accident site can help prevent pain and further injury to the injured area. This is important and should be done as a first aid measure. Improvised splints made out of available material at the site of injury can be used. Special light weight splints/air inflatable splints if available makes the task easier. One should not waste time in applying external fixators or complicated splints at the site of accident. Patient must be strapped well on stretcher or boards without pillow in spine position and handled as if he has sustained spinal injury till he reaches hospital setting and spinal injury has been ruled out.

Spine immobilization is the standard criteria incorporated in all prehospital protocols. Adverse effects which has been pointed out by few investigators are:

- Increased risk for aspiration,
- Airway compromise
- Delay in transport
- Patient discomfort.

It is estimated that 20% of spinal cord injury patients die before reaching the hospital and 25% of spinal cord damage may occur or worsen after an initial event.

Eviscerated Viscera

Eviscerated viscera not only gives a ghastly look but also increases the shock, bleeding and subsequent infection. Clean sterile towel is enough to cover these and bandage is loosely wrapped around it but no attempt is made to push back the intestines and tight bandaging as these measures may produce intestinal twisting and strangulation.

Administration of Analgesics/Antibiotics/Tetanus Prophylaxis

Tetanus and antibiotics can wait till the patient reaches hospital but morphine/pentazocine, if not contraindicated not only will make transportation easy but by reducing pain it also reduces the shock state.

Transportation

Depending upon the resources of the society patient may be transported by ground transport, by helicopters, or by fixed wing aircrafts (Fig. 2.1). Whatever may be the means, the aim is to decrease the time lag between the accident and definitive care. The availability of the resuscitation and sustenance facility during transportation reaches its zenith when the transport times are long. Standard list of equipment which has been found to be useful is as follows:

- Equipment for airway; laryngoscope, oropharyngeal airway, endotracheal tubes, OEA tubes, combitube, laryngeal airway.
- Oxygen cylinder, face mask, Ambu bag, nasal oxygen catheter
- Suction apparatus
- Intra caths, intravenous lines and fluids, crystalloids
- Defabs, cardiac monitor, pulse oximeter, BP apparatus

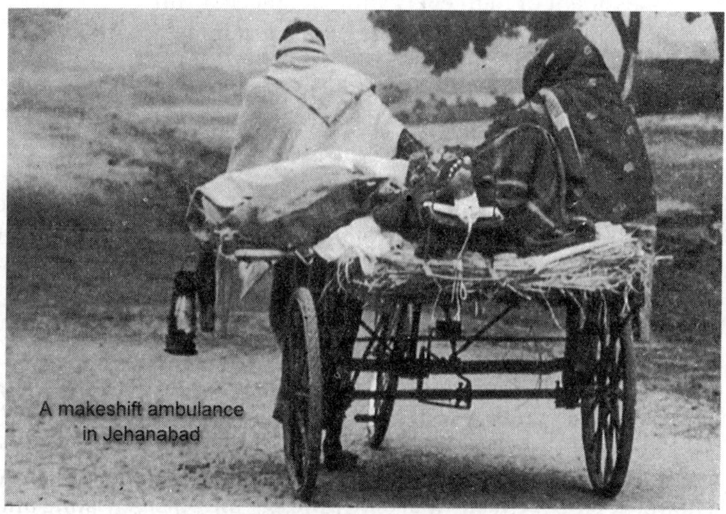

Fig. 2.1: Makeshift ambulance

- Bandages, dressing gauge, elastoplast and gloves
- Splints, cervical collar, stretchers
- Analgesic, inotropics, etc.

Triage

The primary goal of military triage was to prioritize care according to the severity of injury and chances of survival. Casualties being many, resources were customized to provide urgent surgical care to the less critically wounded in order to hasten their return to battle. With the advances in trauma care and delivery systems becoming operative in more and more places, a new dimension has been added to the concept of civilian triage, the goal being rapidly and accurately to identify those trauma victims whose severity of injury warrants the resources of a trauma center or those hospital where trauma care facility exists. It is well established that the chances for survival improves when major trauma are treated in trauma centers.[17] It is important to define major trauma victim.

- Recommended triage scheme involves a 4 step evaluation process (Table 2.1).
- Impaired vital signs and GCS
- Evaluation of critical injury pattern
- Assessment of high energy impact mechanism
- Assessment of special patient considerations
- Extremes of age
- Pregnancy
- Anticoagulation
- Burns
- End stage renal disease.

Major trauma victim: Patient whose magnitude of injury requires resources of trauma center. To define it in terms of severity of injury ISS score of 15 has been accepted the norm. However, for triage trauma score of <11 has been used for evacuation to trauma care facility. Since the primary objective of a trauma system is to decrease mortality and morbidity from injury, it is essential that the criteria used in the system be sufficiently sensitive to identify the vast majority of victims at risk for life-threatening injuries. The prehospital triage decision scheme recommended by the American college of Surgeons[18] provides an excellent algorithm for triage, using multiple components.

Table 2.1: Triage decision scheme[18]

Measure vital signs and level of consciousness		
Step 1	Glasgow coma scale	<14 or
	Systolic blood pressure	< 90 or
	Respiratory rate	<10 or>29 or
	Revised trauma score	< 11
	Pediatric trauma score	< 9
	Yes	No
	Take to trauma center; alert trauma team	Assess anatomy of injury
Step 2	• All penetrating injuries to head, neck, torso, and extremities proximal elbow and knee	
	• Flail chest	
	• Combination trauma with burns	
	• Pelvic fracture	
	• Limb paralysis	
	• Amputation proximal to wrist and ankle	
	Yes	No
	Take to trauma center	Mechanism of injury
Step 3	• Ejection from automobile	
	• Death in same passenger compartment	
	• Extrication time > 20 min	
	• Fall > 20 feet	
	• Roll over	
	• Initial speed > 40 mph	
	• Major autodeformity > 20 inches	
	• Intrusion into passenger compartment >12 inches	
	• Autopedestrian/autocycle impact	
	• Pedestrian thrown or run over	
	• Motorcycle crash > 20 mph	
	Yes	No
	Consider trauma center	
Step 4	• Age <5 or>55	
	• Cardiac disease, respiratory disease	
	• Insulin dependent diabetes, cirrhosis, or morbid obesity	
	• Pregnancy	
	• Immunosuppressed patients	
	• Patient with bleeding disorder or patient on anticoagulants	
	Yes	No
	Consider trauma center	Re-evaluate with medical control
When in doubt, take to trauma center		

REFERENCES

1. The Edwin Smith Papyrus, case 36, XII 8-14, Classics of surgery Library, Gryphon Edition, Ltd. Brimingham, AL, 1984, pp 354-56.
2. Larry DJ. Memories of a military Surgeon, Willmont R (trans): Classics of Surgery Library. Brimingham, AL, Joseph Cushing, 1984.
3. Cowley RA, Hudson F, Scarilan E, et al. An economical and proved helicopter program for transporting the emergency critically ill and injured patient in Maryland. J Trauma. 1973;13:1029-38.
4. Frey CF, Huelke DF, Gikas PW. Resuscitation and survival in motor vehicle accidents. J Trauma 1969;9:292-310.
5. Turnkey DD. Controversies in Trauma Management, Dailey RH and Calhan (Eds). Churchill Livingstone, New York. 1985;p 199.
6. Dailey RH, Calhan M. Editorial comments, controversies in trauma management. Churchill Livingstone, New York. 1985; p 189.

6a. Bulgger EM, Maier RV. Prehospital care of the injured: What's new. Surg Clin N Am 2007;37-53.

7. Ramenofsky ML, et al. Advanced Trauma Life Support Course Chicago, IL, American College of Surgeons. 1993; p 77.
8. Lewis FR. Prehospital intravenous fluid therapy: Physiologic computer modeling. J Trauma 1986;26:804.
9. Wear RL, Winton CN. Load and go versus stay and play: Analysis of prehospital intravenous fluid therapy by computer simulation. Ann Emerg Med 1990;19:163.
10. Aprahamian C, et al. Traumatic cardiac arrest: Scope of paramedic services. Ann Emerg Med 1985;14:583.
11. O'Corman M, et al. Zero time prehospital intravenous. J Trauma 1989;29:84.
12. Trunkey DD. Organised trauma regions and the American college of surgeons categorisation of centres. In Controversies in Trauma management, Dialey RH and Calhan M (Eds), Churchill Livingstone, New York, 1985; p 200.
13. Kochar SK. Prehospital Trauma Care: An Evaluation. MJAFI 1989;45:218-22.
14. Maheshwari J, Mohan D. Road traffic accidents in Delhi: A hospital based study. Journal of Traffic Medicine 1989;17:23-27.
15. McSwain NE Jr. Prehospital care in Trauma, Moore EE, Mattox KL, Feliciano DV (Eds), Appleton and Lange, California, 3rd ed 1995; 107-121.
16. Roberts BG. Machine CPR vs Mechanical CPR in a moving vehicle. Proc Am Assoc Auto Med 1978;22:154.

17. Kilberg L, Clemmer TP, Claussen J. Effectiveness of implementing a trauma triage system on outcome: A prospective evaluation. J Trauma 1988;10:1493.
18. American College of Surgeons, Committee on Trauma, resources for optimal care of the injured patient. American College of Surgeons, Chicago, 1993.

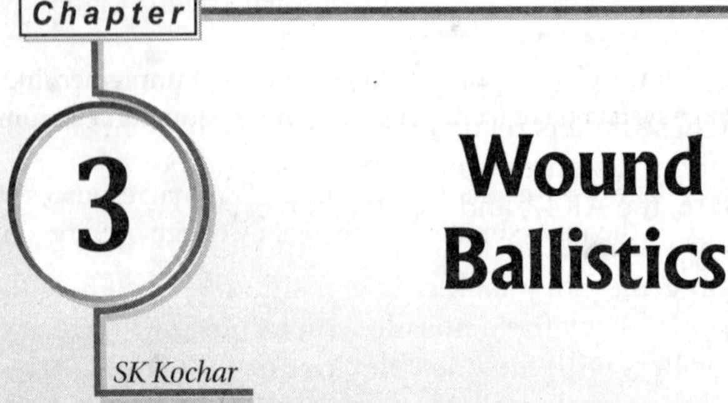

Wound Ballistics

SK Kochar

A basic knowledge of wound ballistics is of tremendous help in managing gunshot wounds. Ballistic is the science of motion of a projectile through a gun barrel and subsequently through a medium, such as air, and eventually through a target. The terminal portion of the trajectory, if the target is a living tissue, is called wound ballistics. A weapon consists of the following:

Barrel: The barrel is the metal tube in which the charge is placed ready for firing and in which it is exploded. This tube compresses the gases developed during combustion and gives the missile direction.

Stock: The stock is that part by which the weapon is held and which supports the barrel. To it are also fixed the lock plate and other accessories.

Lock: The lock contains the lock and trigger mechanism, i.e. the apparatus for the discharge of the weapon.

Types of Weapons

Handguns are typically low-energy weapons with muzzle velocities less than 1400 feet per second. They are the most frequently used firearms in gunshot injuries, and there are three basic types: single-shot pistols, revolvers, or semiautomatics. Examples include the .38 caliber, 9 mm, and the .45 caliber semiautomatic pistols.

Rifles are named for their rifle barrel which consists of a series of helical grooves within the bore of the firearm which impart spin to the bullet providing more stability. These weapons are grouped as single-barrel sporting, double-barrel sporting, or high-powered military assault-type rifles; and common types include the single-shot automatic and the lever, bolt and pump action. Assault rifles typically shoot a higher velocity projectile and are mainly used in the military. These bullets retain over two-thirds of their original muzzle velocity at distances up to 300 yards. Common examples include the M16, the AK47, and also the newer AK74.

Shotguns are similar in appearance to rifles; however, as their name suggests, they lack rifling inside the barrel with a smooth bore only. They fire a missile which consists of a fuse of hundreds of pellets with muzzle velocities of 1,000 to 1,500 feet per second. So, even though they are technically considered low-velocity weapons, at close range they are definitely the most destructive of all small arms. Common types include the single-shot, double-barrel, and also the automatic and pump action. There are several terms used when talking about shotguns. The first is choke, which refers to a partial constriction of the bore at the muzzle that condenses and controls the shot pattern. So a tighter choke would make a smaller spread of the pellets and a greater length of the shot column. The term gauge is actually an archaic term which is still used to describe shotguns today. It refers to the number of lead balls of a given bore diameter required to weigh one pound. Common examples include .12, .16, and .20 gauge. The load of a shotgun is the actual pellet contained within a plastic shell which is thrown forward out of the barrel and, as stated before, can consist of several hundred pellets known as bird shot, to just a few pellets known as buckshot. The wadding is the material which fills up the dead space in the shell, protecting the powder from the shot. It also seals the bore during firing to keep the gas behind the pellets and accelerating forward. It is produced using either paper, felt, cardboard, plastic, or composite materials.

Classification of Weapons

Weapons have been classified according to their muzzle velocity.

Low velocity: These have muzzle velocity less than 1200 f.p.s. Pistols, revolvers, etc. comes in this category.

Medium velocity: These weapons have muzzle velocity above 1200 f.p.s and less than 2500 f.p.s. Stengun and rifles falls into this categories.

High velocity: These have muzzle velocity more than 2500 f.p.s. AK 47, AK 74 and Swedish assault rifle 5.56 are example of this.

Ultra high velocity: These have muzzle velocity greater than 1.5 km per second. These weapons are under experimental stage and may be introduced soon.

Ammunition (Bullet)

Different types of bullet have been used for shot gun, rifles and revolvers. Basically a bullet consist of lead shot with gunpowder encased in a jacket. In order to increase the potential of wounding, bullets have been designed not to exit, thereby delivering all their energy to the victim. Dumdum bullets, hollow-point and explosive bullets are various explosive rounds. Deforming bullets have been banned in military conflict following Hague convention in 1906.

Characteristics of Bullet in Flight

Bullets in flights have been shown to display variation in their orientation. Yawing is the deviation of a bullet in its longitudinal axis from the straight line of it's flight, while tumbling is the action of its forward rotation around the center of motion. Precession is a type of circular yaw, closely resembling the motion of a football in the flight. Nutation is another circular variation in the orientation of the bullet in flight (Fig. 3.1).

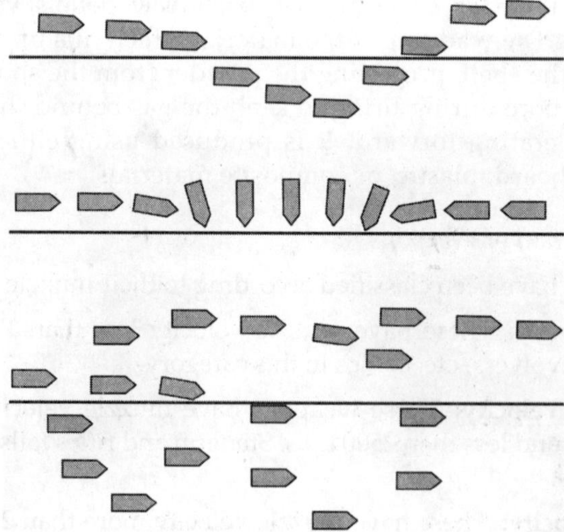

Fig. 3.1: Different characteristics of bullet in flight, viz. yaws, tumbling

Wounding Capacity

Many theories have been advanced to explain wounding capacity of bullets but the theory of kinetic energy appears to explain the observed phenomenon.

$$\text{Kinetic Energy} = \tfrac{1}{2}\,\text{Mass} \times \text{Velocity}^2$$

At low velocity, the rate of dissipation of kinetic energy is proportional to velocity squared. As the velocity approaches and exceeds the speed of sound the rate of dissipation of kinetic energy becomes proportional to velocity cubed or to even higher power of velocity. This has been the guided principle for efforts to increase the bullet velocity to increase the wounding potential.

Pathophysiology and Wound Profile

A bullet striking tissue produces wounding by several mechanisms (Fig. 3.2). Immediately preceding the passage of a higher velocity projectile is a sonic shock wave traveling from the point of impact at the speed of sound through the tissue before the bullet arrives. No tissue displacement or damage has been shown to result from this phenomenon. As the bullet passes through the tissue, it produces a path of destruction slightly larger than its own diameter. Tissue in the path of the bullet is injured directly by crush. Low velocity bullets generally produce this type of damage alone. The penetration depth of a projectile, the size of the hole it makes, and any unusual

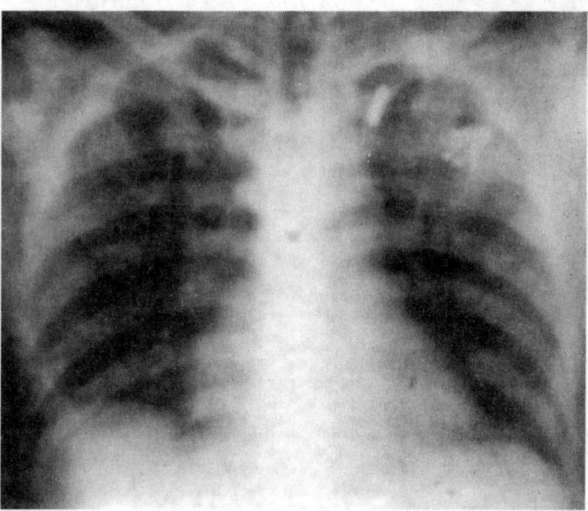

Fig. 3.2: Bullet and shrapnel in the left chest

deviation in course of direction through tissue are the characteristics that best allow us to predict its potential tissue disruption. This is the hard data of wound ballistics and are largely responsible for the leaks in the circulatory or gastrointestinal systems that threaten the life of the wounded.[1] Immediately following the passage of a high velocity projectile through tissue, kinetic energy is dissipated, in part, by the creation of a temporary cavity along the track of the bullet. Tissue accelerates forward and laterally away from the track, generating a cavity filled with water vapor at subatmospheric pressures. The cavity forms within microseconds, only to collapse and reform again multiple times at rapidly diminishing amplitudes. The resultant stretching, compressing, and shearing of tissue may cause damage several centimeters lateral to track. Foreign material, such as clothing, may be sucked into the wound. The stretch of temporary cavitation is better tolerated by relatively elastic tissues (lung, bowel wall, muscle) than it is by the nonelastic solid organs (liver)[2] (Fig. 3.3). The size of permanent cavity (Fig. 3.4) (tissue crushed by the penetrating projectile) can be increased by three mechanism:

1. *Yaw:* As the bullet's long axis makes a greater angle with the bullet path a wider area of tissue comes in contact with the bullet and is crushed.
2. *Bullet deformation:* Mushrooming or flattening of the bullet tip with an increase in bullet diameter.

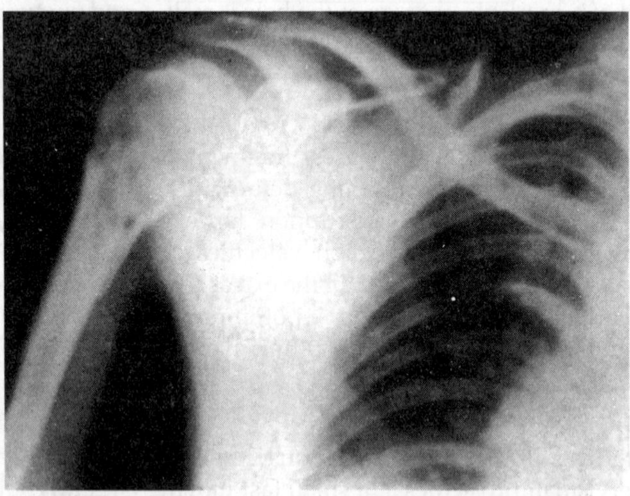

Fig. 3.3: Fractured bone adjacent to the missile track

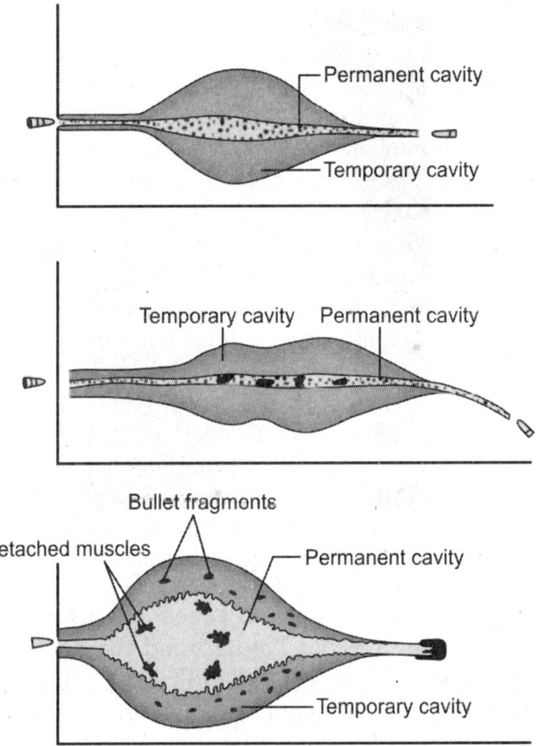

Fig. 3.4: Diagrammatic representation of the temporary cavity at different velocity

3. *Bullet fragmentation:* As velocity of the soft point or hollow point type bullet increases, fragmentation of the bullet is added to the mushrooming deformation and at levels over 900 m/s the tissue disruption far exceeds that of other mechanism.[3] At very high velocities, the entrance wound may actually be larger than the exit as the cavity tends to form earlier and closer to the point of impact.[4] The bullet may exit at maximum (180) yaw, resulting in a large ragged exit.

Wounding Capacity of Shot Gun

Shotguns are smooth-bore weapons designed to discharge a load of very small projectiles at a small fast moving target. Wounding capacity with shot gun shells consists of a spectrum ranging from wounds caused by a solitary pellet to those in which the entire

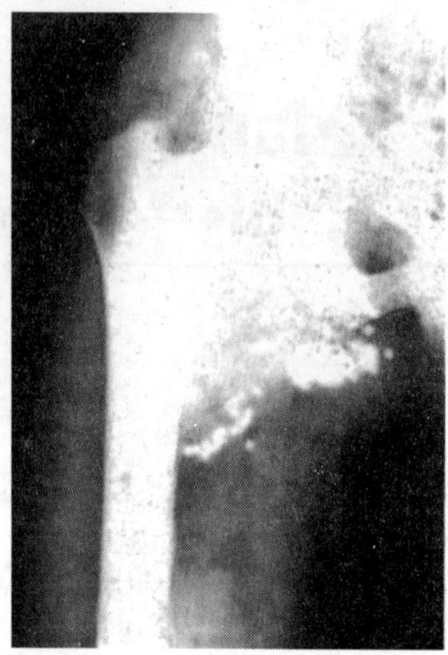

Fig. 3.5: Entire charge of pellets in shot gun wound at short range

charge strikes the target. At six to 12 feet, the wound consists of a central blast with a minor halo around the dense confluence of the major defect. At 24 feet, the bulk of the shot is well away from the center but is still contained within a six inch circle. In wounds where the entire charge has struck so as to be contained in a circle of one foot or less, the striking velocity can be assumed to be muzzle velocity. The critical factor in the kinetic energy formula when considering shot gun wounds is "mass". With the poor ballistic characteristics of the individual pellets most of the load will also stay within the victim, favoring full dissipation of the kinetic energy with the shot (Fig. 3.5).

REFERENCES

1. Fackler ML, Bellamy RF, Malinowski JA. The wound profile: Illustration of the Missile-tissue interaction. J Trauma 1988;28:S21-29.
2. Fackler, ML, Surinchak JS, Malinowski JA, et al. Wounding potential of the Russian AK 74 assault rifle. J Trauma 1984;24:263-6.
3. Fackler ML, Surinchak JS, Malinowski JA, et al. Bullet fragmentation: A major cause of tissue disruption. J Trauma 1984;24:35-9.
4. Sykes LN Jr, Champion HR, Fouty W. Wound ballistics: An Update. Contemporary Surg 1986;29:23-29.

Management of Ballistics Injuries

VK Sinha

The history of human race is the history of wars. Wars have been fought for different reasons but basically an expression of human desire of enforcing his philosophy on others. From spear to nuclear devices, the injuries sustained by these objects were traditionally the domain of military surgeons. With widespread and easy availability of firearms and unlawful exercise of random, ruthless violence to innocent people by terrorists; the war has extended beyond its traditional theater to become a real threat to all and one. With this upsurge in violence, it is imperative that all those involved in the surgical disciplines of health care system should be well versed with ballistics, pathophysiology and nature of wounding and principles of care.

INJURING AGENT

Practically anything can be made to cause injury. In a war like situation, the injuries may be classified as:

a. Blast injuries
b. Missile injuries (Gunshot injuries and secondary blast injuries)
c. Thermal burns
d. Crush injuries
e. Chemical injuries
f. Radiation injuries

Blast Injuries

Blast and blast related injuries are the most common injuries encountered in war and terrorist incidents. No part of the world is immune to this type of injury. In Gulf war about 75 percent of the allied casualties[1] and in IPKF operations in Sri Lanka 68 percent of Indian casualties[2] were a consequence of bomb blasts. Similar figures relate to death of US troops (around 4,000) and Iraqi civilians (around 1,50,000) till Apr 2009 (Associated press data). To understand the nature of injuries caused by blasts, it is imperative to analyze the blast and understand the biomechanics of the blast. The blast can cause damage to the animate and inanimate alike by both its primary effect (the blast wave) and secondary effect (mass movement of air).

A blast is caused by sudden increase in volume. Detonation is a process of passing a shock wave through an explosive substance. The rapidity with which this shock wave passes through the explosive substance determine the effect for a given charge. In conventional explosive like nitroglycerin or TNT (trinitrotoluene) the detonation velocity is about 4 x 105 cm per second whereas in the more modern plastic explosives like semtexH this rate is twice as much. This sudden detonation causes an instantaneous rise in pressure and temperature resulting in tremendous increase in volume which results in a blast wave. The positive high pressure blast wave is followed by a front of negative pressure lasting for a duration much longer than the blast wave itself. This negative pressure causes what is known as a mass movement of air or a blast wind. The sudden extreme rise in pressure produced by the blast causes blast wave. A very minor form of this has been experienced by most of us during festive fireworks when a powerful cracker is blown nearby. The blast wave has the following characteristics:

- It travels like sound wave through and around the objects in its path.
- The effect in a given medium decreases in direct proportion to the distance from the blast.
- The severity of blast wave at a given distance from the source will depend on the acoustic impedance of the medium in which the wave is traveling. Water has got a lower acoustic impedance as compared to air. Therefore, the effect of blast wave is more and for a longer distance in water.
- On reaching an object of a different acoustic impedance, part of the wave is reflected from the surface and reinforces the original shock wave. The bodies receiving this reinforced wave are likely to sustain more damage even if the distance from the blast is more. Cooper et al[3] and Katz et al[4] have described this phenomenon by studying the injury patterns

in blast. That is why the effect of a blast is more in the closed space of a building or a vehicle.

- The effect of blast wave depends on its intensity as well as its duration. Of these two factors, duration determines its effect on human bodies. Blast wave of the duration less than 2 msec are supposedly harmless to human beings. The duration of shock waves in extracorporeal shock wave lithotripsy is 0.002 msec and therefore it does not cause any tissue damage.
- Blast of a higher charge produces shock waves of a longer duration.
- The effect of the blast wave cannot be prevented by body armour.
- The blast wave effects are termed as the primary injuries of the blast.

The negative phase of the high pressure blast wave is responsible for mass movement of air or the blast wind. This has the following features:

- The effects of blast wind depends on the density of air and its velocity.
- Being wind, its effects cannot be transmitted across a solid immovable barrier like a wall. The wall, however, may collapse under its effect.
- In its most intense form it can cause a total disintegration of human life. It can cause amputation of different parts of the body.
- Human beings can fly off under its effect and experience protean types of injuries due to hit and falls.
- The direct and indirect injuries caused by the blast wind are termed as the tertiary injuries of blast.

Causation of Injuries in a Blast

The blast produces injury in one or more of the following ways:

- The injuries caused by the blast wave or the primary injury.
- The injuries caused by missiles-the bomb casing, the sharpnels or other objects energised/propelled by the blast, e.g. flying debris, glass, stones, pieces of concrete, etc. These injuries are termed as the secondary injuries.
- The injuries caused by the blast wind either directly or indirectly. They are termed as the tertiary injury.
- Burns caused in the immediate vicinity of the blast or sustained in the ensuing fire.

- Crush injuries caused by the collapse of building, bunker or a bridge.
- Injuries caused in the inevitable stampede.

It is important to appreciate that most of the salveagable cases amongst the blast victims are the ones having suffered injuries other than primary and tertiary injuries. A great majority of salvageable injuries are caused by missiles on persons outside the lethal zone of the blast. All bodies within the lethal zone die of the effects of blast wave itself. This lethal zone depends on the size of the charge. Zuckermann[5] in his experiments found its zone to be about 4 meters in a 32 kg charge. In a nuclear explosion this may be in kilometers. The burns, crush injuries caused by stampede are no different from the ones encountered in nonblast accidents.

The Effect of Blast Wave—The Primary Injury

The high pressure, high energy blast wave on entering the human body is transmitted in three forms.

Stress waves: These are longitudinal pressure waves traveling like the speed of sound. They cause small rapid distortion of the tissue (stress), which in itself may not be detrimental but the effect is most pronounced at the interfaces of acoustic impedance. Therefore, the maximum damage is expected in air filled viscera like ear, lungs and gastrointestinal tract. The wave reflection within the body causes reinforcement. The reflection from mediastinum and rib cage is responsible for greater damage near these structures.

Traumatic brain injury (TBI) results from mechanical loads in the brain, often without skull fracture, and causes complex, long-lasting symptoms.

Shock waves: These are similar to stress waves in being longitudinal but have a higher velocity and therefore, causes greater damage.

Shear waves: These are slow transverse waves which cause greater distortion of the tissues as opposed to the previously described waves. Because of this greater distortion of tissues, they cause greater tissue damage. They can cause gross movements of tissues in relation to each other. They are responsible for disruption of various vascular pedicles.

The important clinical effects of these waves can be summarized as follows:

Ear: The tympanic membrane being diaphragmatic in nature and having been placed such as to have two acoustic interfaces, i.e. air/tissue and tissue/air makes it specially vulnerable to injury by blast waves. Notwithstanding the minor variations caused as a result of position of the ear in relation to the blast, a healthy tympanic membrane would rupture at a pressure of 100 kpa/ cm^2 applied for a duration of 10 msec or more. However, a previously scarred tympanic membrane ruptures at pressures as low as 15 kpa per cm^2. This vulnerability of the delicate tympanic membrane to incident pressure wave has importance in the overall management algorithms. In absence of the direct symptomatology of lung injury, if the typanic membrane are intact, it is extremely unlikely that lung has suffered the effect of the blast. Besides the ear drum injury, other injuries include-disruption of the ossicular chain, damage to the organ of Corti, and vestibular damage.

Lungs: Lungs, being air filled organs, are particularly susceptible to the effects of blast waves. A pressure loading of 175 kpa for 4 msec may cause minor damage to the alveoli. With high pressures such as 500 kpa severe fatal lung damage is likely. Blast waves produce damage to the alveolar interface which results in blood and extracellular fluid leak into the alveoli. This effect is more pronounced in areas of lungs which are subjected to the effects of reflected waves from the rib cage and the mediastinum. This results in shunting of blood across the fluid filled alveoli. Depending upon the magnitude of this phenomenon, the clinical picture of acute respiratory distress syndrome is produced. In addition, the shear wave traversing the lung may cause 'shearing off" of the lung tissues from its bronchial attachment resulting in bronchopleural fistulae.

Heart: Blast injury effect on the heart may vary from minor abnormality of ECG to more serious cardiac arrhythmia. Blast effect may cause direct cardiac contusion. In addition, the lungs damage may cause indirect changes like right ventricular stress and coronary air embolism.

Gastrointestinal tract: Shock wave may cause damage at the air tissue interface in the gastrointestinal tract. This usually is in the form of ecchymosis which, when extensive may result in paralytic ileus. The shear waves may produce mesenteric disruption. Gastrointestinal tract injury is rare in the absence of lung injury. The only exception to the rule is an underwater explosion in which a partially submerged body would sustain more damage in the lower submerged parts than on the chest lying above water level.

Nervous system: The effects on the nervous system include transient concussion, conduction disorders, disturbances of the blood-brain barrier, axonal degeneration and air sinus fractures.

Effect of the Flying Missiles–The Secondary Injuries

The blasts invariably produce a large number of flying missiles. The missiles may emanate from the bomb itself like pieces of its casing, the various substances kept in the bomb to act as sharpnels, or any object in the immediate vicinity of the blast may be energised to act as sharpnels. These are usually high energy, high velocity missiles. The kinetic energy of these missiles depends on the mass and velocity expressed by equation, $KE = \frac{1}{2} mv^2$. The factors governing the energy transfer to the victim from these missiles are discussed at greater length in the Chapter 3 "Wound Ballistics". As a rule the wounds caused by these missiles are heavily contaminated. The secondary missiles cause injury much beyond the range of the blast wave and blast wind. The commonly used grenade of Indian Army (HE 36) with a very small charge has a very small area of lethal range due to blast itself. However, the effective lethal range due to sharpnels is up to 9 meters. It, therefore, implies that the secondary injuries are the most common ones in any blast.

Effect of Blast Wind–The Tertiary Injury

The commonly used expression "blown to pieces" in the blast is the effect of blast wind. Blast wind generally has a much longer duration and considerably less pressure. The effect is purely mechanical. If the wind is strong enough it can cause amputation of the exposed parts or even total disintegration of the body. These types of injuries carry a prohibitively high mortality. Amputations caused by blast wind perhaps remain the only valid indication for use of a tourniquet. Adams[6] studied the effects of mine blast in a naval base in Cuba and classified them into two types:

Type I: The injuries involving the head, neck, trunk and upper limbs. This group constitute the bulk of the unsalvageable injuries carrying an extremely high mortality. It has been suggested that these cases be given a low priority in evacuation.

Type II: The injuries involving the lower limbs constitute the salvageable group.

Frykberg[7] studied the injury and mortality pattern in major blasts worldover. He studied a total of 3357 casualties and found 87% immediate survivor, out of whom 30% needed hospitalization, 19% were classified as critically ill and 12.4% of those critical ill succumbed to their injuries. In a major bombing in a crowded place immediate deaths are always more than the deaths among hospitalized survivors. Region wise injury pattern has been studied[8,9] and it has been noted that among hospitalized patients, injuries to lower limbs were most common (44%) followed by upper limbs 24%, head and neck 19% and torso 13%. Almost half of the patients had polytrauma and about one quarter had orthopedic injuries.

The distribution of hospitalized patients with regard to ISS was found to be as follows:

1-10	20%
10-20	45%
21-30	12.5%
31-40	07.5%
41-50	07.5%

Needless to emphasize those with higher ISS had higher rate of fatality.

Russian experience in Afghanistan (1979-1988) lead to better understanding of land mine injuries. There are three areas of injury. First, there is an area of mangling or avulsion (traumatic amputation) that occurs at the midfoot or distal tibia (Zone-1). Next is an area in which the soft tissues are separated from bone along fascial planes in the leg. The tissue is compromised but it may heal. The area extends from below the knee to the level of avulsion injury of the foot or lower leg (Zone-2). More proximally, injuries may occur from fragments or debris propelled from the land mine but not necessarily from direct effects of the blast itself (Zone-3). The degree of injury is dependent on the size and shape of the individual's limb, the type of footwear and clothing worn, the amount and type of soil overlying the land mine, and the size of the land mine itself.[10]

Gunshot Injuries

Gunshot wounds have become more frequent in the recent decades due to easy availability of firearms to terrorist groups and criminals. In wars the casualties caused by gunshot wounds are around one-fourth of the total casualties (Gulf war allied casualty rate due to GSW was 19%, Indian casualties in Sri Lanka due to GSW were 32%, Vietnam war-30%). In comparison the incidence of GSW in civilian life has become alarmingly high. It is a cause of death in 22% of all unnatural deaths in USA.[11]

Biomechanics of Gunshot Wounds

This has been discussed in detail in the Chapter 3 "Wound Ballistics". Missile injuries, unlike primary blast injuries don't affect particular organ systems. By law of probability they may damage any part of the body. But certain parts of the body do have a higher share of injuries. Regional distribution of injuries in various wars due to bullets are outlined in Table 4.1.[12]

Higher percentage of injuries to limbs is partly due to extensive use of antipersonnel mines and partly due to the fact that injuries to other body regions have a higher percentage of 'killed in action'. Figures from Korean war are illustrative of this Table 4.2.

Management of Bomb Blast Injuries

The bomb explosion is a particularly devastating and increasingly common form of terrorist violence. These incidents are unpredictable in their timing and location and typically result in large numbers of casualties with distinct pattern and complexity of injuries. Organized prehospital and inhospital trauma care has definite role to play. Aims of prehospital and inhospital trauma care should be to

Table 4.1: Regional distribution of injuries in various wars

Regions	*Korean war (%)*	*Indo-Pak war 1965(%)*	*IPKF-Sri Lanka (%)*	*Gulf-War (%)*
Head	15	1	2	6
Neck	3	2	-	-
Thorax	19	12	8	12
Abdomen	11	13	15	11
Upper limbs	25	22	10	44
Lower limbs	27	69	56	75

Table 4.2: Regional distribution of injuries in Korean war

Regions	Killed in action (%)	Injured in action (%)
Head	41	15
Neck	05	03
Thorax	35	19
Abdomen	10	11
Upper limbs	02	25
Lower limbs	07	27

minimize the time interval between injury and definitive surgery. Triage, rapid evacuation and basic life support; advance life support if the evacuation is going to be time consuming; and trauma care facility have all contributed to the decreased mortality and morbidity recently. History of the bomb blast is obvious but what is more important to know is the situation, whether it was in open or closed space and the position of the patient. In prehospital phase the problem may not be of airway but of ventilation. Typically a patient of blast injury is apprehensive, anxious, confused, breathless, with no signs of external injury and complains of deafness, hemoptysis, colicky abdominal pain, and hematemesis or melena. Clinical examination not only entails auscultation of chest and physical examination of abdomen but also auroscopy as the tympanic membrane reflects the blast load in the individual and serves as a screening examination.

Management of Blast Injury Lung

The incidence of primary blast injury in the lung has varied from 8-8.4%. The diagnosis of blast injury lung is based on symptoms and signs such as dyspnea, cynosis, hypoxia and bloody tracheal secretions. Radiological features on X-ray chest are linear or patchy diffuse infiltrates, pneumothorax and or hemothorax. Pulmonary insufficiency may manifest shortly after exposure to the explosion or may develop during the first or second day thereafter. Patients are very sensitive to intravenous fluids which may precipitate pulmonary edema. Hypovolemia if present due to other injuries should be treated with colloids predominantly. These patients stands general anesthesia badly unless assisted with positive pressure ventilation. Early management of blast injury consists of propped position, intravenous furosemide, oxygen, very small doses of morphine (0.01 mg%/kg body wt). Role of steroids is still not clear and it is better avoided in polytrauma. Clinical respiratory insufficiency/blood gas analysis may indicate the need for assisted positive pressure ventilation with positive end expiratory pressure mode. All victims of blast should be kept under surveillance for forty-eight hours for the late onset of pulmonary insufficiency.

Management of Abdominal Injuries

Injuries to the abdomen (Figs 4.1 and 4.2) may be penetrating or nonpenetrating. Management of penetrating injuries is no different as that of gunshot wounds while for nonpenetrating injuries it is important to establish the presence or absence of intraperitoneal hemorrhage or perforation of hollow viscus. The injury to the bowel, most often involves the ileocecal region. There may be serosal tears, subserosal or intramural hemorrhage as well as perforations. The perforations occur either acutely or develop in areas of ischemic necrosis of the contused bowel a few hours to several days after the forceful impact of the airwaves that accompanies an explosion. The concomitant existence of the rupture of the ear drum or primary blast injury of the lung should raise the suspicion and the patient be repeatedly examined for

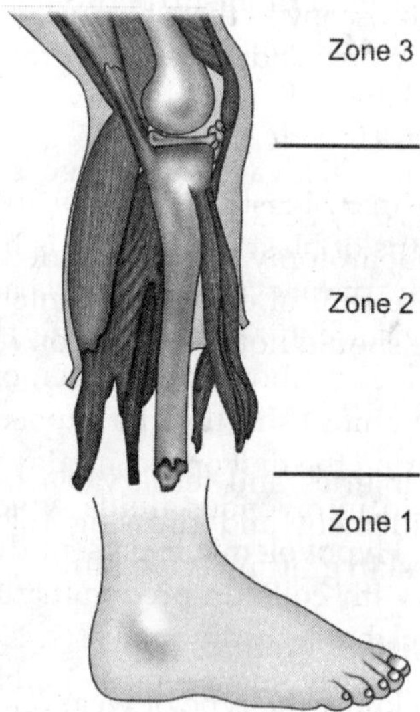

Fig. 4.1: Wound of entry in a case of gunshot wound abdomen

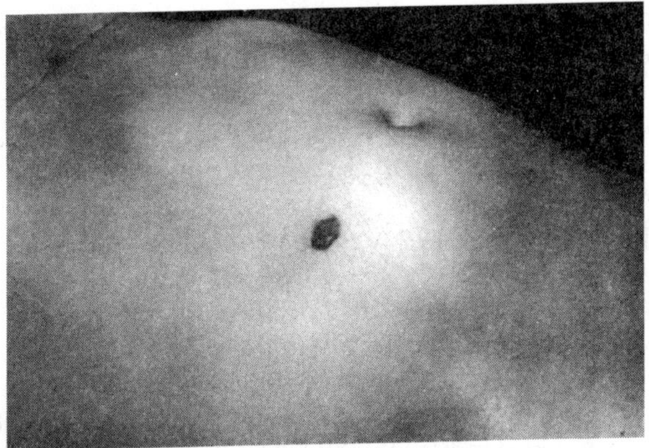

Fig. 4.2: Point of exit of bullet in Figure 4.1 case
(For color version, see Plate 1)

signs of peritonism. Evidence of intraperitoneal hemorrhage, perforation of viscus can be obtained by:

- Presence of shock
- Blood aspirate in nasogastric tube
- Blood on PR/proctoscopy/sigmoidoscopy
- Gas under the diaphragm
- Clinical evidence of peritonism/peritonitis
- Focussed abdominal sonography for trauma (FAST) evidence of blood/solid organ injury
- USG/CT scan
- Diagnostic peritoneal lavage is no longer poular due to wider availability of FAST/USG.

Once indicated laparotomy must be carried out at the earliest. In those cases where clinical evidence of internal hemorrhage is present undue time should not be wasted on resuscitation.

Shell Wounds

Secondary missile injuries and tertiary blast injuries should be treated with debridement and dressing followed by delayed primary sutures or skin grafting (vide infra).

Management of Gunshot Wounds

It is very helpful to know the type of weapon, its caliber, muzzle velocity, range and bullet type. When possible, inquire as to what position the patient was in when the wound was received—

whether sitting, lying flat or kneeling, whether walking or running. All wounds are contaminated by the dirty clothing which may be carried inside by the missile or by dirtying of the wounds by the surroundings. Contamination becomes an invasive infection in about 6 hours before which the wound must be excised in ideal circumstances.

The primary objectives in management of war and warlike wounds are:

a. Removal of all foreign substances and devitalized tissues.
b. Maintenance of blood supply to the part.
c. The management of soft tissue injury is routinely a two-stage procedure. In the first stage, a thorough debridement is done and wound is left open (with certain exceptions mentioned later). The second stage is a delayed primary closure (5-7 days later) or a secondary closure. War wounds, as a rule, are not closed primarily. The first stage is performed as soon as the patient is stabilized after reaching the surgical aid. The golden period of debridement is within 6 hours of wounding. The guidelines to be followed for debridement are:
   - In limb debridement a tourniquet is placed, if possible to be inflated when needed.
   - Antibiotics are started before surgery.
   - The procedure is done under anesthesia.
   - Preliminary X-rays must be displayed in the operating room.
   - A wide area is cleaned and draped around the wound while the wound is kept covered with a pad.
   - Liberal incisions are used.
   - All blood clots, foreign bodies and debris free in the wound must be removed. Liberal lavage with normal saline (tap water is as good)[13] is mandatory.
   - All dead and devitalized muscles must be excised till bleeding and contracting muscle is encountered.
   - Neurovascular structures must be carefully preserved.
   - Repair of major blood vessels must be undertaken promptly.
   - Detached but clean large bony fragments must be retained.
   - Though all foreign bodies must be removed, it is not necessary to waste time in locating all metallic foreign bodies seen in X-rays.
   - Soiled, frayed tendons must be resected without any attempt to restore their continuity at this stage.
   - Hemostasis must be precise.

- Repeated irrigation with saline is beneficial and keeps the field clean.
- At the conclusion of procedures, all blood vessels, nerves and tendons must be covered. It may necessitate an additional reconstructive procedure at an early date.
- Joint capsule should be closed. If this is not possible, at least synovium should be closed.
- Liberal fasciotomy to prevent compartment syndrome must be done.
- Suction drains (Vacuum assisted closure devices are better) are used liberally wherever a closed space is there. Drains are not a substitute for good hemostasis or for good surgical technique and should not be left in place too long. They are usually left in place only until the situation which indicated insertion is resolved.[14]
- Occlusive packing of wound is contraindicated. Only light fluffed gauge is used. Paraffin impregnated gauge is no longer advocated as dressing. Normal saline may be used instead.
- No constrictive dressings are used. Complete plaster casts are discouraged, and if used they should be cut along the entire length down to the skin.
- The following wounds may be closed primarily:
  - Facial wounds
  - Sucking chest wound—Even here the skin should be left open after closing the muscle
  - Scalp wounds
  - Hand wounds especially on palmar surface
  - Wound communicating with joint.

Primary closure of the wound in open fractures is increasingly being advocated[15] and may be done in civil ballistic wounds if following conditions are fulfilled:[16]

1. Patient and surgeons are not a transient population, i.e. definite and complete treatment is being carried out by the same surgeon at the same hospital.
2. Good hemostasis can be obtained following wound debridement.
3. Patient is subjected to surgery before colonization of the wound.
4. Patient general condition is stable.
5. Wound can be closed without tension.
6. Suction drain is used.
7. Expertise is available and the patient can be closely monitored.

Role of Skeletal Stability

Skeletal stability relieves pain by quite simply preventing unnatural movements at abnormal sites. This not only reassures the patient but facilitates easy transportation, good nursing care, permits adjoining muscle and joint rehabilitation, and early ambulation. Near anatomic position realigns neurovascular structures, providing optimal circulation to the injured extremities and reduces the risk of peripheral nerve compression. Restoration of such anatomy improves venous and lymphatic drainage thereby reducing tissue edema. At a cellular level it is now undisputed that such stabilization helps in ingrowth of capillaries and this capillary proliferation not only helps in the process of repair but also improves local tissue resistance to infection; helps in diffusion of nutrients, antibodies and white cell migration. The ultimate aim of any immobilization is to provide good stable alignment, and preservation of limb length without compromising the injured soft tissues.

Techniques for Skeletal Stability

For the occasional surgeon who handles polytrauma in mass casualties, the simpler the method chosen, the better it is. In fact the method the surgeon knows best is the best method. Surgeons at peripheral hospitals must select simpler and rapid methods of immobilization, leaving the surgeons at larger set up to select more complicated procedures.

External fixators have been in existence in clinical practice over the last 150 years and have become popular since world war II. Presently they are the method of choice for treatment of all Type III open fractures of limb bones and most pelvic fractures. The versatility of frame configuration, rapidity and ease of application, with stability as of an internal fixation, and ease of local tissue handling and dressings are its major advantages. External fixators help in early ambulation and rehabilitation. Despite the disadvantages which include pin tract infection, loosening, joint stiffness and occasional neurovascular complications, the external fixators are well in place in modern management of open fractures. Recently there are reports that suggest wane in the use if external fixators.[17]

The place of primary internal fixation in massive compound injuries is not safe because of the fear of infection and its serious long-term sequelae. However, clinical situations such as followings do call for primary internal fixation:[11]

a. Intra-articular fractures requiring anatomical reduction especially in weightbearing joints.
b. Fractures associated with vascular injuries.
c. Certain diphysical fractures.

Fracture Fixation—Damage Control Orthopedics

There is increasing acceptance of internal fixation in open fractures. The beneficial effects of fixation of open fractures, including improved wound care, tissue healing, preventing further soft tissue damage and reduction in infection rates have been well documented. However certain caveats have to be entertained. The injury *per se* leads to release of inflammatory mediators which has effect on pulmonary capillary endothelium and other organs. This may contribute to hypoxia (especially if associated with chest injury) with further cascade of events. If the patient's immune status is good a generalized inflammatory response is mounted resulting in systemic inflammatory response syndrome (SIRS), organ dysfunction and failure as a possible end result. If, on the other hand, the immunity is low there is a singular lack of inflammatory response (anergy) making the patient prone to sepsis. At a stage when the level of these inflammatory markers are high a surgery of some magnitude (definitive internal fixation or complex reconstruction as a part of endeavor to salvage the limb) leads to further release of the same substances resulting in what is called a second hit. The current recommendation is to do the minimum to stabilize the fracture by what has been termed as damage control orthopedics (DCO). DCO provides systemic benefits of reduced operative trauma (avoiding the second hit'), less sustained inflammatory response and improvement in the clinical status in multiple injured patient. The intent of this principle is not to postpone fracture stabilization but to allow immediate fracture stabilization in patients who are not cleared for definitive fracture care.

The current literature suggests that the favored tool for DCO in lower limbs is the application of external fixators. External fixations as a prime modality for the application of damage control. Orthopedics provide the advantages of decreased operating time, decreased blood loss and does not increase local complications besides not impairing the quality of definite osteosynthesis. Pin sites in external fixation do not represent a significant additional source for infection as the small bacterial inoculum inherent to the pin sites is often not sufficient to overcome host defenses to cause deep septic complications.[18] Further definitive fixation is to be done at higher levels of care but the optimal timing is still controversial. It may, however, be worth remembering that in nonpolytrauma situations there is increasing acceptance of a definitive internal fixation (esp. interlocking nail) even in open fractures up to type IIIA. The application of interlocking intramedullary nailing for patients with no infections and ring fixators with indicators of infection is the definitive management. For most open humerus and forearm fractures, the use of splint immobilization placed at forward surgical centres and transition to open plate osteosynthesis after soft tissue closure is recommended.[19]

Compartment Syndrome

Fractures, tissue loss and vascular injury caused by missiles and explosions place extremities at risk for compartment syndrome. Acute extremity compartment syndrome (ECS) is defined as "a surgical emergency characterized by raised pressure in an unyielding osteofascial compartment" that can be caused by trauma, revascularization procedures or exercise.[20] Specific events that may lead to ECS after trauma include hemorrhage from a fracture or arterial injury into an intact compartment, myocyte edema after ischemia-reperfusion injury or resuscitation. Use of tight external dressings may be another cause. The most common sites of ECS are the lower leg (53-62%), followed by forearm (24-26%), thigh (4-15%), foot (4-5%) and hand.[20]

A clinical diagnosis of ECS may be made when one or more signs and symptoms are present: pain out of proportion to the injury with or without pain on passive stretch, sensory changes, weakness, or paralysis. Combat surgeons should have a high index of suspicion of this entity and have a low threshold to perform 2-incision, 4-compartment fasciotomy of the distal extremity. Also extending the skin incision beyond what is needed for compartment release at the time of initial surgery may be advisable to allow progression of muscle edema, as inadequate skin incisions prevent complete compartmental decompression. In addition to surgical technique, timing of fasciotomy is critical, because after 8 hours of total ischemia irreversible damage occurs in the muscle and peripheral nerve.[21] Delayed ECS is another clinical situation where ECS manifests after large volume resuscitation, delayed effects of primary blast injury or air evacuation. Delayed fasciotomies in such clinical scenario have been questioned by many surgeons, because of increased morbidity in the face of little to no functional benefit. However, it is advisable still, for a combat surgeon to err on the side of performing a fasciotomy when faced with such problem.

Management of penetrating injuries abdomen and penetrating injuries chest are detailed in the respective chapters.

Management of Shot Gun Wounds

Shot gun wounds are smooth bore weapons designed to discharge a load of very small projectile at a small, fast moving target. Wounding capacity with shot gun shells consist of a spectrum ranging from wounds caused by a solitary pellet to those in which the entire charges strike the target (Fig. 4.3). At 1-3 meter, the wound consists of a central blast with a minor halo around the dense confluence of the major defect. At 7 meters, the bulk of the shot is well away from the center but is still contained within a six inches circle. Shot gun wounds have been classified according to the distance from the muzzle.

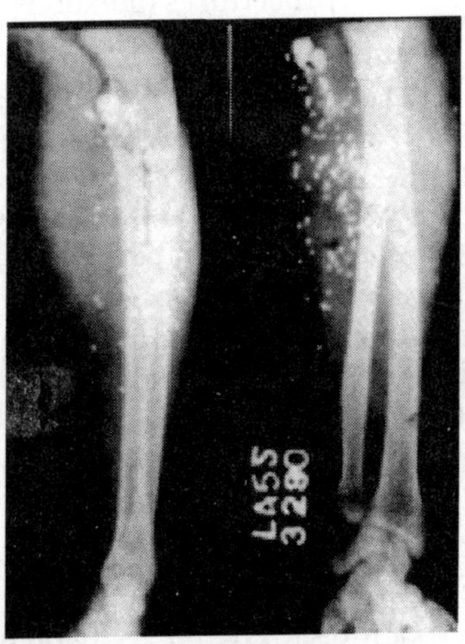

Fig. 4.3: Shot gun injuries demonstrating pellets

Type I injuries are sustained from long range (more than 7 meters) and are generally associated with deep penetration of only subcutaneous tissue and deep fascia. Type II injuries are from intermediate distances, and structures deep to the deep fascia can be assumed to have been penetrated. Type III injuries are sustained from close range (less than three meters) and are associated with extensive destruction. Management of shot gun wounds is dependent on the types of wounds. Type I wounds are generally managed with cleansing, sterile dressing and antibiotics. Type II injuries should be managed as other penetrating wounds in similar areas. Type III wounds need extensive debridement and achievement of hemostasis.

To summarize, the warlike injuries cause a great strain on the health care resources besides devastating the individual and the community psychologically. An insight into the causation of these injuries might help in better management under these stressful situations.

REFERENCES

1. Spalding TJW. Penetrating missile injury in Gulf war. Brit J Surg 1991;78:102-4.
2. Tyagi A. Personal communication, 1993.
3. Cooper GJ, Taylor DEM. Biophysics of impact injury to chest and abdomen. Jr Army Med Corps 1989;135:58-67.
4. Katz E, Oflex B, Adler J, et al. Primary blast injury after a bomb explosions in a civilain bus. Ann Surg 1989;209:484-8.
5. Zuckermann S. Experimental study of blast injury to lungs. Lancet 1940;11:219-24.
6. Adams DV. 21 years experience with landmine injury. J Trauma 1988;28:159-62.
7. Frykberg ER, Tepas JJ, et al. Terrorist bombings. Lessons learnt from Belfast to Beriut. Ann Surg 1988; 208:569-76.
8. Rignault DP, Deligny MC. The 1986 terrorist bombing experience in Paris. Ann Surg 1989;209:368-73.
9. DOE/Lawrence Livermore National Laboratory. "Blast Waves May Cause Human Brain Injury Even Without Direct Head Impacts." ScienceDaily 27 August 2009. 2 October 2009 <http://www.sciencedaily.com/releases/2009/08/090826152713.htm.
10. Necchaev EA, Gritsanov AI, Fomin NF, et al. Mine blast trauma (Experience from the war in Afghanistan). Stockholm, Sweden: Falths Tryckeri, 1995.

11. Hyot DB. In Greenfield's surgery: Scientific principles and practice, Philadelphia, JB Lippincott and Co. 1993 p 252.
12. Sinha VK, Luther ME. Injuries of war and civil disturbances. In Recent Advances in Orthopaedics, Vol I, New Delhi, Jaypee Brothers, 1993, p136-162.
13. Fernandez R, Griffiths R. Cochrane Database Syst Rev. 2008 Jan 23;(1):CD003861. Reviw.
14. World Health Orgainsation. Essential Surgical care manual
15. Moola F, Jacks D, Reindl R, Berry G, Harvey EJ. Safety of primary closure of soft tissue wounds in open fractures. JBJS (B) Vol 90B (suppl 1) 2008r EJ.
16. Kochar SK. Management of gunshot wounds. Proceedings of Annual Conference of Associations of Surgeons of India 27-30 Dec New Delhi, 1988.
17. Rowley DI. The management of war wounds involving Bone. J Bone Joint Surg (Br) 1996;78-B:706-9.
18. McHenry T, Simmons S, Alitz C, et al. Forward surgical stabilization of penetrating lower extremity fractures: circular casting versus external fixation. Mil Med 2001;166:791-5.
19. Clinton K Murray, Joseph R Hsu, Joseph S Solomkin, John J Keeling, Romney C Andersen, et al. Prevention and management of infections associated with combat-related extremity injuries. J Trauma 2008; 64:S239-S251.
20. Pearse MF, Harry L, Nanchahal J. Acute compartment syndrome of the leg. BMJ 2002;325:557-8.
21. Amber E Ritenour, Warren C Dorlac, Raymond Fang, et al. Complications after fasciotomy revision and delayed compartment release in Combat patients. J Trauma 2008;64:S153-S162.

Chapter 5

Injury Severity Score

Siddharth Pramod Dubhashi

INTRODUCTION

In 1971, The Association for the Advancement of Automotive Medicine (AAAM) developed the Abbreviated Injury Scale (AIS).[1] This was intended for use in grading the severity of anatomic injury in one group of trauma patients, i.e. automobile accident victims. The AIS is a list of several hundred injuries, each assigned to a severity value from 1 (minor) to 6 (nearly always fatal). In 1974, AIS became an integral part of a scale developed to grade the severity of injury the Injury Severity Score (ISS).[2] Injury scoring and prognostication has been pursued to achieve goals in four areas:

- Patient care
- Scientific tool
- Administrative and assessment goals
- Trauma care research.

Patient Care

Rapid assessment of magnitude of injury would allow prehospital and emergency department triage of patients for the allocation of specific facility hospital and also appropriate facility within the hospital. The score will indicate the severity of injury, thus identifying individual in need of urgent resuscitation and restoration of homeostasis. Optimal management requires that changes in injury score status should be followed. Injury score provides some means of considering probabilities of outcome. This is crucial in this era of consumer protection act and also where managed care is being practiced.

Scientific Tool

The effectiveness of various treatment regimens comparing patients with similar injuries or severity of disease can be analyzed. It may be used to identify patients as appropriate for incorporation into prospective randomized studies. Quantification of injury is a teaching exercise for medical students, residents and paramedicos. Scoring systems give us a formal framework for stratification and require objective assessment of degree of injury or illness.

Administrative and Assessment Goals

The score can be used for assessment of quality of patient care and for evaluation of management by comparing it with published studies of patients with similar disease or injury. It is an accurate method to assess the quality assurance issues because it allows comparisons with published standards.

Trauma Care Research

Scientific study of the epidemiology of trauma and trauma outcomes will not be possible without trauma care research. Injury severity scoring is indispensible in stratifying patients into comparable groups for prospective clinical trials. It can be used retrospectively to identify and control for differences in baseline injury severity between patient populations.

Classification of Scoring Systems

Anatomical Scores

1. Abbreviated injury scale (AIS)
2. Injury severity score (ISS)
3. Anatomic profile (AP)

Physiological Scores

1. Trauma score (TS) for adults
2. Revised trauma score (RTS) for adults
3. Trauma score for children
4. Glasgow coma scale (GCS) for adults
5. Glasgow coma scale (GCS) for children
6. APACHE scores

Combined Physiological and Anatomical Scores

1. Trauma injury severity score (TRISS)
2. Trauma index score
3. Circulation, respiration, abdomen/thorax, motor and speech score (CRAMS)

Anatomical Scoring Systems

1. Abbreviated injury scale (AIS): Since the introduction of AIS, it has been modified in 1990 (AIS-90), as a simple numerical method for grading and comparing injury severity. Although originally intended for use with vehicular injures, its scope has increased for use with other injures.

For calculating the AIS, the body is divided into 6 regions and each is weighted according to injury severity up to 6 degrees. (Table 5.1).

2. Injury severity score: It was developed by Baker and associates in early 1970.[2] The index is based on specific anatomic injuries. Each injured area of the body is assigned a score on a scale of 1 to 5. The three highest regional scores are then squared and added together for a maximum score of 75. A score of 75 denotes the worst patient outcome. If an injury is assigned an AIS of 6, the ISS score is automatically assigned to 75 (Table 5.2).

Table 5.1: Abbreviated injury scale

Division of the body into 6 patient:
i. Thorax
ii. Abdomen and viscera
iii. Head and neck
iv. Face
v. Bony pelvis and extremities
vi. External structures
Severity scoring in each body region:
0 = no injury
1 = minor injury
2 = moderate injury
3 = serious injury
4 = severe injury
5 = critical injury
6 = lethal injury (incompatible with life)

Table 5.2: An example of the ISS calculation

Region	*Injury description*	*AIS*	*Square Top three*
Head and neck	Cerebral contusion	3	9
Face	No injury	0	
Chest	Flail chest	4	16
Abdomen	Minor contusion of liver	2	
	Complex rupture spleen	5	25
Extremity	Fractured femur	3	
External	No injury	0	
	Injury severity score		*50*

The injury severity score (ISS) system has provided a method for quantitating injures and correlating it with outcome, but it can only be done after thorough evaluation of the patient to assess specific injures and their magnitude.

The most obvious limitation of the ISS is that it limits the total number of contributing injuries to only three, which impairs the usefulness of the score in penetrating injuries. It weighs the injuries to each body region equally, ignoring the seriousness of head injury due to trauma.[3] The assignment of scores is subjective.

Oster et al[4] in 1997 has reported a modified ISS or a new ISS (NISS), based on the three most severe injuries regardless of the body region. This simple but significant modification of the ISS avoids an important limitation. By preserving the AIS as the framework of injury severity, the NISS remains a user friend, and becomes a more accurate predictor of mortality than the ISS, particularly in penetrating injuries. Balogh et al[5] in 2000 reported the ability of the NISS to predict post injury multiple organ failure.

3. Anatomic profile (AP): This is a four valued (A<B<C<and D) description of injury.[6] The first-three values summarize all serious (AIS>2) injures to the head/brain and spinal cord (A), to the thorax and front of neck (B), and all remaining serious injuries (C). D is a summary measure of all nonserious injuries. AP component values are the square roots of the sums of squares AIS score of all associated injures. This scaling method attributes diminishing contribution to injuries other than the most severe in a particular body area. Component values suggest the presence of multiple injuries and distinguish among injuries in body regions; thus B=0 if no serious thoracic injuries were sustained (Table 5.3).

Physiological Scoring Systems

1. Trauma score for adults: This was based on an original scoring system depending on respiratory effort, capillary refill and GCS. For improving this 3 parameter triaging score, Champion et al[7] elucidated the Trauma Score by adding two other parameters–the respiratory rate and systolic blood pressure (Tables 5.4 and 5.5).

Table 5.3: Anatomic profile (AP) component definitions

A. Head
- AIS severity 3-5, Region 1.
- Spinal cord
- AIS severity 3-5, Regions 1,3,4.

B. Thorax
- AIS severity 3-5, Region 3.
- Front of neck
- AIS severity region 1.

C. All others
- AIS severity 3-5, Regions 1,2,3,4,5,6.

D. All others
- AIS severity 1-2, Regions 1,2,3,4,5,6.

Table 5.4: Trauma score for adults

Variables		*TS Points*
Respiratory rate	10-24	4
	25-35	3
	<35	2
	<10	1
Respiratory effort	Normal	1
	Shallow	0
Systolic blood pressure (mm Hg)	>90	4
	70-90	3
	50-69	2
	<50	1
	No carotid pulse	0

Contd...

Contd...

Capillary refill	Normal	2
	Delayed	1
	Absent	0
Glasgow coma scale		
Eye opening	Spontaneous	4
	To voice	3
	To pain	2
	None	1
Verbal response	Oriented	5
	Confused	4
	Inappropriate words	3
	Incomprehensible words	2
	None	1
Motor response	Obeys command	6
	Localizes	5
	Withdrawal	4
	Abnormal flexion	3
	Abnormal extension	2
	None	1
Total GCS	14-15	5
	11-13	4
	8-10	3
	5-7	2
	3-4	1
Total	1-16	

Table 5.5: Survival rate from trauma score for adults

Trauma score	*Survival(%)*
16	99
13	93
10	60
7	15
4	2
1	0

The TS for adults included 1-16 points and is of prognostic value with decreasing the chance of patient survival at 12 point or less. The TS for adults is also of value for comparing the performance of different trauma centres or the same trauma center over time.[7]

2. Revised trauma score for adult: The trauma score has been revised to try to limit some of the subjective measures like capillary refill, respiratory expansion. It includes only the variables of systolic blood pressure (SBP), respiratory rate (RR) and GCS. It includes a complex calculation combining coded (C) factors of the parameters multiplied by weighting values which are coefficients derived from a large database through regression analysis.[8] These values aim to emphasize the increased impact of head injury on the total score (Table 5.6). The coded RTS is calculated as follows:

$$RTSc = 0.2908\ RRc + 0.7326\ SBPc + 0.9368\ GCSc$$

The RTS ranges between 0 and 7.84, with a lower score denoting a more serious injury. A patient with score less than 4 needs an urgent transport to a trauma center. The score is useful for prehospital triage, outcome assessment and quality assurance of critical care service.

However, the RTS is unable to accurately score patients who are intubated and mechanically ventilated, as determining the verbal component of the GCS and the RR are difficult in these patients.

3. Trauma score for children: Anatomical differences make the TS unsuitable for children. Children are more prone to head

Table 5.6: Revised trauma score for adults

Variables		*RTS Points*
GCS	13-15	4
	9-12	3
	6-8	2
	4-5	1
	0-3	0
SBP	>89	4
	76-89	3
	50-75	2
	1-49	1
	0	0
RR	10-29	4
	>29	3
	6-9	2
	1-5	1
	0	0

Table 5.7: Trauma score for children			
Component	*+2*	*+1*	*-1*
Size (kg)	>20	10-20	<10
SBP (mm Hg)	>90	50-90	<50
Airway	Normal	Can be maintained	Difficult to maintain
CNS	Awake	Obtunded	Coma/Decerebrate
Skeletal system	None	Closed fracture	Open/Multiple fractures
Cutaneous system	None	Minor	Major/Penetrating

SBP = Systolic blood pressure, CNS = Central nervous system

injuries because of the relative disproportion of their head and body sizes and because of their relatively loose ligaments of their cervical spines.

Jubevirer et al[9] have designed the TS for children which includes 6 variables and 12 points (Table 5.7). A score of less than 8 points denotes more probability of death.

4. Glasgow coma scale (GCS) for adults: The Glasgow coma Scale for adults monitors behaviors of eye opening (4 points), verbal responses (5 points) and motor responses (6 points), of the injured patient (Table 5.8). The total score ranges between 3 and 15 points. Mild, moderate and severe head injuries are accounted for by 13-15, 9-12 and 8 or less scoring points, respectively.

Table 5.8: Glasgow coma scale for adults		
Behavior	*Response*	*Points*
Best eye opening response	Spontaneous	4
	To speech	3
	To pain	2
	Nil	1
Best motor response	Obeys command	6
	Localizes pain	5
	Withdrawal from pain	4
	Abnormal flexion to pain	3
	Extends to pain	2
	Nil	1
Best verbal response	Fully oriented	5

Contd...

Contd...

	Confused conversation	4
	Inappropriate words	3
	Incomprehensible words	2
	Nil	1
	Total	*3-15*

5. Glasgow coma scale (GCS) for children: The children version of the GCS was designed by Reilly et al,[10] where verbal responses were reported as appropriate words, or social smiles, cries, irritability or restlessness and agitation with the same numerical description for the severity of head injury as in adults (Table 5.9).

6. APACHE scoring systems: The original APACHE scoring system was developed at the George Washington University Medical Centre as a way to measure the disease severity.[11]

Physiologic and chronic health evaluation (APACHE) is a classification system used for all patients in an intensive care unit (ICU). APACHE II, is based on 12 physiologic measurements; patient age, and prior severe deficiency in an organ system.[12] Values for APACHE II variables may be assessed either at ICU admission or as the worst values measured during the first 24 hours after admission. Trauma patients are considered coarsely in APACHE II. First, they are classified into postoperative and nonoperative groups, and then having multiple trauma or head trauma. The basic components in APACHE II are included in (Table 5.10). The APACHE II system has been found to correlate

Table 5.9: Glasgow coma scale for children

Variable	*Score*
Best verbal response	
Appropriate words or social smiles	
Fixes on and follows objects	5
Cries but is consolable	4
Persistently irritable	3
Restless, agitated	2
Silent	1
Eye and motor responses	Scored as in scale for adults

Table 5.10: Components of APACHE II scoring system

Acute physiology score		
Temperature	Mean arterial pressure	Heart case
Respiratory rate	GCS	PaO_2
Arterial pH	Hematocrit	WBC count
Serum sodium level	Serum potassium level	Serum creatinine level
Age score		
Chronic health score		

with outcome in several groups. Its ability to accurately predict outcome for individual cases is limited.[13] The APACHE III system[14] represents an improvement over its predecessor, but its utility with respect to trauma patient has yet to be proven.

Combined Physiological and Anatomical Scores

1. Trauma injury severity score: The TS and ISS from the physiological and anatomical components of the TRISS respectively. Age of the traumatized patient is a third component, and each of the three components is assigned a coefficient. The probability of survical of the traumatized patient can be estimated using a special TRISS chart.[15]

The TRISS is considered to be a good prognostic tool for the evaluation of the traumatized patient outcome. It is also considered valuable for patient triage. It has its limitations.[16] It includes no information about the patient condition as a cardiovascular disease. It cannot include intubated patients where RR and verbal responses cannot be evaluated. It includes the TS, not its revised version.

2. Trauma index score (TIS): The TIS was developed by Kirkpatric and Youmans.[17] It considers physiological organ grades and anatomical regional components. It also escalates the type of injury (Table 5.11). Each parameter of the score is divided into 1 to 4 scoring points. The maximum score is 20 points with less than 7 points denoting a mild condition and less than 18 points denoting the severest condition.

Table 5.11: Trauma index score

Score	*1*	*2*	*3*	*4*
Region affected	Skin/ extremity	Back	Chest/ abdomen	Head/ neck
Type of injury	Laceration/ contusion	Stab	Blunt	Missile
Cardiovascular	Hemorrhage Present/ chest pain	BP<100 HR>100	BP<80 HR>140	Pulseless
CNS	Drowsy	Stupor	Focal	Coma
Respiratory		Dyspnea/ hemoptysis	Aspiration	Apnea/ cyanosis

BP = Blood pressure, HR = Heart rate, CNS = Central nervous system

3. Circulation, respiration, abdomen/thorax, motor and speech (CRAMS) score: The CRAMS score has been developed by Gormicon.[18] It includes a mixture of physiological and anatomical parameters with a maximum of 10 scoring points (Table 5.12). A traumatized patient with a lower score has a more serious condition. The score can discriminate between survivors and non-survivors and is useful for patient triaging. It can compare different trauma centers and different locations or the same center over time.

Table 5.12: CRAMS score

Variable	*Score*
Circulation	
Capillary refill, normal or BP >100 mm Hg	2
Capillary refill delayed or BP 85 to 100 mm Hg	1
No capillary refill or BP<85 mm Hg	0
Respiration	
Normal	2
Labored or shallow	1
Absent	0
Abdomen/thorax	
Abdomen and thorax, nontender	2
Abdomen and thorax, tender	1
Abdomen rigid, flail chest or penetrating injury	0

Contd...

Contd...

Motor	
Normal	2
Responds only to pain	1
Decerebrate or no response	0
Speech	
Normal	2
Confused	1
No intelligible words	0
Total	*10*

Evaluation of Trauma Outcome

There is a general consensus within the trauma care community that patient's injury severity should be characterized by both physiologic and anatomic measures. Such combinations meet a variety of needs, ranging from the evaluation of prehospital protocols to epidemiological evaluation. TRISS introduced in 1981[15] is used in Major Trauma Outcome Study (MOTS) and most trauma registries. TRISS can be used to estimate probabilities for survival of survival for trauma patients from a retrospective database, using a logical model:

$$Ps = 1/(1+e^{-b})$$

Where Ps is the probability of survival and e = 2.7183 (base of Nepierian logarithms), and

$$b = b_0 + b_1\ (RTS) + b_2\ (ISS) + b_3\ (A)$$

Where b_0, b_1, b_2 and b_3 are weights derived from study data (Table 5.13), RTS is the revised trauma score on admission, ISS is the injury severity score, and A = 1 if the patient is over 54 years, and A = 0 if the patient is 54 years or less.

ASCOT: A severity characterization of trauma (ASCOT)[19] was developed to improve on the predictive ability of TRISS. ASCOT combines emergency department admission values of the Glasgow

Table 5.13: MOTS—Controlled site coefficients based on AIS -90[20]

	b_0	b_1 (RTS)	b_2 (ISS)	b_3 (A)
Blunt	–0.4499	0.8055	–0.0835	–1.7430
Penetrating	–2.5355	0.9934	–0.0651	–1.1360

coma scale (G), systolic blood pressure (S), and respiratory rate (R) as coded for RTS with AP components and patients age. ASCOT values are related to Ps (Probability of Survival) by the logistic function:

$$Ps = 1 / (1+e-k)$$

Where $k = kq + k_1G + k_2S + k_3R + k_4A + k_5B + k_6 6 + k_7AGE$ and A<B< and C are AP components. AGE is a variable used to compute patient's survival probability (Table 5.14).

Coefficients for the ASCOT logistic modes are given in Table 5.15. Patients with extremely severe (AIS 6/RTS 0) or very minor injuries are not evaluated with ASCOT logistic model and these set aside patients group are defined and their retrospective probabilities have been given.

Unexpected deaths (Ud) are the object of analysis of trauma care quality. On the other hand, the unexpected survivors (Us) are welcomed and reflect trauma care above the standards. Unexpected deaths (Ud) often correspond to insufficient trauma care.[21]

Definitive outcome-based evaluation (DEF) methodology was established by Flora JD in 1978, is the method used to compare survival probability with the standard database.[22,23] This method

Table 5.14: ASCOT patient AGE characterization

Age	*Ages (years)*
0	0-54
1	55-64
2	65-74
3	75-84
4	>85

Table 5.15: ASCOT model weights (design set)

Variables	*Blunt*	*Penetrating*
Constant	–1.1570	–1.1350
G	0.7705	1.0626
S	0.6583	0.3638
R	0.2801	0.3332
A	–0.3002	–0.3702
B	–0.1961	–0.2053
C	–0.2086	–0.3188
Age	–0.6355	–0.8365

was used for burn patients and then extended to trauma patients by MTOS. It is composed of 3 statistics-W-statistic, Z-statistic and M-statistic.[23]

W-statistic is used to indicate the difference between the predictive number of survivors (given by summing the predicted survival probabilities for each patient) and the actual number of survivors; divided number of excess survivors per 100 patients, compared with the prediction.

$$W = \frac{\text{(actual number of survivors-predicted number of survivors)}}{\text{(number of patients/100)}}$$

A positive value of W indicates that the institute has more survivors than predicted, and so its performance is above the standard in the prediction database.

Z-statistic is used to assess whether the W-statistic is significantly different from zero, and hence if the institution's performance is significantly different from that defined by the prediction database.[24,25]

$$Z = \frac{\text{(number of survivors-predicted number of survivors)}}{\sqrt{\text{sum of } [Ps \times (1-Ps)]}}$$

M-statistic is used to examine the similarity in the mix of severities in the observed data, compared with the prediction data set.[23,24]

M = Summing of minimum (Fi, Fj)
Fi = Fraction of prediction database cases in interval i
Fj = Fraction of observed cases in interval j

The value of M is between 0 and 1, with value close to 1 indicating a very similar mix of severities.

When any scoring system is used to predict outcome or evaluation based on predicted outcome, the determinations must be tempered by inaccuracy of the system. These methods have unavoidable limitations because of the variability in biology, as well as the mathematical assumptions in the statistical analysis. Decision making cannot depend on a numerical score only.

Preventable trauma deaths are clinical reality, but the ways for identification of preventable trauma deaths still are not standardized and need to improve.[26]

REFERENCES

1. Committee on Medical Aspects of Automotive Safety. Rating the severity of tissue damage. The Abbreviated Injury Scale. JAMA 1971; 215:277-80.
2. Baker SP, O'Neill B, Haddon W Jr, et al. The injury severity score: evaluating emergency care. J Trauma 1974; 14(3): 187-96.
3. Consulting Staff, Department of Surgery, Trauma Services, St. Anthony Hospital. Trauma Scoring Systems. Medicine 2004. http://www.emedicine.com/med/topic 3214. htm.
4. Oster T, Baker SP, Long W. A modification of the injury severity score that both improves and simplifies scoring. J Trauma 1997; 43(6):922-6.
5. Balogh Z, Offner PJ, Moore EE. NISS predicts post injury multiple organ failure better. J Trauma 2000;48(4):624-7.
6. Copes WS, Champion HR, Sacco WJ, et al. Progress in characterising anatomic injury. Proceedings of the 33rd annual meeting of the association for the advancement of automotive medicine. Baltimore, MD, October 2-4, 1989.
7. Champion HR, Saccow J, Carnazzo AJ. Trauma Score Crit Care Med 1981;9:672-5.
8. Champion HR, Saccow WJ, Copes WS. A revision of the trauma Score. J Trauma 1989; 28: 623-9.
9. Jubevirer RA, Agarwal NN, Beyer FC. Paediatric Trauma Triage: a review of 1307 cases. J Trauma 1990;30:1544-90.
10. Reilly PL, Simpson AD, Thomas LA. Paediatric version of GCS. Childs Nervous System 1988;4:30-3.
11. Knaus WA, Zimmerman JE, Wagner BP. APACHE. Acute Physiology, Age and Chronic Health Evaluation, a physiologically based classification system. Crit Care Med. 1981;16:470-8.
12. Knaus WA, Draper EA, Wagner DP. APACHE II: A severity of disease classification system. Crit Care Med. 1985;13:818-23.
13. Civetta JM. The clinical limitations of ICU scoring systems. Probl. Crit 1989;3:681-92.
14. Knaus WA, Wagner DP, Draper EA, et al. The APACHE III prognostic system. Crit Care Med 1991;100:16-19.
15. Boyr C, Tolson M. Evaluating the trauma care: The TRISS method; The Trauma Injury Severity Score. J Trauma 1987;27:370-5.
16. Cayten CG, Stanl VVM, Murphy JG. Limitations of the TRISS Method. a multihospital study. J Truama 1991;31(4):471-82.
17. Kirkpatric JR, Youmans RL. Trauma Index: an aid in the evaluation of injured victims. J Trauma 1971;11:711-3.
18. Gormicon SP. CRAMS Scale: Field triage of trauma victims. Ann Emerg. Med 1982;11:132-5.

19. Champion H, Copes W, Sacco W, et al. A new characterization of injury scoring 1990;30:539.
20. Champion H, Sacco W, Copes WS. Injury severity scoring again, Editorial Comments. J Trauma 1995;38:94-5.
21. Llullaku SS, Hyseni N, Bytysi CI, Rexhepi SK. Evaluation of trauma care using TRISS method: the role of adjusted misclassification rate and adjusted W-statistic. World J Emerg Surg 2009;4:2.
22. Champion HR, Copes WS, Sacco WJ, et al. The major trauma outcome study: establishing national norms for trauma care. J Trauma 1990; 30:1356-65.
23. Hollis S, Yates DW, Woodford M, Foster P. Standardized comparison of performance indicators in trauma: a new approach to case-mix variation. J Trauma 1995;38:764-6.
24. Boyd CR, Tolson MA, Copes WS. Evaluating Trauma Care: The TRISS Method. J Trauma 1987;27:370-78.
25. Thanapaisal C, Wongkonkitsin N, Seow OTS, et al. Outcome of In-Patient Trauma Cases. J Med Assoc Thai 2005;88(11):1540-44.
26. Chiara O, Cimbanassi S, Atessio Pitidis A, Vesconi S. Preventable trauma deaths: from panel review to population based studies. World J Emerg Surg 2006;1:12.

Chapter

6 Management Protocols in Polytrauma

SK Kochar

Trauma presents the surgeon with a confusing and rapidly changing situation. In a typical case, the patient appears suddenly in the midnight with multiple injuries that are not immediately apparent but may be life-threatening and is unable to communicate meaningful information because of associated head injury or intoxication. The surgeon must respond so that resuscitation is begun immediately, life-threatening injuries are treated, and all other injuries are identified. These many variables conspire to create fertile soil for overlooked injuries (Table 6.1).

Reasons injuries may be missed are:

- Hemodynamic instability
- Alteration in consciousness
- Intubated
- Paralysis
- Inexperience (low index of suspicion)
- Radiological error
  - Failure to perform the study
  - Inadequate film
  - Misinterpretation
- Technical errors
- Admitted in inappropriate service

Table 6.1: Incidence of missed injuries in trauma cases

Chan et al 1980[1]	Blunt injury	327	39 (12%)
Hamdan 1989[2]	Penetrating	—	25
Albertson and Thomson 1989[3]	Blunt	218	75 (34%)
Enderson et al 1990[4]	Blunt	399	36

Established well thought out protocols helps in organizing the resuscitation and assessment of the trauma patient and minimizes the chances of missing injury. Classically, two surveys for the trauma patient have been described. The primary survey is designated to identify all immediately life-threatening injuries and to treat these injuries in the emergency department as they are discovered. The secondary survey is designated to be "head to toe" search for all other injuries the patient has sustained.[5] However, even this approach does not ensure that all injuries will be discovered. A recent study demonstrated that 9 percent of multiple trauma patient sustained injuries that were not discovered during the primary and secondary surveys.[4] Tertiary survey is carried out after life-threatening injury has been investigated and managed.

FIRST PRIORITIES PROTOCOLS

Objectives are to detect cardiovascular and respiratory instability and initiate therapy to minimize tissue hypoxia, identify immediately life-threatening injuries and prevent damage to spinal cord.

a. Airway maintenance and cervical spine control
b. Breathing and ventilation
c. Circulation
d. Disability: neurological status
e. Exposure/environmental control.

1. Clinical examination to evaluate airway, breathing, circulation by inspecting the patients for skin color, chest wall motion, and extremity movement. Agitation is frequent sign of hypoxia and compromise of the airway. Noisy breathing, cyanosis, and the use of accessory muscle of respiration are all strongly suggestive of obstruction of the airway. Unconscious, obtunded patients with facial trauma, facial burns, laryngeal injury and those with hemorrhage into the soft tissue of the neck are at particular risk and need to have airways cleared and secured.
2. Clear the airway of blood, saliva, loose teeth, foreign body, vomitus and fallen tongue. Keeping the cervical spine in neutral position perform the jaw thrust/chin lift maneuver and place the oropharyngeal airway. Occasionally, there is need

for endotracheal (orotracheal or nasotracheal) intubation. Indications for this definite airway include apnea, inability to maintain an airway, need for protection of an airway, need for hyperventilation in patients with injuries to the brain, and inability to maintain oxygenation with face mask. Rarely, intubation may be difficult and depending upon the emergent situation one may have to perform cricothyroidotomy/tracheotomy. Availability of laryngeal airways and combitube have decreased the need for surgical airways. A word of caution, always protect cervical spine while attempting intubation.

3. See and watch the breathing effort. Adequacy of ventilation and oxygenation may be assessed with pulse oximetery. Auscultate the chest for air entry, any rhonchi or crepts. Tension pneumothorax, flail chest, pulmonary contusion, sucking chest wound, massive pneumothorax need ruling out. Tension pneumothorax and sucking chest wound must be addressed in primary survey. In tension pneumothorax, important clinical features are a sense of impending death, marked respiratory distress, deviated trachea, distended neck veins, unilateral absence of breath sounds, cyanosis, and hypotension. Needle thoracocentesis using a 14-gauge catheter over needle inserted into second intercostal space in midaxillary line and connected to a under water seal will tide over the crisis and the same after secondary survey should be converted into tube thoracostomy. The diagnosis of sucking chest wound is obvious and its prompt closure with occlusive dressing using Gamchee pad and elastoplast will improve the breathing.
4. Palpate the pulse, note its volume, rate and rhythm and measure the blood pressure. The most common type of shock in trauma patient is hypovolemic due to hemorrhage but cardiogenic (cardiac tamponade, tension pneumothorax, and myocardial contusion), neurogenic shock (spinal cord injury) may occasionally occur.
5. Establish intravenous access, collect the blood for blood grouping and cross matching. Collect the blood for baseline investigations and start the intravenous infusion of crystalloid till the blood is obtained.

LAC-USC trauma transfusion protocol[5a]
Rapid uncontrolled hge shock

Hge control surgical/ endovascular
Send type and cross match, aPTT, INR and platelet count
Autotransfusion of shed pleural blood
Hypothermia control (warm fluids and vent gases, remove wet clothing, dry patient, (Bair hugger)

1. Start with O Rh negative PRBC
2. Switch to type specific or cross matched blood as soon as it is available.

Component therapy triggers
Empirical

6 units of PRBC; history of coumadin
Request trauma cooler
6 units type specific FFP
1 unit ABO/Rh matched apheresis platelets

Targeted

Abnormal aPTT/ INR
Platelet <50 × 103
Fibrinogen <100
Request trauma cooler
6 units type specific FFP
1 unit ABO/Rh matched apheresis platelets
cryoprecititate
Diffuse nonsurgical bleeding
Recombitant factor VIIa 100 mcg/kg, additional doses as required (best if pH>7.1 and T>350

Recommendation

Ideal fluid for resuscitation should be safe, efficacious, cheap, easy to store and transport have the capacity to carry oxygen and nutrients to the cells protect the cell from, resuscitation injury.

6. Cardiac tamponade when present must be addressed during primary survey. It is usually associated with penetrating trauma to the parasternal area, upper abdomen, and rarely the neck, while blunt cardiac rupture as a cause is extremely rare. Patients usually have a grey death like appearance, extreme anxiety, tachycardia, hypotension, distended neck veins, and muffled heart sounds. The hypotension may partially respond to infusion of fluids but these patients may need pericardiocentesis in emergency room and definitive emergency sternotomy/thoracotomy in operation theater.

7. Establish cardiac monitoring.
8. Control extremity hemorrhage. Pressure dressing suffices most of the time but if bleeding is profuse consider shifting to operation theater for control of bleeding but before that one should complete the secondary survey to rule out internal hemorrhage. Note the size of pupil, level of consciousness and record GCS. Pupillary size, symmetry, and reaction to light are important diagnostic tools to aid in lateralization of intracranial injury.
9. Stabilize the neck with cervical collar.
10. Pass the Foley's catheter. If a male patient has blood at urethral meatus/suspicion of urethral injury, a retrograde urethrogram is performed after secondary survey prior to insertion of catheter.
11. Pass the nasogastric tube and note the color of the aspirate.
12. Obtain X-ray chest, pelvis and lateral view of cervical spine.

SECONDARY SURVEY

The objective of the secondary survey is to detect cardiovascular, respiratory, or brain pathology, which is an imminent threat to the patient's life, and identify potential or actual spinal cord or cerebral injury that may cause significant morbidity. To rule out blunt or penetrating trauma to the abdomen and to detect the presence of abdominal pathology, which requires therapeutic interventions at the earliest possible point to minimize morbidity and mortality.

The secondary survey is not performed until the primary survey is completed, resuscitation has been initiated and revaluation of the vital functions has been performed.

The check list consists of the following:

- Obtain a brief history.
- Perform a brief external examination of the head, neck, chest, abdomen, back, pelvis, and extremities.
- Perform a more complete neurological examination.
- Obtain thoracic and lumbar spine X-rays, if indicated.
- Indicate specific therapy for spinal cord injury.
- Institute medical treatment for severe brain injury.
- Perform diagnostic peritoneal lavage, local wound exploration or physical examination of the abdomen as appropriate.

- Special studies like USG abdomen, CT scan, arteriogram and laboratory test as relevant.
- Insert an arterial line, central line, Swan ganz catheter, when indicated.
- Administer prophylactic antibiotic.
- Consider tetanus prophylaxis in all trauma patients.

History

Details of the accidents may not be forthcoming as the patient may be unconscious due to head injury, impaired sensorium due to alcohol, drug or shock. The mnemonic AMPLE developed by Freeark and Baker at Cook county hospital, Chicago[6] is excellent for obtaining a history of the trauma patient.

A. Allergies
M. Medications currently being taken by the patient
P. Past illness and operations
L. Last meal
E. Events/environment related to the injury.

Knowledge of mechanism of injury provides valuable information because of expected patterns of injury. Blunt injury is more common in vehicle accidents while penetrating injuries are invariably by stab wounds or as a result of gunshot. Crushing injuries are often due to fall or vehicle accidents.

Systemic Physical Examination

Head

Scalp lacerations and hematoma may be detected easily, but small wounds may be hidden within the hair. A laceration or hematoma of the scalp or a skull fracture should alert the surgeon to the possibility of significant underlying intracranial injury.[7] Fractures of the cranial vault may be seen or palpated through scalp or facial lacerations. A Battle's sign, Panda eyes, CSF rhinorrea or otorrhea epistaxis, hemotympanum or hemorrhage from the ear may signify the presence of a basilar skull fracture. A facial fracture should be considered whenever a facial laceration or contusion is present and may be identified by palpating the orbital rims, zygomatic arches, mandible, or nose or by grasping the mandibular or maxillary teeth to detect instability.

Signs of a jaw fracture are the presence of malocclusion, intraoral ecchymosis, loose teeth, preauricular pain, excessive mobility, and a palpable deformity through a jaw laceration. Signs associated with an orbital fracture are deformity, swelling, ecchymosis, diplopia, and subconjunctival hemorrhage. A zygomatic fracture is suspected if the patient has infraorbital hypoesthesia, a subconjunctival hemorrhage, or deformity or ecchymosis in the region of the zygoma. Epistaxis, CSF rhinorrhea, telecanthus, or deformity should suggest the presence of a nasal fracture.

The oral cavity is evaluated for the presence of a laceration, bleeding or a hematoma. Any laceration of the cheek should be assessed for the possibility of injury to the facial nerve or parotid duct. The presence of a periorbital laceration or swelling or an orbital fracture suggests the possibility of an eye injury. Enophthalmia or dysconjugate gaze may represent extraocular muscle entrapment. When possible, the patient is checked for visual acuity and pupillary response to light. The eye should be carefully observed for the presence of extrusion of intraocular contents. Fundoscopic examination is performed to detect the presence of a vitreous hemorrhage or retinal detachment. The eye is examined for the possibility of a corneal abrasion or dislocation of the lens.

Neck

Before examination of neck, injury to cervical spine must be ruled out clinically and confirmed by radiological examination. Immobilization of the spine should be maintained until the injury has been treated or excluded. The neck is evaluated for hoarseness, airway obstruction, cervical subcutaneous emphysema, and hemoptysis, which commonly reflect injury to the larynx or cervical trachea. Cervical esophageal or pharyngeal injuries may be suggested by the presence of dysphagia, hematemesis, oral bleeding, or subcutaneous emphysema. Injury to the carotid or vertebral artery should be suspected if the patient has a pulse deficit, cervical hematoma, impaired level of consciousness, hemiparesis, or bruit. The external wound/hemorrhage may suggest the possibility of major vascular injury. Wounds that penetrate the platysma demand further investigations.

Chest

The chest is re-examined to find out occult injuries and assess the injuries that require treatment during the primary survey and resuscitation. Inspection for contusions and deformity, palpation for crepitus and tenderness, percussion for hyperresonance, tympany or dullness, and auscultation for decreased breath sounds, and heart sounds all are redone. The aim is to detect or rule out the presence of fracture ribs, pneumothorax, hemothorax, pneumohemothorax, flail chest, pulmonary contusion and injury to trachea, bronchus, and esophagus. A tracheal or bronchial injury is suggested by the presence of progressive massive subcutaneous emphysema, hemoptysis, or tension pneumothorax and should be suspected in a patient who has a transmediastinal penetrating wound.[8] Findings that suggest the possibility of an esophageal injury are the presence of hematemesis, chest pain, transmediastinal penetrating wound, bloody gastric aspirate, or cervical subcutaneous emphysema.[9] An injury to the aorta or its tributaries should be considered if the patient has a carotid, brachial, or femoral pulse deficit; interscapular, precordial, or cervical bruit; or impaired level of consciousness. A rupture of the diaphragm with intrathoracic evisceration is likely in a patient who has a diminution in breath sounds, bowel sounds during auscultation of the chest, tracheal shift, tachypnea, or cyanosis.

The current literature indicates that in blunt trauma patients with abnormal physical examination, abnormal conventional radiography, or abnormal ultrasonography of the chest, CT was likely to reveal relevant chest injuries. However, there was no strong evidence to suggest that CT could be omitted in patients without these criteria, or whether these findings are beneficial for patients.[9a]

Abdomen

The abdomen is inspected for contusions, brusie, ecchymosis, abrasions, laceration, or any penetrating injury. No attempt should be made to remove the stabbing instrument till the patient is in operation theater as it may Herald severe bleeding. Both the front and the back of the abdomen, perineum, and lower chest need to be viewed. Careful logrolling of the patient must be done to examine the back. Abdomen palpation may detect localized and generalized tenderness, guarding or rigidity and signs of peritoneal irritation such as rebound tenderness. The presence or absence of bowel sounds is important but nonspecific as this may be absent in fracture of ribs, pelvis or vertebra. Examination of the perineum, rectum, vagina and external genitalia should be done. Perineal or scrotal hematoma, a high riding prostate, lacerations and obvious open injuries to the pelvic ring are all important diagnostic signs mandating further workup or immediate surgery. Flank ecchymosis, pain, or hematoma may be associated with a retroperitoneal vascular or renal injury. Hematuria usually signifies an injury to the kidney, ureter, bladder, or urethra. A urethral injury should be suspected if blood is found at the urethral meatus; if an ill defined, mobile or elevated prostate is noted on rectal examination; or if there is a perineal hematoma, pain, or ecchymosis. A rectal injury is suspected if blood is found on rectal examination or the patient has penetrating wound of the lower abdomen, pelvis, or upper thighs. A uterine injury is suspected if there is bleeding through the cervix or a pelvic hematoma present on bimanual examination especially if this is identified in association with penetrating trauma. Vulvar or vaginal lacerations or hematoma are identified on internal examination.

Musculoskeletal and Peripheral Vascular Assessment

Extremity fractures, ligamentous instability, or joint capsule disruption should be suspected when there is local tenderness, crepitus, excessive motion or impaired motion (Figs 6.1 and 6.2). To detect arterial or venous injuries, the neck supraclavicular fossa, groin, and extremities are carefully evaluated. Decreased or absent pulse is strongly suggestive of an arterial injury, but the presence of a pulse doesn't exclude such a possibility.[10] External hemorrhage or the presence of a hematoma suggests the likelihood of a vascular injury. Other findings that may indicate the presence of a vascular injury are a bruit, thrill, pallor, impaired capillary refill, cyanosis, paresthesia, hypoesthesia, or extremity hypothermia. A compartment syndrome should be suspected if the patient has a palpable muscular tension and hypoesthesia, paresis, or pain with passive motion. Leg edema, cyanosis and dilated superficial veins are suggestive of the presence of a transected or thrombosed vein or an arteriovenous fistula. A peripheral nerve injury should be suspected when there is a sensory or motor deficit, fracture, dislocation or laceration.

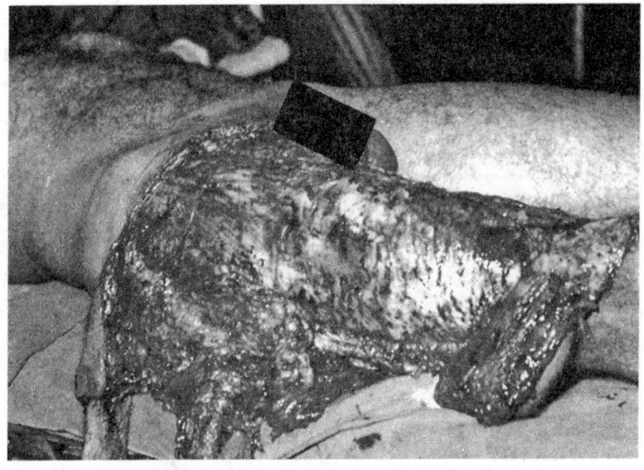

Fig. 6.1: Extensive degloving injury in RTA
(For color version, see Plate 1)

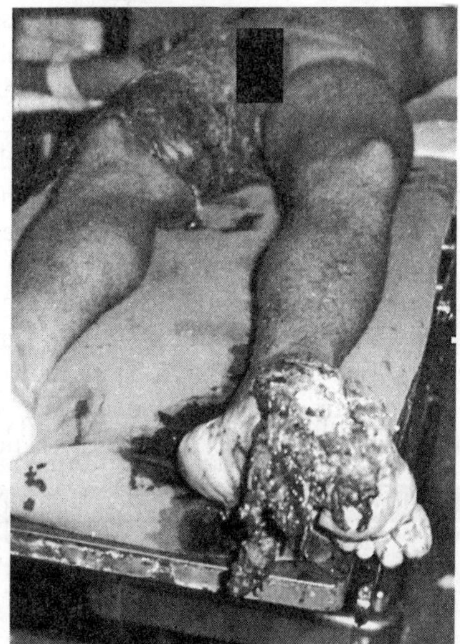

Fig. 6.2: Extensive injury in a rail accident victim
(For color version, see Plate 2)

Neurologic Assessment

The neurological examination during secondary survey is a complete one and includes GCS, reassessing the pupils for size and reactivity, and evaluation the function of the cranial nerves, motor and sensory function, coordination, and reflexes. Any abnormality must be investigated with early CT scan of the head and spine as indicated.

TERTIARY SURVEY

During all phases of trauma care, frequent re-evaluation is performed to detect and treat any deterioration in the patient condition. Certainly, once the secondary survey has been competed, continuing re-evaluation of the patient is necessary that occult injuries have not been overlooked. Often this late appearing lesions or sequelaes are detected.

Decision Making

Following the initial survey and resuscitation an overall assessment of the patient is made (Table 6.2) to decide the life-threatening/limb threatening injuries and to prioritise these to address in a definitive fashion. In a case of polytrauma cluster analysis/pattern perception is more logical than algorithms. Example of cluster analysis adapted from Trunkey DD[11] is given in the (Table 6.3).

Surgical priority: It is important to understand that the patient who is hemodynamically unstable or stable patient who become unstable must have surgical priorities established within 15-20 minutes of arrival in the emergency department. There may be requirement of more than one operating team in those patients with more than one life-threatening process or limb threatening process. For example, a patient may need a neurosurgeon and a general surgeon operating simultaneously. The sequential priorities are head, torso, vascular, orthopedic, and maxillofacial

Table 6.2: An example of the ISS calculation

Region	*Injury description*	*AIS*	*Square top three*
Head and neck	Cerebral contusion	3	9
Face	No injury	0	
Chest	Flail chest	4	16
Abdomen	Minor contusion of liver	2	
	Complex rupture spleen	5	25
Extremity	Fractured femur	3	
External	No injury	0	
	Injury severity score		*50*

Table 6.3: Example of cluster analysis

Immediate information	*After 5 min of assessment and resuscitation*	*Immediate management and operative decision*	*Secondary management and operative decision*
Coma Dilated unreactive pupil Right hemiparesis	Coma and pupillary dilatation, right hemiparesis persists Cold calorics positive (tonic deviation to side of cold injection)	Simultaneous left craniotomy and laparotomy	After craniotomy and laparotomy, a right femoral arteriogram is obtained. If the arteriogram is abnormal, vascular repair is done, followed by operative fixation of the femur
Clinical shock Systolic BP 80	Chest X-ray normal	Sterile dressing and traction splint to right leg during the above procedures	
Compound right femur fracture No pedal pulse right foot	Shock worsens Systolic BP 60		

Rationale: This paient had two life-threatening processes and one potential limb threatening process. The neurological examination at 5 min strongly suggests there is a left sides mass lesion, with the brainstem intact. CT scan is not indicated because the patient is bleeding to death, with the most likely source in the abdomen. The life-threatening processes are treated simultaneously and the potential limb threatening process as soon as possible.

injuries. Brain injuries always take first priority. The critical decision during the initial assessment and resuscitation is whether or not the patient has a mass lesion. Majority of neurosurgeons will prefer to perform a CT scan before operating and if the facilities are not available, localizing/lateralizing signs and strong clinical suspicion form the basis of exploration. Deterioration of neurological signs during resuscitation is also presumptive for a mass lesion. During initial resuscitation one should be careful to prevent secondary injury to brain from hypoxia or hypovolemia. In torso injury, abdomen takes priority over chest. X-ray chest shows into which hemothorax the blood loss is occurring. Chest injuries can be managed nonoperatively in almost 85 percent of cases as the lung parenchyma is low pressure system. Aggressive bleeding in the chest is mostly as a result of a mediastinum injury. Sometimes a massive hemothorax comes from rupture of the diaphragm, with decompression of blood from the abdomen into the pleural cavity. In patients with multiple injuries and a widened mediastinum (X-ray), a mass lesion within the cranial vault still takes the number one priority. The other injuries can be dealt with concurrently. Arrives in shock, the shock is not caused by the widened mediastinum, and other sources must be sought.[11] Most often the bleeding is into the peritoneal or retroperitoneal space. Exploratory laparotomy gets priority over arch arteriogram. If the patient is stable and arch arteriogram confirms contained rupture of aorta in a case of polytrauma one must rule out abdominal bleeding by diagnostic peritoneal lavage, USG abdomen, CT scan or by laparotomy before attempting repair of the contained ruptured aorta.

Pelvic hemorrhage can be massive and must be addressed almost simultaneously with associated torso hemorrhage (Fig. 6.3). At the same time it is necessary to rule out significant arterial injuries by arteriography as it occurs in approximately 15 percent of pelvic fractures. Compound pelvic fractures are difficult to manage. Strong consideration must be given to diversion of the fecal stream to minimize soiling of the pelvic wound by stool in the post injury period. In general, all orthopedic injuries should be fixed at the first operation after head and torso injuries have been dealt with. Next, comes the peripheral vascular injury. Some surgeons feel that peripheral vascular injury takes priority over the ortho injury as peripheral vascular repair will not be disrupted by a careful orthopedic surgeon. Maxillofacial injuries usually take last priority in operative management. The only maxillofacial injury that takes immediate priority is one associated with an airway problem.

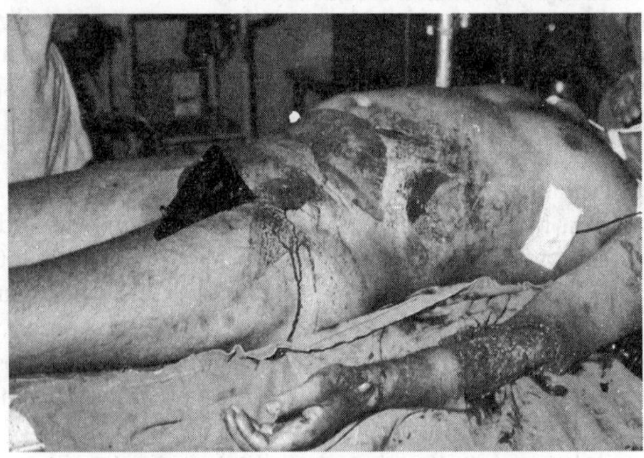

Fig. 6.3: Polytrauma in road traffic accident
(For color version, see Plate 2)

REFERENCES

1. Chan RNW, Ainscow D, Sikoski JM. Diagnostic failures in the multiply injured. J Trauma 1980;20:684.
2. Hamdan TA. Missed injuries in casualties from Iraqui-Iranian war. A study of 25 cases. Injury 1987;18:15.
3. Albrektesen SB, Thomson JL. Detection of injuries in traumatic death. The significance of medicolegal autopsy. Forces Sci Int 1989;42:135.
4. Enderson BL, Stevens SL DeBoo JM, et al. Occult pneumothorax in blunt trauma. South Eastern Surgical Congress. Napples 1990.
5. Initial assessment and management. In American College of Surgeons Committee on Trauma. Advance Trauma Life Support Program, 1989; p9.

5a. Alam HB, Rhee P. New development in fluid resuscitation. Surg clin N Amer 2007;(87):55-72.

6. Krantz BE. Initial Assessment. In Trauma Ed Moore EE, Mattox KL, Felicianno DV. Apple & Lange, California 3rd ed, 1995;p123-39.
7. Gurdjian ES, Gurdjian ES. Acute head injuries. Surg Gynaecol Obstet 1978;146:805.
8. Richardson JD, Flint LM, Snow NJ, et al. Management of transmediastinal gunshot wounds. Surgery 1981;90:671.
9. Symbas PN, Hatcher CR, Vladis SE. Oesophageal gunshot injuries. Ann Surg 1980;191:703.

9a. Brink M, Kool DR, Dekker HM, Deunk J, Jager GJ, van Kuijk C, Edwards MJ, Blickman JG. Predictors of abnormal chest CT after blunt trauma: a critical appraisal of the literature. Clin Radiol. 2009;Mar;64(3):272-83. Epub 2008 Nov 13.

10. Gelberman RH, Menon J, Fronek A. The peripheral pulse following arterial injury. J Trauma 1980;20:948.
11. Trunkey DD. Surgical priorties. In Progress in Trauma and Critical Care Surgery. Ed Najarian JS and Delaney JP, Mosby Year book, St. Loius, 1992;p 79.

Trauma Care: Echelon Concept and Its Relevance

SK Kochar

During the times of Mahabharata, the war used to stop at the sunset. Early hours after the sunset were utilized for collection and treatment of the wounded soldiers. Over the passage of time swords have been replaced by guns and the stab wounds by gunshot wounds. Injuries inflicted by modern weapons are devastating in nature and need urgent care and attention and cannot wait till the sunset. Influx of the casualties due to shell wounds as a result of bomb blasts adds to the quantum of the load. Thus, care of the wounded during the war needs collection, stabilization, evacuation, treatment and finally rehabilitation. As is obvious fighting soldier cannot be given more than the first aid during the thick of battle and he has to fallback or is to be brought back. How far he falls back, how does he get evacuated and where he gets treated, these questions have evolved over the years. The concept of Forward dressing lines → Regimental aid post → Advance dressing station → Field hospital → General hospital → Base hospital was being practiced till the Vietnam war, where it was observed that when the casualties were taken directly from the battlefield to corps. surgical hospital bypassing the regimental aid post and MASH the mortality rate was reduced to 1.7 percent. However, this is possible during the day, and in those limited conflicts where the air evacuation of the casualties can be done. As it often happens movements are restricted during the day and difficult during the night. In view of the long transport hours the design of medical care for military casualties involves delivering them through a continuum of progressively more definitive care.

First echelon of care: The goal at this level are rapid treatment for evacuation from the field or return to duty if physically possible, based on triage decisions made by these initial medical providers. The injured are taken to a regimental aid post, where fluid resuscitation and advance trauma life support or basic life support care is provided by a medical officer.

Second echelon of care: Patients flow continuous from the first to the second echelon of care, which may be an advanced dressing station/forward surgical center/forward treatment center or may be even border static hospital. These facilities are staffed by medical officer and/or surgical team to provide more definitive resuscitation measures such as airway control, fluid resuscitation including blood transfusion, and in some situations, immediate surgery. Patients are again triaged for further evacuation, as indicated, to the next echelon of care.

Third echelon of care: Base hospitals/general hospitals/zonal hospitals comprise of the third echelon of care and are staffed by both general and specialist medical providers. These facilities can provide definitive resuscitation and surgical treatment for life and limb threatening injuries. Patients are provided with postoperative surgical intensive care as needed. Patients are retained for further evacuation if required.

Fourth echelon of care: Fully equipped and staffed hospital forms the final echelons of care in the military triage system. Patients evacuated to these facilities can receive both definitive operative and nonoperative care as well as long-term care and rehabilitation.

Every casualty need not pass through every echelon of care depending on the situation prevailing and the theater of war. Following important principles of trauma care are to be kept in mind.

- The time interval between injury and definitive care has got direct bearing on the mortality and morbidity.
- In mass casualties triage is very important and it affects the quality of care within the resources available.
- The right place for definite care of the wounded is the hospital settings.

FIRST ECHELON OF CARE

Care is divided into three distinct phases.

Care Under Fire

It is the care rendered by the medic or corpsman at the scene of injury while he and the casualty are under effective hostile fire.

Available medical equipment is limited to that carried by the individual operator or by the corpsman or medic at the medical pack. It consists of first field dressing and shell dressing for tying over the wound and tubonic morphine for the pain relief. Keeping the casualty from being wounded further is the first objective. Wounded soldiers who are unable to participate further in the engagement should lie flat and still if any ground cover or trench is available. If no cover is available the casualty if possible is moved to safety and left there till the situation improves to evacuate. No immediate management of the airway should be anticipated at this time because of the need to move the casualty to cover as quickly as possible. It is very important, however, to stop major bleeding as quickly as possible, since injury to major vessel may result in very rapid onset of hypovolemic shock. The importance of this step requires emphasis in light of reports that hemorrhage from extremity wounds was the cause of death in more than 2,500 casualties in Vietnam war who had no other injuries.[1] These are preventable deaths. Although the use of tourniquet has been condemned in the past; if applied by paramedic judiciously can be life saving. In fact it should form a part of essential medical aid available with the soldier and they should be trained in its use. This may enable them to quickly put a tourniquet on themselves if necessary without sustaining further blood loss while waiting for medical assistance.[2]

Transport of the casualty will often be most problematic aspect of providing tactical combat casualty cover. Situation may not permit the stretcher or these as such may not be available at the action area. Quite often than not transport of the patient is currently accomplished with a shoulder carry or improvised litter. Protection of the spine takes the back seat as various studies have demonstrated that gunshot wounds of neck are rare and even in penetrating injuries of neck, it possibly would have been of some benefit in only 1.4 percent of patients.[3]

Role of paramedic:

- Return fire as directed or required
- Try to keep yourself from getting hurt
- Try to keep the casualty from sustaining additional wounds
- Stop any life-threatening external hemorrhage with a tourniquet
- Take the casualty with you when you leave

Tactical Field Care

This is rendered at the regimental aid post where a medical officer is available and certain equipment and medicines are positioned. This phase is distinguished from care under fire phase by more time with which to render care and a reduced level of hazard from hostile fire. The amount of time available to render care may be quite variable but there is need to avoid undertaking non-essential diagnostic and therapeutic measures. If a victim of blast or penetrating injury is found to be without pulse, respiration, or signs of life, cardiopulmonary resuscitation will not be successful in the battlefield and should not be carried. On the battlefield, the cost of attempts to perform cardiopulmonary resuscitation on casualties with what are inevitably fatal injuries will be measured in additional lives lost as care is withheld from patients with less severe injuries. Attention is first directed to evaluation of airway, breathing, and circulation. There should be no attempt at airway intervention if the patient is conscious and breathing on its own. If the patient is unconscious, the cause will most likely be hemorrhagic shock or penetrating head trauma. The airway should be opened with the chin lift or jaw thrust maneuver without worrying about cervical spine immobilization. If spontaneous respiration is present and there is no respiratory distress, an adequate airway may be maintained in an unconscious patient in most cases by insertion of a nasopharyngeal airway though we have always used oropharyngeal airway. Should an unconscious patient develop an airway obstruction, the nasopharyngeal/oropharyngeal airway may need to be replaced with a more definite airway. Endotracheal tube is the preferred airway techniques and in advanced countries paramedical are trained in its skill. In our country neither in civil nor in army paramedics are confident enough to pass a endotracheal tube in the field settings. This job has to be handled by the medical officers and thus there is requirement of easier techniques to be developed for paramedics. Esophageal obturator airway had its own list of complication and at present laryngeal airway or combitubes seems to be the answer. Though yet not introduced for general use it will be introduced shortly. Cricothyroidotomy is the other airway option. Here again paramedics in civil or armed forces in developing countries are not trained in its techniques. If required to be performed the onus is going to be on the medical officer who probably are better trained in tracheostomy than cricothyroidotomy. If blood or other obstruction are present in the oropharynx, they should be removed by hand or battery powered suction/foot suction. A useful adjuvant and easy to carry is MR syringe. It can be effectively used for oropharynx suction.

Attention should next be directed towards the patients breathing. Only two conditions need recognition and management and these are: tension pneumothorax and sucking chest wound. Sucking chest wound is obvious while tension pneumothorax should be suspected in a patient who has got unilateral penetrating chest trauma and progressive severe respiratory distress. Sucking chest wound is sealed with a petroleum jelly gauge and a battle dressing with three sides sealed with adhesive plaster leaving one side open to avoid tension pneumothorax. Tension pneumothorax is to be tackled by the medical officer as paramedics can not diagnose it and even if they reach some conclusion, cannot treat it. The thorax should be decompressed with a 14-gauge needle with a finger stall at the other end with a hole in it to act as a one way valve. Tube thoracostomy is not attempted. Bleeding site should be addressed next. Here again stress should be on pressure control or use of tourniquet. Intravenous access should be obtained next. Though it has been hotly debated and the benefit of prehospital fluid resuscitation in trauma patient has not been established[4-8] in field conditions with long or rather indeterminate transport hours fluid resuscitation does have a role to play. As recently as operation desert storm, transport time to medical facility was found to range from 2-4 hours.[8] Types of fluid again have generated a lot of controversy but in field conditions and at first echelon care level, crystalloids should see the patient through to the second echelon where colloids/blood may be supplemented. Next being pain relief and morphine is still the trusted one. Intramuscular route should be avoided due to erratic absorption in shock conditions. Antibiotic should be started and antitetanus prophylaxis instituted and patient evacuated to second echelon for definitive care.

Checklist for Management Plan

1. Airway management

- Chin lift or jaw thrust
- Unconscious casualty without airway obstruction

- Naso-/oropharyngeal airway
- Unconscious casualty with airway obstruction
  - Cricothyroidotomy
- Cervical spine immobilization not mandatory

2. **Breathing**
   - Consider tension pneumothorax—Unilateral penetrating chest injury
   - Progressive respiratory distress
   - Decompress—needle thoracostomy
3. **Bleeding**
   - Control-pressure dressing/tourniquet
4. **Intravenous**
   - Start an 18-gauge intravenous or saline lock
5. **Fluid resuscitation**
   - Controlled hemorrhage without shock: no fluid necessary
   - Controlled hemorrhage with shock: 1L isotonic saline followed by 500 ml Haemaccel. Draw blood for grouping before Haemaccel
6. **Inspect and dress wounds**
7. **Check for additional wounds**
8. **Analgesia as necessary**
   - Morphine 5 mg intravenous, wait 10 min: repeat as necessary
9. **Splint fractures and recheck pulse**
10. **Antibiotics**
    - Cefoxitin 2 gm slowly intravenous/Ciprofloxacin intravenous infusion
11. **Cardiopulmonary resuscitation**
    - Not attempted if no pulse, respiratory or sign of life.

Faculty at RAP: Medical officer, nursing assistant 2/3, ambulance assistant/equivalent.[4]

Facility: Stretcher, oxygen, splints, intubation set, ambu bag, suction apparatus, cut down set, tracheostomy/cricothyroidotomy set, nasogastric tube, catheterization set, splints dressings, analgesics/antibiotics, few general instruments.

Capability: Every ambulance assistant is well trained in basic life support, which consists of the following: extrication of casualty, clearing and securing the airway with oropharyngeal airway, stoppage of external bleeding, application of air splints and Thomas splint.

Every nursing assistant has got the additional capability of: venous access, ambubag ventilation, monitoring of pulse, respiration, blood pressure and pulse oximetry.

Medical officer has got additional capability of: endotracheal intubation, management of: sucking chest wound, tension pneumothorax, cardiac tamponade. He can perform if reqd: cut down, tracheostomy/cricothyroidotomy, catheterization.

SECOND ECHELON OF CARE

Second echelon of care may be forward surgical center (FSC) or forward treatment center (FTC) or a field hospital or a border static hospital. With whatever name it goes basically it has got a surgical team. It is at this place patient comes in contact with the surgeon for the first time and resuscitation can be performed and life and limb saving surgery can be under taken. It is at this place the initial examination goes beyond primary survey and X-ray facility is available and blood transfusion facility exists. Limited laboratory investigations can be done. Patients can be hospitalized for/up to 6-7 days.

Well defined areas are reception, resuscitation, evacuation, ward, operation theater, radiology department, lab and blood transfusion department. Resuscitation department of a field hospital must be able to deal with large number of seriously injured casualties arriving simultaneously or in quick succession. Each casualty must be assessed, resuscitated, and stabilized in preparation for life saving surgery or evacuation as quickly as possible in order to prevent any delays developing in the system.

Departmental SOPs

General

- Allocate primary and secondary survey responsibilities to team members by team leader on the basis of skills abilities.
- Priorities are allotted for resuscitation, operative intervention and for radiological investigations, so that patient does not over crowd any particular facility.

- All casualties to receive oxygen (10 l/min) during resuscitation.
- Don't transfer casualties from resuscitation trestles to preoperative area unless all parameters are stable.
- Hold unstable patients needing immediate operation on the resuscitation trestles until the next operating table is available.
- All casualties referred from other hospital areas to be assessed in the resuscitation department prior to transfer for surgery.
- Patients needing orthopedic surgery, neurosurgery, cardiothoracic surgery evacuated to third echelon after stabilization.

Battlefield Trauma Life Support[9]

Primary and secondary survey is practically the same as in polytrauma protocols but with little modification with majority of injuries being gunshot wounds.

Primary Survey

Airway

- Is the airway patent.
- If the answer is no, apply suction, chin lift, jaw thrust or insert oral or nasopharyngeal airway as appropriate.
- Assess the response to each maneuver. If inadequate, use advanced airways techniques (endotracheal intubation or cricothyroidotomy) after preoxygenation.
- If the casualty has sustained blunt injury, beware of cervical spine injury and protect the spine.

Breathing

- Look for equal chest movement, tracheal deviation, wounds, and cyanosis.
- Listen for breath sounds and percussion abnormalities.
- Feel for crepitus, surgical emphysema, and pain.
- Record respiratory rate.
- Insert a chest drain in all casualties with penetrating chest wounds.

Circulation

- Assume all hypotensive casualties have hypovolemic shock until proved otherwise.
- Control external hemorrhage.
- Record pulse rate, blood pressure, and capillary refill.
- Assess patency of existing intravenous lines and replace if necessary. If percutaneous intravenous cannulation fails, perform cut down, or if trained, use central lines.
- Take blood for grouping and cross matching and baseline investigation.
- Give all shocked casualties 1 liter crystalloid and 500 ml of Haemaccel as quickly as possible. Reassess pulse, blood pressure, and capillary refill. If no improvement, repeat 1 liter of Ringer's lactate and 500 ml of colloid stat.
- If no response, get type specific blood, start transfusion, and consider urgent surgery.

Disability of Neurological Function

- Prevent secondary brain injury remember the ABCs
- Isolated head injury does not cause shock: Don't withhold intravenous fluid
- Use AVPU (A=alert, V=vocalizing, P=response to pain only U= unresponsive) and pupil assessment.
- If abnormal, search for small fragment injury

Exposure

- Beware of weapons and ordinance concealed by clothing particularly grenades attached to webbing.
- Expose all patients prior to secondary survey. Cover with blankets as soon as possible to minimize hypothermia.
- Bag and label all clothing's and personal effects.
- Remember to examine the back of the casualty. Log roll the casualty if you suspect spinal injury.
- Perform urinary catheterization, if indicated, only after rectal examination.
- Insert nasogastric tube if indicated.

Secondary Survey

- Start secondary survey after completion of primary survey and patient is hemodynamically stable.
- Document all findings.

Head

- Check head and neck carefully for small wounds.
- Look for bruising, swelling, or asymmetry.
- Identify any fractures and look for cerebrospinal fluid, rhinorrhea, otorrhea, or hematotympanum.
- Inspect the teeth for breakage or altered bite. If fracture or hemorrhage, can it compromise the airway during evacuation?
- Look for ocular injury.
- Gently palpate all scalp wounds to assess for skull fracture or fragments.
- Skull X-ray for all penetrating head wounds after resuscitation.
- Perform Glasgow coma score if indicated.

Chest

- Re-evaluate breathing and palpate entire chest wall including clavicles and sternum.

Abdomen

- Is there any evidence of intra-abdominal injury?
- Consider diagnostic peritoneal lavage if the casualty has equivocal abdominal signs, spinal cord injury or patient is unconscious.

Pelvic, Genitourinary, Rectal Examination

- Examine carefully for entry wounds and assess integrity of pelvis.
- Perform rectal examination looking for blood, bone fragments, integrity of the rectal wall, and the presence of anal sphincter tone.
- Scrotal hematoma, meatal blood, or high riding prostate may suggest urethral damage. Don't pass a urethral urinary catheter.

Limbs

Look for wounds, deformity, swelling, abnormal movement, pain, absence of peripheral pulses, and local neurological deficit. Restore the limb to anatomical position if possible, recheck pulse.

Drugs

- Initiate all drugs as per protocol, antibiotic, antitetanus and analgesics.
- Record fluid intake/output.

Casualty Notification

Dangerously ill/seriously ill listing by medical officer only.

An Evaluation

The Faculty

- Surgeon, anesthetist, physician, radiologist.

The Facility

- Casualty department
- Operation theater
- Trauma ward
- Blood transfusion
- X-ray, USG

Capability

- Life and limb saving surgery.

Relevance for Civilian Set-up

Subdistrict hospital can easily organize the trauma care on the similar pattern as the facilities available to these hospital are similar though the trauma load is far less. For the civil set up the next echelon will be district hospital/city hospital.

THIRD ECHELON OF CARE

This hospital receives casualties from second echelon. Surgical teams and other discipline like eye, ENT, medical specialist, radiologist, pathologist are available. Intensive care unit is available and orthopedic and emergent neurosurgery facility exists. Ultrasonography and CT scan are available. Physiotherapy department is an additional benefit. Definitive treatment is provided to all patients except those needing thoracic, spinal, neuro and reconstructive surgery and rehabilitation.

The Faculty

- General surgeons
- Orthosurgeons
- Physician
- Anesthetist
- Ophthalmologist
- Otorhinolaryngologist
- Radiologist
- Pathologist

The Facility

- Casualty department
- Trauma ward
- ICU
- Surgical wards
- ENT and EYE department
- Radiology department
- Laboratory
- Blood bank
- Physiotherapy department
- Mortuary.

Trauma Care Ambulance

The ambulance is well equipped with the following:

- Laryngoscope, endotracheal tube, Ambu bag
- Suction apparatus
- Oxygen cylinder
- Pulse oximeter
- Intravenous fluids, intracaths
- Splints and cervical collars
- Cardiac monitor and defab
- IC drains and dressings

Departmental SOP's

These are the same as are followed at second echelon except that a tertiary survey is carried out after 24 hours of admission to rule out any important minor injury. Hospital stay is limited to 30 days and the evacuation is to tertiary care center or back to work/ sick leave.

Management Protocols

Trauma care has been organized into Protocol "A" and Protocol "B" (Flow chart 7.1). Protocol A is followed when casualties are 1-5 and Protocol B when these are 6-30.[10]

Protocol A

Patients are brought to casualty department where reception and resuscitation are started. It consists of initial examination, clearing of airway, securing of the airway with endotracheal tube if required, respiratory support with IPPV if required/indicated, setting up of intravenous drip with venous access, collection of blood for grouping and crossmatching, hemoglobin estimation and leukocyte count, allotting the priority and initial resuscitation to the extent that patient can be sent to operation theater if urgent surgery is required or to ICU if further resuscitation is necessary. Radiological investigations are done in casualty department. For special investigations and ultrasonography patients are taken to radiology department if the condition of the patient permits and these investigations are of vital importance in management.

Flow chart 7.1: Communication channel of protocols

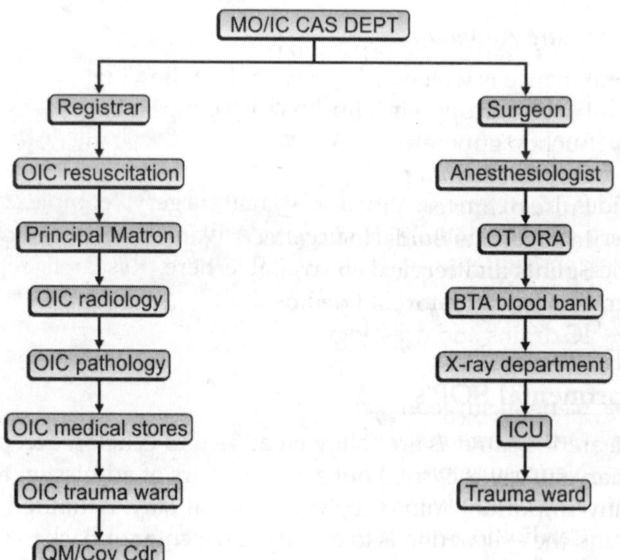

Protocol B

It is to be followed whenever there are 6-30 casualties. Sequence of action is: mobilization of men and material: space for thirty casualties; activation of OT and surgical team; mobilization of blood bank and lab; gearing up of diagnostic facilities and mobilization of ambulances. Reception, resuscitation and information section is housed in specially earmarked/trauma ward. ICU caters for 5 beds and 25 beds are kept earmarked in trauma ward for casualties. Besides the technical backup, certain administrative actions and jobs are part of the plan. Personal belongings are to be collected. Security of the equipment and arms will be required. Traffic control is to be monitored. All these actions are time scheduled for the better functioning. Communication channel is as follows:

Procedures in protocol II is no different than protocol I except that the suturing and dressings of the wounds (minor) and plastering are done in trauma ward at the bed side, thus decreasing the work load on the operation theater. A separate team of medical officers and assistants accompanies the surgeon for documentation of injuries and other medicolegal documents. Priorities are allotted not only for operation theater but also for radiological investigations, so that these facilities are not overcrowded.

FOURTH ECHELON OF CARE

This hospital is equivalent to level I trauma center and during peace time it is equivalent to university/medical college hospital. This hospital primary role is that of tertiary care center and provides treatment facility for spinal surgery, complex neuro surgery and cardiothoracic surgery. Advanced orthopedics prosthetics, rehabilitation are all available here. Research, registry, and training is imparted in this hospital.

The Faculty

- General surgeon
- Orthosurgeon
- Neurosurgeon
- Reconstructive surgeon
- Cardiothoracic surgeon
- Urologists

- GI surgeon
- Ped surgeon
- Anesthetist
- Physician

The Facility

- Casualty
- ICU
- Trauma ward
- Operation theater
- Imaging
- Laboratory
- Blood bank
- Mortury

The Ability

Casualty Department

- Reception and resuscitation
- Treatment and investigation
- X-ray and USG
- Casualty OT
- Documentation

ICU

- Resuscitation and monitoring
- Life support systems
- CVP lines, arterial lines, blood gas analysis, ventilators, glucometers, oxygen saturators, noninvasive BP, cardiac monitors, barrier nursing, critical care, plasma pheresis, pulse oximeter, end tidal capnometry.

Trauma Ward

- Reception resuscitation
- Treatment and preparation for surgery
- Investigation and intermediate care

OT

- Emergency OT

Imaging

- USG
- 500 mA set
- C T scan
- MRI
- Vascular radiology

Laboratory

- Blood gas analyzer
- Autoanalyzer

Blood Bank

- Rare blood Gp
- FFP
- Platelet concentration

Trauma Care Ambulance

- Suction apparatus
  - Oxygen cylinder
  - Intravenous fluid
  - Airway access, laryngeal airway, etc.
- Cardiopulmonary resuscitator
- Pulse oximetry
- Cervical collar
- Air splints
- Paging devices-Medical control.

Options for Developing Countries

Problems of rural India are distinct from urban India and problem of urban area again differ from metropolitan but emergencies do occur in rural/urban/metros and the response and reactions involved remain the same. Problem of trauma care at all level remain the same, may be the magnitude of quantum and type may differ. Existing system of primary health center → Sub-district hospital → District hospital → City hospital/Medical college hospital can work very well if trauma care organized on the pattern of echelon concept be followed. Recenly echelon concept has been evaluated and it was observed that this does not increase mortality though the morbidity is marginly increased.[11]

EDITORIAL

Prehospital Devices, Dressings and Drugs

Knowledge in the safe removal of the body armour and safe disarmament and storage of weapon remains of paramount importance in protecting the casualty and the health care provider from grave injury.

Prehospital tourniquet use plays a central role in the hemorrhage control on the modern battlefield. Current military doctrine mandates use of tourniquet as a first line of treatment for casualties who have extremity hemorrhage when care is administered under hostile fire. Once the casualties are removed from hostile fire, the need for the tourniquets may be reassessed to determine if a lesser form of hemorrhage control will suffice.[12] Casualties who sustain traumatic amputations, mangled extremities, or major vascular injuries may have had substantial hge before first responder treatment and tourniquet application. Bleeding may have slowed or stopped spontaneously because of hypotension combined with vessel spasm and retraction. The cue the medic look for to know if a tourniquet has been tightened enough may not be present (cessation of bright red blood). The tourniquet thus may not be tight enough to control hemorrhage once resuscitation is begins and higher blood pressure are restored. To avoid this, tourniquet must be replaced by pneumatic tourniquet once the casualty reaches hospital.

Current military practice is to have intravenous access established in the field with no or minimal fluid administration. The practice of permissive hypotension is designed to decrease the incidence of rebleeding from quiescent or partially controlled hemorrhage sites. Receiving physicians must be aware that casualties may have received little or no resuscitation. These patients if present with hypotension will need massive transfusion protocol.[13]

Hemostatic Dressings

Two products have been deployed by the united state military in to battlefield setting. Zeolite, a granular mineral based product, causes an exothermic reaction when exposed to water or blood, thereby concentrating blood clotting factors and accelerating homeostasis. Compared with standard gauze dressings zeolite has been demonstrated to provide superior homeostasis, decrease blood loss, decrease resuscitating requirement in animal studies. Few concerned area are the heat generated by the dressing and its stability during movement and transport of casualties.

Chitosan is a nontoxic biodegradable, complex carbohydrate derivative of chitin, a naturally occurring substance. In its acid salt form Chitosan has mucoadhesive properties that augment homeostasis. Both the liquid forms of Chitosan and the dressing that has been deployed in the battlefield settings have demonstrated superiority in hemorrhage control over standard dressings in multiple animal mode and battlefield casualties.[14]

Needle Thoracostomy

Although paramedics may be well trained to treat tension pneumothorax, the identification of a tension pneumothorax in field may be nearly impossible. Most common mechanism of trauma in the field is penetrating injuries. Tactical situation and other factors may delay transportation of these patients to treatment facilities capable of diagnosing and definitely treating the tension pneumothorax. All patients with chest trauma and hypotension may benefit with placement of needle in the chest.

Intraosseous Access

The entire concept of intraosseous infusion is extremely attractive in a combat setting given the potential number of casualties and long evacuation times allowing for a stretching of the envelope of resuscitation when minutes are a matter of life and death because of exsanguating hemorrhage.

Pain Medication and Antibiotics

With newer availability of oral transmucosal fentanyl citrate or fentanyl lollipops up to 1600 microgram of fentanyl may be self administered by a casualty and provide rapid analgesia. Side effects include nausea and vomiting.

Although single injection of broad-spectrum long acting antibiotic has been recommended with in few minutes of injury, us army carry fluoroquinolone for self administration.

IV Fluid

Hextend has replaced Ringer's lactate as the fluid carried by medics in the field. It is effective in hypotension resuscitation and potentially has the benefit as the dole resuscitation fluid after severe traumatic brain injury by reducing fluid requirement and eliminating the need for manifold without affecting the coagulation profile.[15]

Hypothermia prevention at every step can be achieved by exposing only the relevant parts, covering with blankets, using warm IV fluids, use of body bag during transportations.

Permissive Hypotension

Small volume resuscitation helps compensate for logistic problems in providing enough fluid on the battlefield to resuscitate a casualty adequately. Hypertonic saline Dextran is an effective resuscitation fluid when used in small volume. It is currently not known whether permissive hypotension would increase the incidence of late complications resulting from incomplete resuscitation. This is absolutely contraindicated in the setting of traumatic brain injury because of a resultant severe cerebral hypoperfusion with a potentially catastrophic outcome.

REFERENCES

1. Maughen JS. An enquiry into the nature of wounds resulting in killed in action in Vietnam. Milit Med 1970;135:8-13.
2. Butler FK Jr, Hagman J, Butler EG. Tactical combat casualty care in special operations. Milit Med 1996;161, Suppl: 3-16.
3. Arishita GI, Vayer JS, Bellany RF. Cervical spine immobilization of penetrating neck wounds in a hostile environment. J Trauma 1989;29:332-7.
4. Bickell WH. Are victims of injury sometimes victimized by attempts at fluid resuscitation (editorial). Ann Emerg Med 1993;22:225-6.
5. Kaweski SM, Sise MJ, Virglio RW. The effects of prehospital fluids on survival in trauma patients. J Trauma 1990;30:1215-8.
6. Deakin CD, Hicks IR. AB or ABC prehospital fluid management in major trauma. Journal of Accident and Emergency Medicine 1994; 11: 154-7.

7. Owen TM, Watson WC, Prough Ds, et al. Limited initial resuscitation of uncontrolled haemorrhage reduces internal bleeding and subsequent volume requirments. J Trauma 1995;39:200-7.
8. Koehler RH, Smith S, Bacaner T. Triage of American casualties; The need for change. Milit Med 1994;159:541-7.
9. Riley B, Mahoney P. Battlefield trauma life support: Its use in the resuscitation department of 32 Field Hospital during Gulf War. Military Medicine 1996;161:542-6.
10. Kochar SK. In Hospital trauma care: An evaluation. MJAFI 1990;46:45-8.
11. Kochar SK, Verma SK, Dash SC, Rai RS. Trauma Care. Echelon concept and its relevance. Second International Conference on Trauma and Critical Care, 17-19 Oct Delhi Cantt, 1997.
12. Marby RL. Tourniquet use on the battlefield. Mil Med 2006;17(5):352-6.
13. Beekley AC, Starnes BW, Sebesta JA. Lessons learned from Modern Military surgery. Surg Clin N Amer 2007;87:157-184.
14. Wetmore I, McManus JG, Pusatcri AE, et al. A special report on Chitosan based haemostatic dressing: experience in current combat operations. J Trauma 2006;60(3):655-8.
15. King DR, Cohn SM, Proctor KG. Changes in intracranial pressure, coagulation and neurological outcome after resuscitation from experimental traumatic brain injury with hetastarch. Surgery 2004:136(2):355-63.

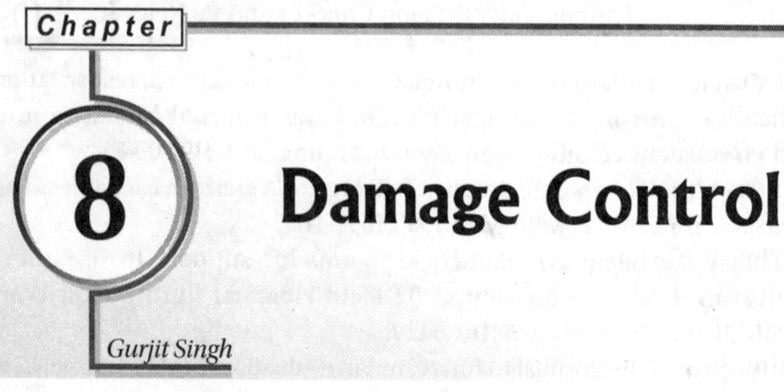

Damage Control

Gurjit Singh

INTRODUCTION

Improvement in prehospital care and trauma resuscitation has increased chances of early survival of injured patients who would have succumbed at the accident scene or enroute to the hospital. Extensive multivisceral damage often requires lengthy and complex repairs in shock patients whose bleeding (often from several sources) is difficult to control. Rapid surgical "bail out" tactics are the only option.[1]

Damage control is a management strategy and has been in vogue for over a century. Although originally introduced as an approach to abdominal injuries the damage control strategy has rapidly extended far beyond its original goal and represent a major paradigm shift in the case of severely injured.[2] Increase in violence and mass causalities has revived interest in this concept so that patients sustaining multiple high energy injuries can be cared for.

The term damage control has its origin from US Navy with reference to "capacity of ship to absorb damage and maintain mission integrity". Such a procedure will allow rapid assessment and temporary repair while on high seas so as to enable the ship to expediently return to a controlled environment in port.

Damage control is a surgical strategy that sacrifices the completeness of the immediate repair in order to address adequately the combined physiological impact of trauma and surgery.

Complex or time consuming procedures are deliberately avoided in hemodynamically unstable patients.[3] Definite repair of the injured organs is postponed until re-operation can be performed on a stable, nonbleeding and warm patient with optimized oxygen delivery.

Damage control surgery is a useful salvage strategy for the most critically injured patients. Such an approach can be conveniently and effectively employed in a scenario like military field surgery, civilian mass casualty events and long haul transfers for rural areas.

The underlying philosophy of a rapid temporary life saving solution followed by delayed definitive repair is being applied to situations in which surgical resources are limited or normal optimal care for multiple causalities is not an option.

The US Army has routinely utilized damage control surgery concepts since at least World War II. Indian Armed Forces also follow the principle of operating on only the most severely injured patients to save life and limb. Postoperative patients are rapidly evacuated because of the very limited availability of surgical personnel, supplies and holding facilities. This type of surgery requires rapid, resource sparing surgical interventions. However, the adaptation of damage control principles to the military setting may be more problematic than initially thought. The concept of damage control has an important role on the battlefield but the precise mode of application must be considered.

Key issue is patient selection followed by availability of critical adjunctive measures commonly required in the immediate post-operative period. Therefore, a patient who would be typical resource intensive in the civilian trauma center probably will be expectant in the military mass casualty situation.

Why Damage Control

Kashuk et al[4] coined the term "bloody viscous cycle" which refers to the progressive deterioration in the patient's physiological parameters, a lethal triad of events including hypothermia, coagulopathy and metabolic acidosis characterizes the cycle.[5] A fourth component was later described by Asensio and colleagues[6] who added dysrhythmia, which usually heralds the patient's death.

Hypothermia has been reported in 21% of all severely injured patients and up to 46% of trauma victims requiring laparotomy leave the operating hypothermic.[7,8]

Thermal homeostasis depends upon factors governing heat loss viz conduction, convection, evaporation, radiation and the body's ability to generate and maintain metabolic energy. Heat loss begins at the moment of traumatic insult and is exacerbated by factors such as shock, low perfusion, prolonged exposure, immobility of the acutely injured patient and extremes of age. Clinically significant hypothermia is considered present when the core temperature is less than 35 °C.[9] Temperature less than 34 °C has been linked with a need for early therapeutic packing.[10]

There are many causes of hypothermia in victims of major trauma.

Hypovolemic shock in the preoperative period adversely affects oxygen delivery and leads to decrease in oxygen consumption and therefore production of heat.[11,12] Vasodilation in an intoxicated patient will further compromise the ability to produce heat. Undressing the patient in a cool resuscitation room, an uncovered patient during resuscitation and infusion of unheated crystalloids and packed red blood cells are all sources of heat loss.

Paralyzing the patient which prevents shivering, administering anesthetic agents which prevent vasoconstriction, failing to cover areas of the body not undergoing operation, opening one or more body cavities in a cold operating room and irrigating body cavities with unheated crystalloid solutions are further sources of heat loss during a thoracotomy or laparotomy. These multiple sources of heat loss cannot be fully compensated for by increasing heat production in the patient in shock, so resuscitation and surgical teams must prevent or reverse hypothermia. Therefore, it is logical to practice damage control and rapidly complete any trauma operation in which patient's initial body temperature is less than 34° to 35°C or the temperature decreases below this level at any time during the operation.[13,14] This is particularly true in patients undergoing thoracotomy or laparotomy because hypothermia will not be correctable until chest or abdomen is closed.

Hypothermia is associated with sympathetic alpha-adrenergic overdrive, peripheral vasoconstriction and end organ hypoperfusion, resulting in conversion from aerobic to anaerobic metabolism and metabolic acidosis. Aggressive fluid resuscitation especially with normal saline exacerbates the situation, predisposing to impairment of the coagulation cascade. The patient remains cold, becomes acidotic and bleeds. Mortality rates of 100% have been reported in trauma patients with core temperature of less than 32 °C undergoing laparotomy.[15]

Dilution of coagulation factors and platelets by fluid resuscitation, decreased total and ionized calcium concentration, hypothermia, the severity of injury, shock and metabolic acidosis may all contribute to the dysfunction of normal hemostatic mechanisms.[16]

Hypothermia in the critically ill patient leads to dysfunction of intrinsic and extrinsic coagulation cascade.[17]

A combination of intrinsic and extrinsic factors are responsible for post-traumatic coagulopathy. **Amongst intrinsic factors most important include:**

- Excessive tissue injury resulting in consumption coagulopathy and activation of inflammatory cascade.
- Activation of the C- reactive protein inflammatory cascade.
- Hemodilution
- Decrease in total and ionized calcium concentration.
- Effects of progressive hypothermia and acidosis.

Important extrinsic factor to be considered is:

- Large volumes of intravenous fluids (Not warmed) leading to further hemodilution and massive transfusion of stored blood (Not warmed) which adversely affect coagulation cascade.

Clinical coagulopathy occurs because of hypothermia, platelets and coagulation factors dysfunction which occurs at low temperatures, activation of the fibrinolytic system and hemodilution following massive resuscitation. Platelet dysfunction is secondary to the imbalance between thromboxane and prostacycline that occurs in a hypothermic state. Hypothermia and hemodilution produce an additive effect on coagulopathy. Presence of continued hemorrhage in this setting is an indication for platelet transfusion even with a normal platelet count.

Anaerobic metabolism starts when the shock stage of hypoperfusion is prolonged, leading to metabolic acidosis caused by production of lactate. Acidosis decreases myocardial contractility and cardiac output. Acidosis also worsens from multiple transfusions, the use of vasopressors, aortic cross clamping and impaired myocardial performance. While acidosis by itself is an unusual reason to terminate a laparotomy being performed for trauma, it often accompanies hypothermia and a coagulopathy.[18] The use of lactate clearance as a marker of successful resuscitation is now widely accepted. Multiple studies have documented the prognostic value of blood lactate as an index of oxygen delivery, morbidity and mortality in hemorrhagic shock.[19]

Patient Selection and Indication

By definition the damage controlled patient is at or near the point of physiologic exhaustion. The goal of damage control approach is to preserve the living patient. Stone et al[20] were the first to describe the "bailout" approach of staged surgical procedures for severely injured patients.

No single model has been able to accurately predict the timings for institution of damage control.[21]

Not all trauma patients require damage control measures.

Physiologic guidelines for institution of damage control have been validated by Asensio et al[22] and are as follows:

- Hypothermia ≤ 34°C
- Acidosis pH ≤ 7.2
- Serum bicarbonate ≤15 meq/L
- Transfusion ≥4000 ml of blood
- Transfusion ≥5000 ml of blood and blood products
- Intraoperative volume replacement ≥ 12000 ml
- Clinical evidence of intraoperative coagulopathy

Patients with exsanguination are perhaps the best candidates to undergo damage control.[23]

However, there are many preoperative and intraoperative states that would suggest the need for damage control.

Preoperative

- Multiple mass casualties
- Multisystem trauma with major abdominal injury
- Open pelvic fracture with major abdominal injury
- Major abdominal injury with need to evaluate early possible extra-abdominal injury
- Need for emergency department thoracotomy
- Presence of sustained hypotension (<90 mm Hg)
- Presence of coagulopathy
- Presence of hypothermia
- Need for the adjunctive use of angioembolization

Intraoperative

- Need for intraoperative thoracotomy
- Major abdominal vascular injuries
- Major thoracic vascular injuries
- Major complex hepatic injuries
- Presence of bowel edema/ischemia

Rotondo MF, Zomies DH have mentioned certain key factors in patient selection for damage control.[24]

Conditions

High energy blunt torso trauma
Multiple torso penetrations
Hemodynamic instability
Presenting coagulopathy and/or hypothermia

Complexes

Major abdominal vascular injury with multiple visceral injuries
Multicavitary exsanguination with concomitant visceral injuries
Multiregional injury with competing priorities

Clinical Factors

Severe metabolic acidosis (pH < 7.3)
Hypothermia (temperature <35°C)
Resuscitation and operative time > 90 minutes
Coagulopathy as evidenced by development of non-mechanical bleeding
Massive transfusion (>10 units packed red blood cells).

The most important goal of early institution of damage control is patient survival. Early pattern recognition is encouraged in that the decision to apply damage control is made early in the patient's course so as to result in improved outcome.

Damage Control Procedure

The widely accepted three stages of damage control are described as follows:

1. Limited operation for control of hemorrhage and contamination. It includes control of hemorrhage from the heart or lung, conservative management of injuries to solid organs, resection of major injuries to the gastrointestinal tract without

re-anastomosis, control of hemorrhage from major arteries and veins in the neck, trunk or extremities, packing of organ or spaces to control the inevitable coagulopathy and use of an alternate closure of a cervical incision, thoracotomy, laparotomy or site of exploration of an extremity.

2. Resuscitation in the surgical ICU. It includes vigorous rewarming of the hypothermic patient, restoration of a normal cardiovascular state by the infusion of fluids and blood and use of inotropic and related drugs, correction of residual coagulopathy after hypothermia is reversed and supportive care for the insulted lungs and kidneys.
3. Re-operation. This relates to completion of definitive repairs, search for missed injuries and formal closure of the incision if possible.

Damage control according to Asensio et al[25] implies immediate control of life-threatening hemorrhage, control of gastrointestinal contamination with rapid resections or closure, the use of intraluminal shunts, and judicious abdominal packing with temporary abdominal wall closures. Specifically in chest injuries one should repair cardiovascular injuries, perform stapled pulmonary thoracotomy, pack if needed, place chest tubes, and close the skin. For abdominal injuries, damage control can involve control of major hemorrhage, hepatic packing, pancreatic drainage, temporary hollow viscus closure, rapid stapled resections, splenectomy, nephrectomy, vascular pedicle clamping *in situ* and the use of intra-abdominal vascular shunts.[25] Frequently patient experience abdominal compartment syndrome. Therefore, the post-traumatic open abdomen with temporary abdominal wall closure is used as an extension of damage control.

Post Damage Control Complications

Given the physiological condition of the patient who require the damage control approach, it is not surprising that the rate of complications and mortality is high. Morbidity includes wound infection (5-100%), intra-abdominal abscess (0-83%), dehiscence (9-25%), bile leak (8-33%), enterocutaneous fistula (2-25%) and abdominal compartment syndrome (2-25%).[26] Multisystem organ failure is described in 20 to 30% of patients contributing significantly to the mortality rate of 12 to 67%.[26]

Reoperation

Reoperation is anticipated to occur during damage control as a planned procedure in a hemodynamically stable, fully rewarmed and physiologically "recaptured" patient. This reoperation cannot occur until after the patient has been aggressively resuscitated to acceptable parameters in the ICU. Conversely emergent reoperation as an unplanned event usually occurs in three types of clinical scenario:

a. Ongoing bleeding
b. Missed enteric injury resulting in systemic inflammatory response syndrome and shock
c. Development of abdominal compartment syndrome.

The aim of the resuscitation at this juncture is to control hemorrhage or contamination and if necessary, decompress the peritoneal cavity.[27] Usually there is a window of 36-48 hours after the initial injury, between the correction of the metabolic disorder and the onset of systemic inflammatory response syndrome and/ or multiple organ failure. In this phase definitive procedures are undertaken. Thorough re-exploration is made for any additional injuries and restoration of gastrointestinal continuity and vascular repair are done. Provisional feeding access and an attempt at definitive closure is made. The patient then returning to the intensive care unit for further care.

CONCLUSION

Damage control is of great value as a life saving maneuver in selected patient with exsanguinating trauma and intra-abdominal injuries. On the basis of the results from several studies up to 60% of patients survive this approach, yet the risk of intra-abdominal abscess and multisystem organ failure are high. These continues to be an ongoing challenge to identify better predictors of outcome; improved means of resuscitation, greater understanding of physiologic derangements and better timing to institute damage control. Delays in decision to perform damage control contribute to higher morbidity and mortality. Therefore, damage control is a vital part of the management of the multiple injured patient and should be performed before metabolic exhaustion.

REFERENCES

1. Hirshberg A, Mattox KL. Planned reoperation for severe trauma. Ann Surg 1995;222:3-8.
2. Holcomb John B. Military; civilian and rural application of the damage control. Military Medicine, June 2001;1-2.
3. Burch JM, Ortiz UB, Richardson RJ, et al. Abbreviated laparotomy and planned reoperation for critically injured patients. Ann Surg 1992;215:476-82.
4. Kashuk JL, Moore EE, Millikan JS, et al. Major abdominal vascular trauma: A unified approach. J Trauma 1982;22:672-9.
5. Rotondo MF, Zonies DH. The damage control sequence and underlying logic. Surg Clin North Am 1997;77:761-77.
6. Asensio JA, Petrone P, O'Shamahan G, Kuncir EJ. Managing exsanguinations: what we knew about damage control/bailout is not enough. Proc(Bayl Univ Med Cont) 2003;16:294-6.
7. Gregory J, Flancbaum L, Townsend M, et al. Incidence and timing of hypothermia in trauma patients undergoing operations. J Trauma 1991;31:795-800.
8. Steinmann S, Shackford SR, Davis JW. Implications of admission hypothermia in trauma patients. J Trauma 1990;30:200-2.
9. Luna G, Maier R, Pavlin E, et al. Incidence and effect of hypothermia in seriously injured patient. J Trauma 1987;27:1014-8.
10. Garrison J, Richardson D, Hilakos A, et al. Predicting the need to pack early for severe intra-abdominal haemorrhage. J Trauma 1996;40:923-9.
11. Weg JG. Oxygen transport in adult respiratory distress syndrome and other acute respiratory problems: Relationship of oxygen delivery and oxygen consumption. Crit Care Med 1991;19:650.
12. Durham CM, Siegel JH, Weiter LG, et al. Oxygen debt and metabolic academia as quantitative predictors of mortality and the severity of the ischemic insult in haemorrhagic shock. Crit Care Med 1999;19:231.
13. Offner PJ, de souza AL, Moore EE, et al. Avoidance of abdominal compartment syndrome in damage control laparotomy after trauma. Arch Surg 2001;136:676.
14. Rutherford EJ, Fusco MA, Nunn CR, et al. Hypothermia in critically ill trauma patient. Injury 1998;29:605.
15. Jurkovich GJ, Greiser WB, Luterman A, Curerri P. Hypothermia in trauma victims: an ominous predictor of survival. J Trauma 1987;27:1019-24.
16. Cosgrif N, Moore EE, Sauara A, et al. Predicting life-threatening coagulopathy in the massively transfused patient: Hypothermia and acidosis revisited. J Trauma 1997;42:857-62.
17. Gubler K, Gentilello L, Hassanthosh S, et al. The impact of hypothermia on dilutional coagulopathy. J Trauma 1994;36:847-51.

18. Eddy VA, Morris JA Jr, Cullinane DC. Hypothermia, coagulopathy and acidosis. Surg Clin North Am 2000;80:845.
19. Toschlog EA, Dulabon GR, Rotondo MF. Shock. In: Puffas TN, Purcell GP EDS. Unbound Surgery. Unbound Medicine, 2004. Available at:http://www.unbound surgery.com.
20. Stone HH, Strom PR, Mullins RJ. Management of major coagulopathy with onset during laparotomy. Ann Surg 1983;197:532-5.
21. Garrison SR, Richardson JD, Hilakos AS, et al. Predicting the need to pack early for severe intra-abdominal hemorrhage. J Trauma 1996;40:923-9.
22. Asensio JA, Petrone P, Roldan G, et al. Has evolution in awareness of guidelines for institution of damage control improved outcome in the management of post-traumatic open abdomen. Arch Surg 2004;139:2009-15.
23. Alicia M Mohr, Juan A Asemio, M Grcia-Nunez Patrizio Petreone, Zliod C Sefri. Guidelines for the institution of damage control Patients. International Trauma Care (ITACCS) Fall 2005.
24. Rotondo MF, Zomies DH. The damage control sequence and underlying logic. Surg Clinic North Am 1997;77:761.
25. Asensio JA, Mc Duffie L, Petreone P, et al. Reliable variables in the exsanguinated patient which indicate damage control and predict outcome. Am J Surg 2001;16:294-6.
26. Micheal BS, Donald H, Jenkins MD, et al. Damage control: collective review. The Journal of Trauma, injury, infections and critical care Nov 2000;49(5):974.
27. Scott C, Sagraves, Eric A Toschlog, Micheal F, Rotondo. Damage control surgery–the intensivist's Role. J Intensive Care Med 2006;21(1):5-11.

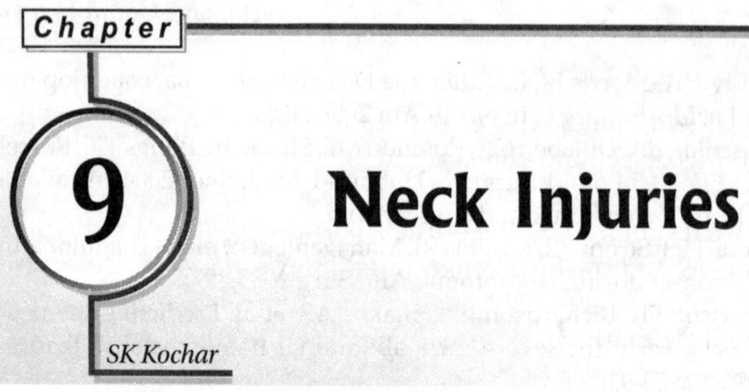

Injuries to neck are important due to two reasons. Firstly, neck contains a large number of anatomical structures, compact in a very small space, and secondly, any injury especially penetrating injury is likely to damage vital structures. Often the signs and symptoms are trivial in the immediate postinjury phase and the injuries are either underestimated or are missed. It is mandatory that one is familiar with the principles of recognizing and managing these potentially lethal injuries. Mortality following blunt and penetrating injuries has been reported to be 10 percent in recent series[1] while the penetrating alone had a mortality of 2-6 percent in most series.[2-4]

ANATOMY

The neck is commonly divided into three anatomical areas. Zone I injuries occur at the thoracic outlet, which is often described as extending from the level of the cricoid cartilage down to the level of the clavicle. This area included the proximal carotid arteries, the subclavian vessels, and major vessels in the chest, lung, upper mediastinum, esophagus, trachea, and thoracic duct. Zone II includes the area above the level of the cricoid to the angle of the mandible. Zone III area is located between the angle of the mandible and the base of the skull.

Mechanism of Injury

Injury may be blunt or penetrating in type. Blunt injury is less common and it could be due to the fact that neck is protected by the head and chest when exposed to blunt injuries. However, in motor vehicle accidents, the neck and head may be hyperextended, rendering the neck vulnerable to a steering wheel, dashboard, or windshield, and midline structures may be crushed between the striking object and the cervical vertebrae. Strangulation and the neck clothe getting trapped in thrasher is other form of blunt injuries. In blunt trauma the brunt is borne either by cervical spine or by larynx and trachea. Penetrating injuries may be due to gun-shot or knife. Occasionally, the "clothes line" or the string of the kite when strike the individual moving on high speed results in penetrating injuries.

Signs and Symptoms

The signs and symptoms will depend on the organ involved. The injury to cervical spine may or may not produce neurological deficit. The local pain and the deformity vary greatly. A potentially hazardous unstable spinal injury can exist in the complete absence of signs and symptoms, and sequelae of iatrogenic spinal destabilization can result in quadriplegia or other major permanent disability. Every patient of polytrauma should have cervical spine well protected till spinal injury is conclusively ruled out. Clinical manifestation of injury to carotid artery are: decreased level of consciousness, hemiplegia, cerebrovascular accident, hematoma, hemorrhage, absent carotid pulse, hypotension and pulse deficit. Jugular vein injury may present with hematoma, hemorrhage, hypotension. Injury to larynx and trachea manifest with strider, subcutaneous air, bubbling wound, hoarseness, dysphonia, hemoptysis. Esophagus and pharynx when injured may present with subcutaneous air, hematemesis, dysphagia, sucking wound. Injury to nerves in the neck produces:

- Recurrent laryngeal nerve: Hoarseness
- Hypoglossal: Deviation of tongue
- Glossopharyngeal: Dysphagia
- Stellate ganglion: Horner's syndrome
- Spinal accessory: Inability to shrug shoulder
- Phrenic: Ipsilateral diaphragmatic paralysis.

Low cervical penetrating wounds may injury intrathoracic structures, viz. aortic arch vessels, parietal and visceral pleurae, esophagus, pulmonary parenchyma. Shock may be present in as many as 37 percent of trauma victims and may develop in another 3 percent after admission.[1]

Initial Evaluation

Maintenance of upper airway patency and protection of the cervical spine share top priority in the immediate management of the trauma victim. The protocol for initial airway assessment and management recommended by the American College of Surgeons Committee on Trauma is given in Flow chart 9.1. Stabilization of neck may be achieved with a cervical collar or in case of penetrating injuries, sand bags securely positioned on either side of the neck. Two large bore (14-gauge) intravenous cannulae are used for administration of fluids and blood. Blood samples are obtained for type and crossmatch as well as chemistries and arterial blood gases. X-ray of cervical spine and chest are done during the initial stabilization period (Figs 9.1 and 9.2). A systemic evaluation of screening lateral film should include the followings:[5]

1. Examination of technical adequacy and visualization of all seven cervical vertebrae and the C7-T1 interspace.
2. Examination of soft tissues, visible airway, and abnormal subcutaneous air.

Flow chart 9.1: Protocol for initial airway assessment and management

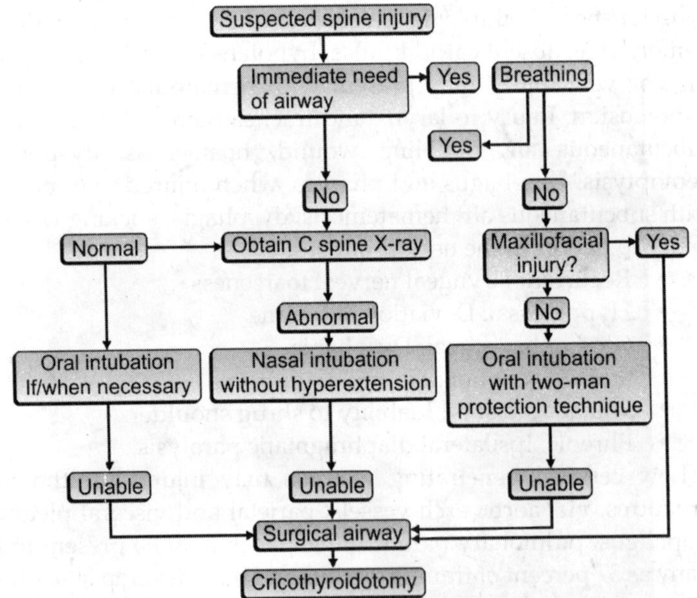

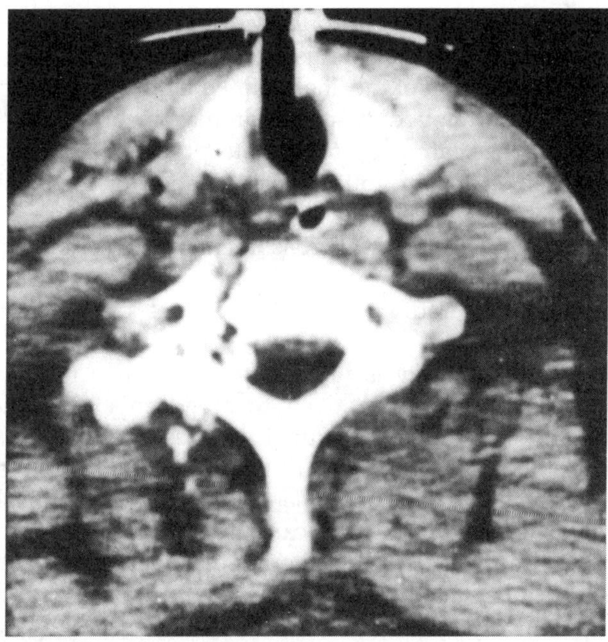

Fig. 9.1: GSW neck. Tracheostomy tube *in situ*, fracture cervical vertebra 7 and fragments lying in the spinal canal

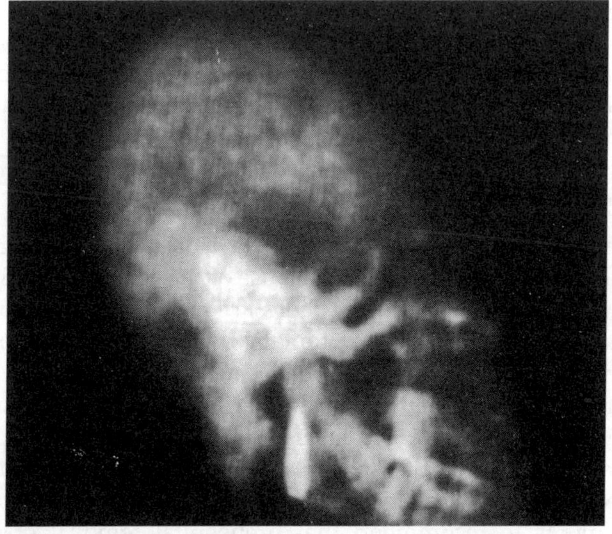

Fig. 9.2: GSW neck. Bullet lying in zone III

3. Measurement of the retropharyngeal airspace to identify abnormal prevertebral soft tissue swelling.
4. Careful inspection of the lines defined by the anterior margin of the vertebral bodies, posterior margin of the vertebral bodies, arches, laminae, and spinous processes.
5. Measurement of any offset or angulation of these lines, if present.
6. Special attention to any encroachment on the vertebral spinal canal.
7. Inspection for radiolucent fracture lines of the vertebrae themselves.

If the study of X-ray is normal, the protective measures to the axial spine can be removed to allow an examination of the posterior neck. The individual spinous process should be palpated with notation of any soft tissue swelling, crepitus, step off, or tenderness. An adequate neurological examination should be done. The neck should be carefully inspected for external evidence of trauma such as discoloration, hematoma, edema, and tenderness. Subcutaneous air may be visually dramatic if massive, or detectable only by palpation if subtle. Any externally evident edema or nematoma of the neck must be observed closely as a potential source of airway compromise. Carotid pulses should be assessed. Abnormality in the contour of the thyroid cartilage by inspection and palpation should be noted. The midline position of the trachea in the suprasternal notch should be confirmed. In penetrating injury whether platysma has been breached or not must be assessed. The examination of upper extremities and chest is important when the injury is in the lower cervical region.

Clinical Clearance of Cervical Spine Injury

Numerous large prospective studies have described the large cost and low yield of the indiscriminate use of cervical spine radiology in trauma patients. Although there are case reports of bony or ligamentous injuries in asymptomatic patients, no asymptomatic patient in the literature has had an unstable cervical spine fracture or suffered neurological deterioration due to the injury. There is no conclusive evidence in the literature that supports clinical clearance of the spine in the prehospital environment. There is enough variation between prehospital and in-hospital assessments to recommend that prehospital removal of spinal immobilization be avoided. Mechanism of injury alone does not determine the need for radiological investigation.

The cervical spine may be cleared clinically if the following preconditions are met:

- Fully alert and orientated
- No head injury
- No drugs or alcohol
- No neck pain
- No abnormal neurology
- No significant other 'distracting' injury (another injury which may 'distract' the patient from complaining about a possible spinal injury).

Provided these preconditions are met, the neck may then be examined. If there is no bruising or deformity, no tenderness and a pain free range of active movements, the cervical spine can be cleared. Radiographic studies of the cervical spine are not indicated.

Canadian C-Spine Rule comprises three main questions: (1) is there any high-risk factor present that mandates radiography (i.e. age >/=65 years, dangerous mechanism, or paresthesias in extremities)? (2) is there any low-risk factor present that allows safe assessment of range of motion (i.e. simple rear-end motor vehicle collision, sitting position in ED, ambulatory at anytime since injury, delayed onset of neck pain, or absence of midline C-spine tenderness)? and (3) is the patient able to actively rotate neck 45 degrees to the left and right? By cross-validation, this rule had 100% sensitivity (95% confidence interval [CI], 98-100%) and 42.5% specificity (95% CI, 40-44%) for identifying 151 clinically important C-spine injuries.[5a]

RADIOLOGICAL EVALUATION

The patient with neck injury may have blunt or penetrating injury. Patient may be alert and stable, may be awake and unstable, may be obtuned and stable. There is no controversy for investigation or management of unstable patient whether it is blunt injury or penetrating injury. It is only awake and stable patient which is subject of controversy regarding investigation and management. Evaluation of these patient has been hotly debated. Evaluation is required to know is it ligamentous injury, injury to vertebra, injury to spine or injury to carotid vessels beside injury to trachea or injury to esophagus.

Ample evidence exists that CT significantly outperforms plain radiography as a screening test for patients at very high risk of cervical spine injury and thus CT should be the initial screening test in those patients with a significantly depressed mental status. There is insufficient evidence to suggest that cervical spine CT should replace plain radiography as the initial screening test for less injured patients who are at low risk for cervical spine injury but still require a screening radiographic examination.[5b]

Newer generation CT continues to miss CS injuries in unreliable patients. MR changed the management in 7.9% of patients having had an admission CT with no acute injury. Use of MR for CS clearance in the unreliable patient has been recommended.[5c]

Management of Penetrating Neck Wounds

Before World War I, observation (unless major hemorrhage occurred) was the mainstay of therapy irrespective the wound has penetrated platysma or not and the mortality was 15 to 18 percent.[6] World war I surgeons adopted the same nonoperative principles with a reported mortality of 11 percent but morbidity was significant.[7] During World War II, the Korean war, and the Vietnam conflict, early intervention, antibiotics, tracheostomy, more rapid evacuation, and better resuscitation lowered the mortality rate to 7 percent.[8] However, the literature of the 1960s and 1970s is divided between operative and nonoperative management, the trend of the 1980s is for a selective approach. Selective exploration has proven to be safe and effective, provided that a prospective comprehensive diagnostic protocol is followed compulsively. In both policies of mandatory exploration and diagnostic evaluation, selective exploration has repeatedly been shown to be effective, and no clear advantage has emerged of one over the other, so either approach is justified.[9]

Mandatory Exploration

With the mandatory exploration approach, all wounds that penetrate the platysma muscle warrant exploration, regardless of vital signs or symptomatology. The rationale behind this policy includes the following points:

Many wounds may hide significant underlying injuries as:

- The mortality and morbidity of the missed injuries is significant.

- The mortality and morbidity of a negative neck exploration is insignificant.
- Length of hospital stay is similar if no injuries are found.
- Mandatory exploration is less time consuming than observation.
- Mandatory exploration requires fewer invasive tests and therefore less costly.

In developing countries like India where all the tests may not be available every where and the cost is a major factor mandatory exploration is the treatment of choice.

The patient is examined as described earlier and evidence of impending airway compromise is treated appropriately. Patient without hoarseness, change in voice, or subcutaneous emphysema may be intubated upon induction of anesthesia, if gas exchange is not compromised. The asymptomatic patient may undergo a superficial wound exploration in the emergency room to confirm penetration of the platysma. If the muscle has not been penetrated, the wound may be treated like any simple wound on an ambulatory basis. If mandatory exploration is to follow, most authors recommend foregoing all further preoperative diagnostic studies because they are unnecessary and no additional useful clinical information is gained. However, arteriography do have a role to play in injuries to certain zone of the neck. Gunshot wounds or stab wounds at the thoracic inlet or base of the neck may require vascular control below the level of clavicles. Conversely, penetrating wounds at the base of the skull can produce an internal carotid artery injury in which extracranial distal control is impossible. Arteriography is helpful in these situations.

Selective Observation

Proponents of selective observation feels that in the absence of specific indication as given in Table 9.1, most patients may be observed. Should signs or symptoms develop, then exploration would be warranted. The rationale is less cost, less hospitalization, and fewer negative surgical exploration, and, therefore, less mortality and morbidity.

The diagnostic evaluation—selective exploration protocol begins with physical examination, assessment of the airway, and local wound exploration, if necessary, to exclude superficial preplatysmal injuries. Prompt surgical exploration is recom-mended

Table 9.1: Absolute indications for exploration of neck wounds

Category	*Indication*
General	All gunshot wounds
	Shock
Vascular	Hemorrhage
	Diminished or absent pulse
	Expanding hematoma
Airway	Difficulty breathing
	Voice change
	Subcutaneous emphysema
Visceral	Difficulty in swallowing
	Subcutaneous emphysema
	Air bubbling from the wound
	Hemoptysis
	Hematemesis
Neurological	Progressive deficit

if absolute indications as mentioned in Table 9.1 are present. In the absence of such findings in the asymptomatic patient, a complete diagnostic evaluation should be undertaken. This include, an arch arteriogram, contrast swallow and triple endoscopy. Any positive finding on these studies mandates surgical exploration. Negative results from diagnostic evaluation— selective exploration averages 10-25 percent.[9, 10]

Specific Injuries Management

Vascular Injuries

Penetrating carotid artery injuries. The assessment of patients with penetrating neck trauma without hard signs suggestive of vascular injuries remains controversial. Many authors believe that physical examination alone is unreliable in identifying serious vascular injuries and some authors advocate[3,11] routine surgical exploration of all wounds that have violated the platysma to identify all vascular injuries. More commonly, routine exploration of zone II injuries is advocated, while zone I and zone III injuries are investigated with angiography because of the greater difficulty of operative exposure. Most centers recommend a policy of liberal or even routine angiography to screen for vascular injury and to minimize nontherapeutic neck explorations.[12,13] Recently it has been observed that a combination of a careful physical examination and color Doppler imaging provides a reliable way to assess penetrating neck trauma and may be safe alternative to routine contrast angiography.[14]

Approximately 47 percent of the injuries involve the common carotid artery, 33 percent involve the internal carotid artery, and 20 percent involve the external carotid artery.[15] The diagnosis of penetrating injuries may be simple (hemorrhage from a neck wound or hemispheric neurologic deficit); however 42 percent of the patients with "clinical evidence" of arterial injury will have negative angiograms, and conversely, angiograms of 20 percent of the "clinically negative" patients will show injuries.[16]

In the absence of obvious arterial injury, precisely performed arteriography is an effective way to evaluate arterial integrity. The use of angiography in stable patients with obvious injury requiring operation is debatable. Arteriography is generally recommended for patients with injuries located in either Zone I or Zone III. Low neck wounds may involve structures in superior mediastinum requiring thoracotomy for control and/or repair. Zone III injuries are located high in the neck and often pose difficult problem with exposure. Precise definition of the location and extent of injury may alter the operative approach. Therapeutic approach mandates.

No neurological deficit: Every one agrees that repair is the treatment of choice, if technically feasible.[15,17]

Mild to severe neurological deficit (not including coma): The resounding theme is to repair the injured carotid artery. If hemorrhage is uncontrollable, obviously ligation is appropriate.

Coma: The literature is divided. Some feels repair seems to offer better results[18] while others agree that ligation and repair are both valuable and that coma is not a contraindication to repair.[19] Few authors rest the decision on prograde flow[20] while other refutes its importance.[17]

Preoperative shock (unable to assess neurological status): In the presence of shock with inability to determine just how much the actual neurological deficit is compounded by decreased oxygen delivery, it is probably best to repair. Obviously, in the face of a carotid artery injury that is surgically inaccessible, ligation should be performed regardless of neurological status.

Injuries to the Larynx and Trachea

Injury to the larynx and trachea may be blunt or penetrating. Blunt trauma are almost always associated with motor vehicle accidents. As a vehicle stops, the hyperextended head hits the windshield and the exposed neck comes into contact with the dashboard. Penetrating injuries to the larynx or trachea are usually due to gunshot wounds or stabbing; most victims are stabbed on the left side.

Signs and symptoms: Hoarseness and stridor are the most common symptoms of laryngeal trauma and flattening of the anterior neck with loss of thyroid and cricoid cartilage contours are common signs with laryngeal trauma. Cervical subcutaneous emphysema, hemoptysis, and pain with swallowing imply laryngeal disruption. Patient may have post-traumatic postural dyspnea.[21]

Diagnosis: In most cases, the definitive diagnosis should be made after securing the airway. Laryngeal-cervical spine X-rays may disclose subcutaneous emphysema that may be contained within the pretracheal fascia and therefore, may be undetected clinically. Chest X-ray may show pneumomediastinum or pneumothorax. Pneumomediastinum from the larynx or trachea would imply bacterial contamination of the mediastinum; antibiotics and drainage should be considered. Laryngoscopy (direct or indirect) may precipitate laryngospasm or cause more trauma to the already traumatized tissue and should be performed after a patent airway is obtained.

MANAGEMENT

If the patient has worsening stridor or other evidence of developing upper airway obstruction, an immediate cricothyroidotomy should be performed without attempt at direct laryngoscopy and intubation. Blind nasotracheal intubation should never be attempted if an upper airway injury is suspected. The additional caveat is to observe for evidence of airway trauma during intubation of patients not previously suspected of harboring such an injury: if a laryngeal fracture, submucous hemorrhage or air, or linear tears of the laryngeal mucosa are seen, intubation through the larynx should not be attempted. Endotracheal intubation or even manipulation by direct laryngoscopy, can aggravate an existing injury and complicate definitive repair. The worst scenario is the patient with blunt transection of the subglottic trachea. Passage of an endotracheal tube can rupture the remaining mucosa and soft tissues, allowing the trachea to retract into the thoracic inlet and rendering all subcutaneous efforts at establishing an airway impossible. The recommended algorithm[22] for management of suspected blunt trauma to the upper airway is given in Flow chart 9.2.

Surgical Management

Tracheostomy may be performed through a vertical incision under local anesthesia or mask anesthesia. If the site of injury is laryngeal or high tracheal, then the tracheostomy should be one

Flow chart 9.2: Protocol for the management of suspected blunt upper airway trauma[22]

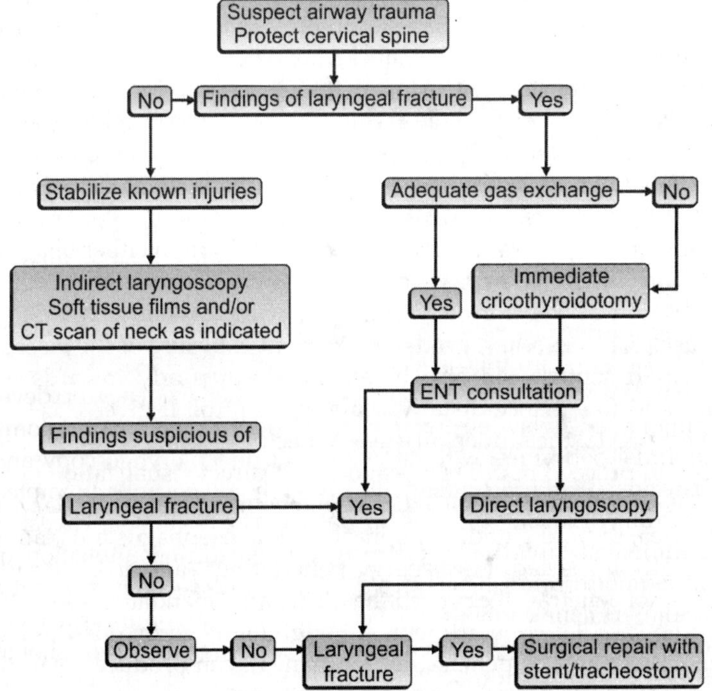

or two rings below the injury. However, if the site of the injury is low cervical, then the tracheostomy may be brought out through the site of injury. The laryngeal mucosa may be repaired with 5-0 absorbable sutures, and the cartilaginous structures with stainless steel wire. Endolaryngeal stenting may be necessary; prefabricated silicone stents or finger cots filled with sponge rubber may be used. Stents are left in place for 6-8 weeks. Tracheal injuries should also be stented with T-tubes to prevent postoperative stenosis.

Surgical Exploration of the Neck

Several surgical approaches can be taken for exploration of the neck for penetrating wounds, but what is more important is that one must be prepared for access to both sides of neck, base of skull, and into the mediastinum and both sides of chest.

Vascular compartment exposure for unilateral injury is approached by anterior sternocleidomastoid carotid incision. Zone I injuries with known or suspected perforations of the innominate artery itself may require extension of this incision, by means of an upper median sternotomy to the fourth interspace. Complete exposure of the subclavian artery for trauma is most easily accomplished with a fourth interspace anterior thoracotomy on the appropriate side. The anterior sternocleidomastoid incision, upper median sternotomy, and thoracotomy can well be combined in an "open book" incision with excellent exposure of all of the arch great vessels.

Bilateral neck trauma may be explored through either bilateral carotid incisions or a transverse "thyroid" incision. Lateral extension of the transverse incision, with division of the strap muscles, if necessary, produces excellent exposure of the visceral compartment. It can also be extended superiorly towards the mastoid to enhance distal vasculature control. It gives excellent exposure to the upper airway. A neck exploration for trauma should proceed in orderly fashion with direct visualization of all structures in the visceral and vascular compartments. The larynx, trachea, thyroid gland, hypopharynx, and esophagus must all be visually inspected. Low energy penetrating trauma that clearly does not penetrate the carotid sheath does not mandate exploration of the vascular compartment, although high energy missiles and complex blunt or penetrating mechanism can produce a carotid intimal flap or pseudoaneurysm despite apparent nonpenetration of the carotid sheath. If there is penetration of the carotid, with or without an obvious hematoma, proximal and distal arterial control should be established prior to exposure of the area of injury. Once the carotid sheath is open, the common, internal, and external carotid arteries, internal jugular vein, and vagus nerve should be visually inspected for integrity, bleeding, or intramural hematoma. In the absence of any injury, the incision should be irrigated and closed without drainage.

REFERENCES

1. Stone HH, Callahan GS. Soft tissue injuries of the neck. Surg Gynecol Obstet 1963;117:745.
2. Golueke PJ, Goldstein AS, Sclafani SJA, et al. Routine verses selective exploration of penetrating neck injuries: A randomised prospective study. J Trauma 1984;24:1010.
3. Roon AJ, Christensen N. Evaluation and treatment of penetrating cervical injuries. J Trauma 1979;19:391.
4. Campbell FC, Robbs JV. Penetrating injuries of the neck:A prospective study of 108 patients. Br J Surg 1980;67:382.
5. Williams CF, Bernstein TW, Jeleko. Essentiality of the lateral cervical spine radiograph. Ann Emerg Med 1981;10:198-204.

5a. Stiell IG, Wells GA, Vandemheen KL, et al. The Canadian C-spine rule for radiography in alert and stable trauma patients. JAMA 2001;286:1841-8.

5b. Holmes JF, Akkinepalli R. Computed tomography versus plain radiography to screen for cervical spine injury: a meta-analysis. J Trauma. 2005 May;58(5):902-5.

5c. Menaker J, Philp A, Boswell S, Scalea TM. Computed tomography alone for cervical spine clearance in the unreliable patient–are we there yet?. J Trauma 2008;64(4):898-903; discussion. 903-4.

6. LaGarde LA. Gunshot wounds, W Wood & Co, Newyork, 1914 p204.
7. Surgeon General's Office. The medical department of the United States Army in the World War. Vol II, Washington DC, Government printing office, 1927;p68
8. Beebe GW, DeBakey ME. Battle casualties: Incidence, Mortality and Logistic considerations, Springfield, Illinois, Charles C Thomas, 1952.
9. Noyes LD, McSwain NE, Markowitz IP. Panendoscopy with arteriography verses mandatory exploration of penetrating wounds of the neck. Ann Surg 1986;204;21-31.
10. Rakeschanadra MR, Bhatti FK, Guadino E, et al. Penetrating injuries of the neck: Criteria for exploration 1983;23:47-49.

11. Apffelsteadt JP, Muller R. Results of manadatory exploration for penetrate cervical injuries. World J Surg 1994;18:917-9.
12. Jurkovich GT, Zingarello W, Wallace J, Curreri PW. Penetrating neck trauma:diagnostic studies in the asymptomatic patient. J Trauma 1985;25:819-2.
13. Wood J, Fabian TC, Mangiante EC. Penetrating neck injuries: Recommendations for selective management. J Trauma 1989;29:602-5.
14. Demetriades D, Theodorou MD, Cornwell III, et al. Penetrating injuries of the neck in patients in stable condition. Arch Surg 1995;130:971-5.
15. Fry Re, Fry WJ. Extracranial carotid artery injuries. Surgery 1980;88: 581.
16. Mc Cormic TM, Burch BH. Routine angiographic evaluation of neck and extremity injuries. J Trauma 1979;19:384.
17. Ledgerwood AM, Mullins RJ, Lucar CE. Primary repair verses ligation for carotid artery injuries. Arch Surg 1980;115:488.
18. Brown MF, Graham JM, Feliciano DV, et al. Carotid artery injuries. AM J Surg 1982;144:748.
19. Unger SW, Tucker WS, Madeza MA, et al. Carotid artery trauma. Surgery 1980;87:477.
20. Liekweg WG Jr, Greenfield LJ. Management of penetrating carotid artrery injury. Am Surg 1978;188:587.
21. Cherry JR, Hammon JE. Transection of the cervical trachea resulting from closed trauma to the neck. J Laryngol Otol 1984;98:97.
22. Schenk WG. Neck Injuries in Moylan JA. Trauma Surgery. Philadelphia, JB Lippincott & Company, 1988.

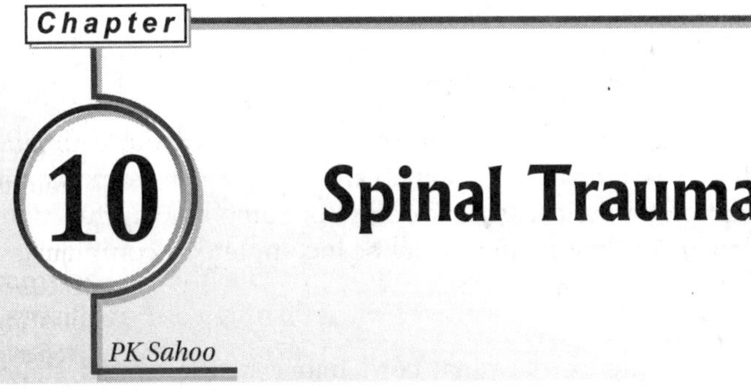

Spinal Trauma

PK Sahoo

HISTORICAL REVIEW AND INTRODUCTION

Spinal cord injury is a mortal condition and has been recognized as such since antiquity. Five thousand years ago, in the Edwin Smith Papyrus, the clinical features of six cases of injury to the cervical spinal cord was described with an advice: "an ailment not to be treated". In the First World War 90% of the patients who suffered a spinal cord injury died within one year of wounding. The vision of a few pioneers–Guttmann in the United Kingdom and Munro and Bors in the United States- has greatly improved the outlook for those with spinal cord injury, although the mortality associated with quadriplegia was still 35% in 1970. Since 1970 there has been a renewed interest in the management of spinal injuries as a whole. The better understanding and management of spinal cord injury have lead to a reduction in mortality and less morbidity in those who survive.

Although the effect of the initial trauma is irreversible, the spinal cord is at risk from further injury by injudicious early management. Such complications must be avoided in unconscious patients by being aware of the possibility of spinal cord injury from the nature of the accident especially in unconscious patients. When spinal injury is suspected the patient must be handled and transported correctly from the beginning at the site of accident.

Ideal management now demands on the spot treatment, immobilization, proper transportation, rapid evacuation from the site of accident. Improved emergency care and effective medical and surgical management at a center where intensive care of the patients can be supervised by a specialist in spinal cord injuries will prevent morbidity and mortality.

Definition of Spinal Cord Injury

Spinal cord injury is defined as an occurrence of an acute traumatic lesion of neural elements in the spinal canal, resulting in temporary or permanent motor deficit, sensory deficit, or autonomic dysfunction. These deficits or dysfunctions may be incomplete or complete.

Incidence

The yearly incidence of spinal cord injury in the united states ranges from 29 to 50 patients per million people. Approximately, 10,000 cases occurring each year.

At present the annual incidence of spinal cord injury is about 15 to 50 per million of the population. The peak age incidence is around 20 to 40 years.[1,2] The sex incidence shows predominance of men with 4:1 male to female ratio.

Etiology

Most injuries occur as result of major vehicle accidents (60%), followed by fall (20%), act of violence mostly gunshot wounds (14%). Motor vehicle accidents are the leading causes in the young. The proportion of injuries occurring due to fall increase with age. Act of violence are fairly distributed up to the age of 60. Some unusual modes of injury seen in India are, due to clothes/hair being caught in machinery, fall from bullock cart and cattle hits. A successful ejection causes injuries to thoracolumbar and cervical spine in 20% cases. The most common site of cervical vertebral body fracture is C5. Neurological injury at this level estimated to be about 30%, which is greater than, at any other level in the cervical spine. Noncontiguous multiple spinal fracture occur in approximately 5% of cases, failure to recognize these injuries may result in devastating spinal cord damage.

BIOMECHANICS OF SPINE INJURY

Spinal injuries are result of movements of the spine beyond the physiological range.[3] The logical understanding of the biomechanics of cervical spine injuries is very useful, in following, management of the patients with such lesions. Numerous classification of cervical spine injuries, based on biomechanical and other factors have been proposed.[4] The classification given below was originally formulated by Allen and associates and found to be an extremely useful classification. However, classification of cervical spine fractures and dislocation based on biomechanics has the following limitations. First, a single injury mechanism may produce different type of traumatic lesions in different individuals. Secondly, in a real clinical setting, complex forces act upon the spine to produce injury and is very difficult to simplify all the forces involved. Additionally the patient may sustain multiple, repetitive injuries to the cervical spine, i.e. in a rollover accident, an individual may be repeatedly and sequentially injured. Here two fundamentals concepts need to be stressed. Firstly, the cervical spine is acted upon by forces, which have vectorial quality. This implies that the forces have magnitude and direction. Predominantly **compressive forces** along the axial direction of cervical spine tend to cause bony injury by **compression**. It produces destruction of cortical end plates and comminuted fractures of the vertebral body. Pure **distractive forces** cause ligamentous injury, avulsion injury to the vertebra and **dislocation** without fracture of the vertebra. A rotational injury produces 360 degrees or global instability of the spine. The second point to be stressed is the three-column concept by Dennis (1983).[5] The column comprises of the anterior, middle and posterior columns. Anterior column has anterior longitudinal ligament, anterior annulus fibrosus and anterior body of vertebra. Middle column has longitudinal ligament, posterior annulus fibrosus and the posterior body of the vertebra. Posterior column comprises of lateral masses, right and left facets joints. In extension injuries, both compressive and distractive forces are coupled. Dennis (1983) differentiated between mechanical and neurological instability. First degree instability is mechanical instability. This does not actually threaten the neural elements. Second degree instability is neurological instability and the neural elements are a risk. Third degree instability is mechanical and neurological instability. Severe burst fracture dislocation is usually unstable third degree instability.

Mechanism of Spine Injuries

The following is a description of the types of injuries commonly seen in neurosurgical practice.

Flexion compression injuries: The mechanism here is loading with the head in the flexed position. Mild injury causes blunting of the anterosuperior cortical end plates without any significant loss of stability. Extreme injury produces tear drop fracture in the anteroinferior part of vertebral body with retropulsion of the vertebral body into the spinal cord causing anterior cord syndrome. Profound neurological loss with posterior ligamentous instability may occur in such a situation. Intermediate injury– Leads to compression of vertebral body and posterior ligamentous instability. Common site is C5-C6.

Vertical compression injuries: In vertical compression injury there is direct axial loading of the cervical spine with very minimal flexion or extension of the spine. Mild injury causes cupping of superior and interior cortical end plates. In severe cases there could be comminuted burst fracture with retropulsion of the fracture fragments to spinal cord and may produce anterior cord syndrome. Individuals who dive head first into shallow water may have burst fracture C4-C5.

Flexion rotation injuries: Flexion rotation injuries typically give rise to unilateral facet dislocation.

Distraction flexion injuries: With combination of distractive and flexion forces there is disruption of the posterior ligaments including intraspinous and supraspinous ligaments, ligamentum flavum and capsule of facet joints. There is minimal or no bony injury to the vertebral body. The upper vertebral body glides over the lower resulting in bilateral facet dislocation. This is a highly unstable injury because all the ligaments in the middle segment as well as the intervertebral disc are generally disrupted.

Compressive extension injury: This is a rare mechanism for cervical spine injury. Usually there is fracture of the posterior bony elements with or without disruption of intervertebral disk, PLL and ALL. In severe injuries there is complete separation with dislocation of vertebral body.

Distractive extension injury: This injury causes disruption of ALL, disc and widening of disc space with a tiny tear drop fracture. This is commonly seen in patients with pre-existing spondylosis and who fall forward striking their face or forehead. It results in central cord syndrome.

Hyperflexion followed by hyperextension injury: Hyperflexion followed by hyperextension results in whiplash injuries.

Penetrating injuries: Penetrating injury can be low velocity penetrating wound with a knife or a high velocity penetrating injury with a bullet.

Pathophysiological Changes in Spinal Cord Following Injury

Huges (1978)[6] described a sequence of events following injury, commencing with swelling of nerve fibers and disintegration of both axon material with myelin. Associated with this is the disruption of the cell bodies, chromatolysis if the axonic damage is remote from the cell bodies. In the first 24 hours reactive microscopic changes are minor, but after that time there is necrosis, swelling, cellular infiltration and breakdown products from the neural degeneration. The neural tissue and particularly the long tracts may be preserved despite clinical evidence of complete cord transection. In late stages there is evidence of regeneration of nerve fibers. The cord lesion may be at some distance from the site of bony injury. Hughes also emphasized the fusiform extent of damage over one or more segments tapering off above and below the level of injury, commonly as a small round area in the posterior column.

The pathophysiological changes that occurs in the first few hours after the experimental spinal cord injury has been studied. The first changes are seen in the gray matter bearing out the clinical experience that the central part of the cord is the most severely affected. The amount of edema and the total amount of tissue destruction are in general, proportional to the severity of the initiating trauma. However, the time sequence of events is uniform regardless of the forces involved. The vasomotor reactivity of the involved segment is lost immediately after the injury and the impaired spinal cord blood flow and hypoxia are possibly the most important ensuing secondary features. While most of the experiments confirm that the severity of the injury is the main determinant of the ultimate deficit, there is abundant work to show that early relief of compression may improve recovery of the spinal cord. As all forms of treatment to date have been shown to have very little effect on the degree of neurological recovery, attention is turning increasingly to the possibility of influencing the repair and regenerative process in the injured cord. Aquayo, classic experiments[7] demonstrated that all axons can regenerate given the right environment and that CNS tissues are inhibitory. Schwab (1991)[8] identified two specific proteins (NI 35 and NI 250), on oligodendrocytic cell bodies that arrested axonal regeneration and he was able to reverse this effect with specific antibodies. Other work on spinal regeneration include nerve growth factors, trophic nervous system factors, Schwann cell factor, fibroblast and epidermal growth factor and electromagnetic fields.[9]

Biology of Acute SCI

Biology of Acute SCI Involves both Primary and Secondary Injury Mechanisms[10-15]

Most traumatic cord injuries occur as a result of rapid cord compression because of a fracture-dislocation or burst fracture.[16] Acute spinal cord distraction, acceleration-deceleration with shearing, and transection from penetrating injuries are additional mechanisms of trauma.[17,18] There is strong evidence[10,11,19] that the primary initial injury initiates a series of events that include the following:

1. Ischemia, impaired autoregulation, neurogenic shock, hemor rhage, microcirculatory disruption, vasospasm, and thr- ombosis.[10,11,14]
2. Ionic derangements, including increased intracellular calcium and sodium, and increased extracellular potassium;[10,12,13]
3. Accumulation of neurotransmitters, including serotonin, cat- echolamines, and extracellular glutamate, which contribute to cellular injury;
4. Arachidonic acid release, free radical and eicosanoid pro- duction, and lipid peroxidation;[10]
5. Endogenous opioids;
6. Edema;
7. Inflammation;
8. Loss of adenosine triphosphate-dependent cellular processes; and
9. Apoptosis.[10,20,21] The development of these secondary injury events, which lead to tissue destruction during the first few hours after injury, is of relevance to the surgical and non- surgical treatment of SCI.

Management at the Site of Accident

All polytrauma patients should be suspected to have spinal injury unless proved otherwise and managed accordingly. Witnesses or paramedical staff or Doctor present at the scene should have adequate knowledge for the management of such patients at the site of accident.

Conscious Patient

The diagnosis of spinal cord injury is made if the individual complaints of neck and back pain, weakness of limbs and sensory disturbances.

Unconscious Patient

It must be assumed that the force that rendered the patient unconscious has injured the cervical spine until radiography proves otherwise. Until then the head and neck must be carefully placed and held in neutral (anatomical) position and stabilized by hard cervical collar or sand bags on each side of the head with forehead tapes. During turning or lifting, it is vital that the whole spine is maintained in the neutral position like log rolling. While positioning the patient, relevant information can be obtained from the witness. Carelessness during turning, lifting and transportation may produce complete lesion in an individual with incomplete cord lesion.

Positioning of the Patient

The spine is best immobilized by placing the patient **supine**, as this position is important for resuscitation and rapid assessment of life-threatening injuries. However, unconscious patients on their backs are at risk of passive gastric regurgitation and aspiration of vomit. This can be avoided by tracheal intubation, which is ideal method of securing airway in an unconscious patient. If intubation is not required or cannot be performed the patient should be "**log rolled**" carefully in to a **modified lateral position** 70–80 degrees from prone with head supported in the neutral position by the underlying arm. This posture allows secretion to drain freely from the mouth and a rigid collar to minimize neck movements.

The log rolling should be performed by a minimum of four people in a coordinated manner ensuring that, there are no unnecessary movements in any part of the spine. One person is responsible for holding the head and neck, one for the shoulder and chest, one for the hip and abdomen, and one for the legs. The **prone position is unsatisfactory** as it may severely embarrass respiration, particularly in quadriplegic patient. The **semi prone coma position is also contraindicated**, as it results in rotation of the spine.

Transportation of the Patient

Proper care must be taken during transportation of the patients so that an incomplete injury should not become complete. Scoop stretchers are available and may be used for transportation to Ambulance. The neck should be immobilized by hard cervical collar or with sand bags on the sides of the neck during transportation.

Aims of Evaluation of Spine Injured Patients are:

1. Simultaneous diagnosis and resuscitation
2. Prevent/limit secondary injuries
3. Recognize and treat associated injuries

Early Management at the Site/Casualty

The Emergency Medical service team should be trained to evaluate and manage the following:

A - Airway
B - Breathing
C - Circulation-Pulse, BP
D - Disability detection and documentation
E - Exposure and evaluation as a whole
F - Fluid administration

Prior to history taking and clinical evaluation in all polytrauma including spine injury patients, proper management of airway, breathing and circulation is vital at the site of accident/casualty.

Airway: Proper management of airway is absolutely vital for good outcome. The oral cavity has to be gently cleaned off all foreign bodies like food particles, broken teeth, blood, vomits, etc.

Breathing: The rate and type of respiration has to be observed. The simplest way to evaluate breathing is to observe the movements of the chest. The front and back of the chest has to be inspected. If the breathing is poor intubation/ventilation/tracheostomy may be required urgently. With care, tracheal intubation is usually safe in patients with injuries to the spinal cord. Intubation may be performed at the site of accident by the attending doctor or paramedic without rotating the neck. The breathing may be poor due to cervical spinal cord injury leading to phrenic nerve and diaphragmatic palsy. Injury to thoracic spinal cord with intercostals muscle paralysis. Associated rib fractures, lung contusion and hemopneumothorax leads to decreased respiratory movements.

Circulation: Once the airway is protected intravenous access should be established for cardiopulmonary support. In high spinal cord injury the patient may be hypotensive due to sympathetic paralysis, peripheral pooling of blood and associated bradycardia due to vagal over activity. Fast Ringer's lactate, atropine and pressure amines are required to be administered.

Disability detection: If respiration and circulation are satisfactory patient can be examined briefly. A basic examination should include measurement of pulse, blood pressure and respiratory rate, level of consciousness, pupillary response and site and extent of spinal injury.

Specific signs of spinal injury should be sought, including local bruising, deformity and tenderness of the spine. The patient must be subjected to a coordinated log roll for proper and safe assessment of the back.

The neurological pattern of cord injury includes complete and incomplete cord lesion.

The clinical effects of complete cord lesion are spinal or neurogenic shock evidenced by marked hypotension and bradycardia. Besides there will be flaccid paralysis of bladder with urinary retention, flaccid paralysis of the bowel with paralytic ileus, loss of perspiration below the level of injury, hypotonia, weakness, sensory impairment and aflexia below the level of injury. Incomplete cord lesions are anterior cord syndrome, central cord syndrome, posterior cord syndrome, Brown-Séquard syndrome, root lesion and cord concussion.

In spinal cord injury the neurological examination must include the following:

- Sensation to pinprick (Spinothalamic track)
- Sensation to fine touch and joint position sense (Posterior columns)
- Muscle power (Corticospinal track)
- Reflexes (including abdominal, anal, bulbocavernosus)
- Cranial nerve function

A more practical approach is to grade the extent of injury according to their functional status rather than neurological finding. By and large, the original Frankel[22] grading system remains the most useful one.

Grade A: Complete motor paralysis and sensory loss.

Grade B: Complete motor paralysis with incomplete sensory loss.

Grade C: Some motor function preserved below the injured segment but of no practical use.

Grade D: Useful motor and incomplete sensory function but not normal.

Grade E: Normal motor and sensory function.

Documentation: A written record of the patient's problems, treatment received and response to treatment should be documented. This information should include patient personal data, medical history, treatment initiated, and the patient's response to the treatment, laboratory and X-ray data. The names of referring hospital should be included. If a patient is transferred, complete records of treatment given during transport should be mentioned.

Exposure and evaluation of associated injuries: After clearing airway, maintaining breathing and arresting any hemorrhage the whole body to be examined from head to toe and any injury has to be noted.

Inspect and palpate the abdomen for any abdominal injury, which should be managed at the earliest. Any flail chest, sucking wound of the chest needs urgent attention. Chest compression test to find out fractures ribs, pelvic compression to find out fracture of the pelvic bones should be carried out.

Palpate/feel all the extremities to detect fractures of upper and lower limbs. Splint the fractures.

Fluid administration: In polytrauma patients with spine injury IV line to be started at the site if possible. Fluid in the form of Ringer's lactate/normal saline solution to be given to maintain any fluid loss.

Investigations

Optimal treatment of patients with spine injury lies on an accurate radiologic assessment of traumatic lesions. Failure to recognize a fracture or instability may result in subsequent development of severe neurological sequel. The bony injuries to the spinal column are best visualized by plain X-ray films and computerized tomography scan which remains the initial imaging modalities of choice in patients with spinal trauma. A translateral plain X-ray film of spine between Cl to T1 detect about 75 to 85 percent of cervical spine injury like compression fracture, comminuted fracture, burst fracture and dislocations (Figs 10.1 to 10.4). The accuracy increases to nearly 100 percent, when AP view, open mouth view for fracture odontoid and Swimmer's view for C7-T1 vertebra fracture is included. Between 15 to 20 percent of patients who have cervical spinal cord injuries will have no overt radiographic findings on plain films. Approximately two-third of these patients will show abnormalities, when thin section of CT of spine is taken. CT scan has the added advantage as it demonstrates the bone and/or disc material in to the spinal canal and presence

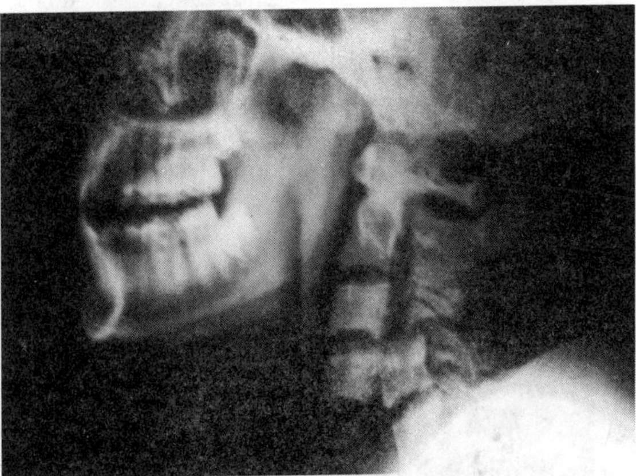

Fig. 10.1: X-ray cervical spine lateral view, showing C4-C5 dislocation

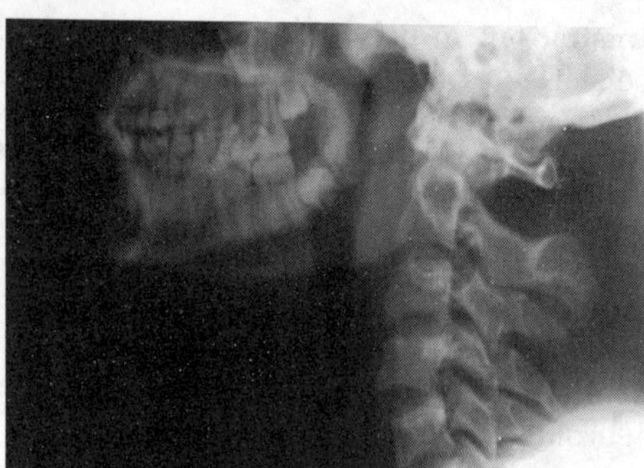

Fig. 10.2: X-ray cervical spine lateral view, after reduction of C4-C5 dislocation

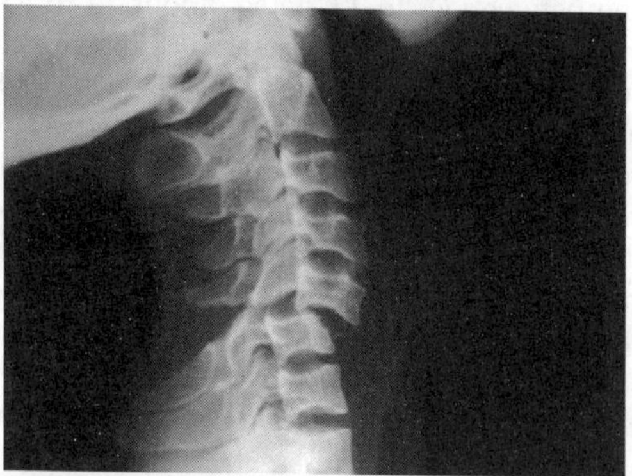

Fig. 10.3: X-ray cervical spine lateral view showing C5-C6 dislocation

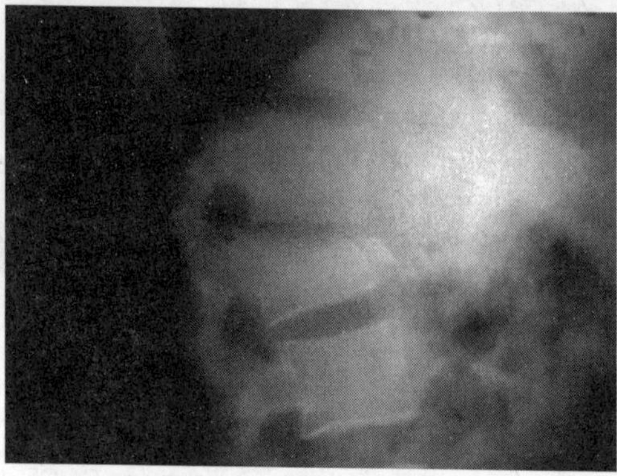

Fig. 10.4: X-ray thoracolumbar spine showing LV2 compression fracture

of fracture of the lamina, pedicle, facets and vertebral body. CT also offers the three-dimensional configuration of fractures by reformatting and there by permits visualization of extent of injury. However, significant cord injuries and neurological deficits can occur in the absence of detectable bony injuries.[23] Till recently the radiographic diagnosis of cord injuries relied on the indirect evidence from myelography or contrast enhanced tomography scan.[24] Today MRI is the imaging modality of choice in evaluation of traumatic cord lesions because of it's ability to visualize the spinal cord directly by sagittal, coronal and axial scans without the need for contrast (Figs 10.5 to 10.8). Cord changes like edema, hematoma, contusion, myelomalacia, atrophy and syringomyelia can only be seen by MRI scans. Besides disk herniation, anterior or

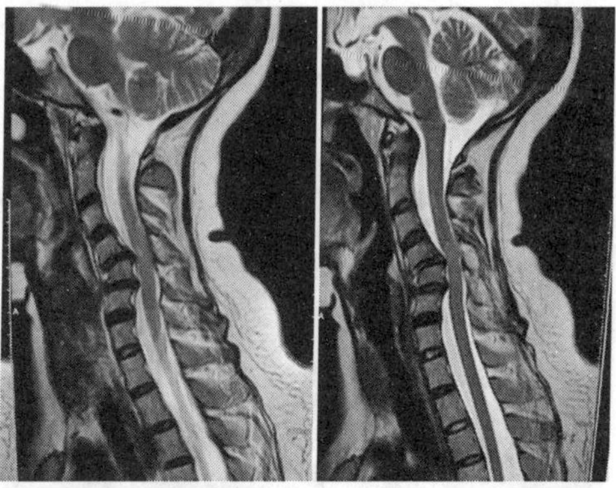

Fig. 10.5: MRI cervical spine sagittal view showing C4-C5 dislocation

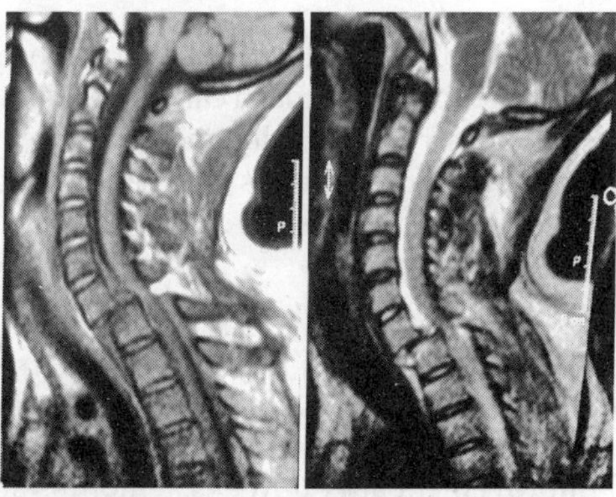

Fig. 10.6: MRI cervical spine sagittal view showing C7-D1 dislocation

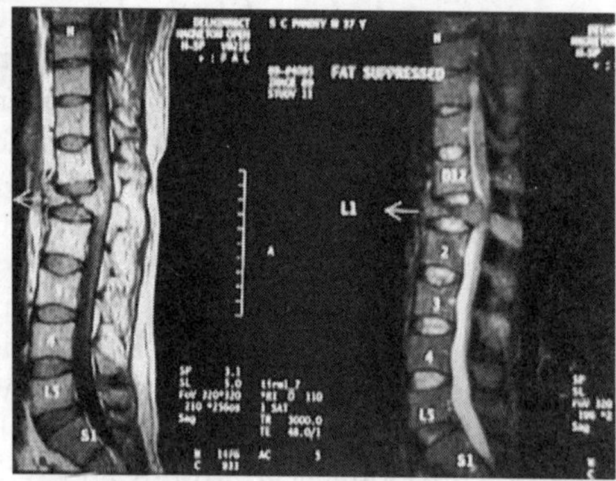

Fig. 10.7: MRI cervical spine sagittal view showing LV1 compression fracture

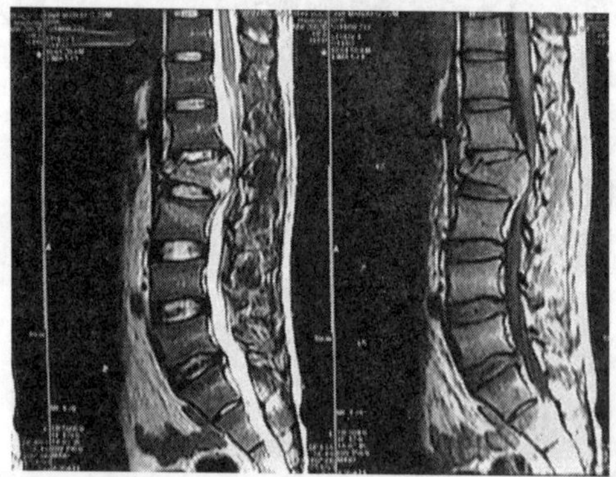

Fig. 10.8: MRI cervical spine sagittal view showing LV2 compression fracture

posterior compression of the cord can be better delineated by MRI and the appropriate surgical approach can be decided. MRI is also the method of choice for imaging ligamentous injury like ALL, PLL, intraspinous and supraspinous ligament and ligamentum flavum.

Medical Management

In 1990 Bracken et al[25] published the multicentric trial of double blind, randomized, clinical trial of massive doses of methylprednisolone which has proved beyond doubt that there has been neurological improvement after 6 weeks, 6 months and one year, if methylprednisolone is given in the first 8 hours following spinal cord injury. If the patient reaches within 3 hours post injury the recommended methyl prednisolone treatment regimen involves the intravenous administration of 30 mg/kg bolus (administered over 15 min), followed by a 45 min pause. This is followed over the next 23 hours by a maintenance intravenous infusion of methyl prednisolone (5.4 mg/kg per h). Thus, the total administration time is 24 hr. The efficacy of this regimen was only established for closed injuries of the spinal cord. The efficacy for penetrating injuries and closed injuries below the conus medullaris is not established. Therefore, it seems prudent not to administer methylprednisolone to these patients as it doubles the wound infection rate and increases the chance of gastrointestinal hemorrhage.

The third national acute spinal cord injury randomized controlled trial of 1997 has proved, that patients with acute spinal cord injury who receive methylprednisolone within 3 hours of injury should be maintained on the treatment regime for 24 hours. When methylprednisolone is initiated 3 to 8 hours of injury, patients should be maintained on steroid therapy for 48 hours. Patients treated with tirilazad for 48 hours showed motor recovery rates equivalent to patients who received methylprednisolone for 24 hours.

Management of bladder function: Despite vastly improved management; urinary tract complications are still the main cause of morbidity and mortality. The aim of bladder management is preservation of renal function and continence. After a severe spinal cord injury, it is safer to put **indwelling** 12 or 14 F Foley's catheter preferably silicone for monitoring the patient. Once the patient's condition improves **intermittent urethral catheterization** should be carried out every 6 hours using 12 or 14 F Foley's catheter under strict aseptic technique. When the patient begins to sit up but continues to be incontinent intermittent clean self-catheterization can be advised. Patients catheterize themselves with the aim of remaining continent between catheterization and therefore avoiding the need to wear urinary drainage apparatuses.

Management of bowel function: The patient should receive intravenous fluid for at least the first 48 hours, as paralytic ileus usually accompanies a severe spinal injury. A nasogastric tube is passed and oral fluids are forbidden until normal bowel sounds return. Acute gastric hemorrhage or perforation is an uncommon but dangerous complication after spinal cord injury, and for this reason H2-receptor antagonists should be started as soon as possible after injury and continued for at least 3 weeks.

Skin and pressure areas: Nursing care and two hourly turning should be instituted to prevent bedsores. When the patient is transferred from trolley to bed the whole of the back must be inspected for bruising, abrasions or sign of pressure on the skin. Manual turning can be achieved on a standard hospital bed. Alternatively, the electrically driven turning and tilting bed can be used. In the Stryker frame, the patient can be turned between supine and prone position by inbuilt circular turning mechanism.

Care of joints and limbs: The joints must be passively moved through the full range to prevent stiffness and contractures. Proper positioning, immobilization aids, and care of the paralyzed limbs will prevent deep vein thrombosis and pulmonary embolism.

Cervical spine injuries are known to be associated with head, chest, abdominal, pelvic and extremity injuries. Associated trauma needs prompt recognization and appropriate management.

The spinal injury—cervical spine: Patients with injury of the cervical spine should initially be managed by skull or cervical traction. Cervical traction creates a longitudinal pull along the cervical spine and reduces dislocation, restores normal anatomical alignment and provides stabilization. This form of treatment is most commonly used for treating injuries from the atlanto occipital joint to T1 (Fig. 10.9). There are essentially three methods of applying cervical traction, the head halter, cranial tongs and halo head ring.

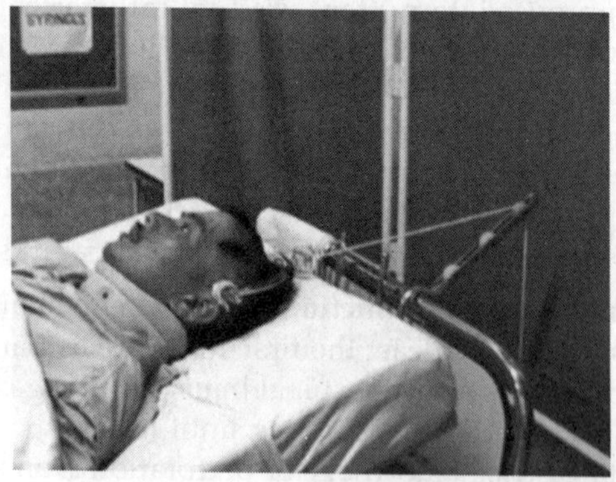

Fig. 10.9: Cervical traction in place

The head halter is easy to apply and is useful only for soft tissue injuries to reduce muscle spasm. It may also be used in cases of cervical spine injury with associated head injury operated patients. Cranial tongs are more invasive because they are embedded in the outer table of the cranium. More traction can be applied to the cervical spine to reduce subluxation or fracture dislocation. The disadvantages of the tongs are they confine the patient to bed and do not provide rigid immobilization. Gardner-Wells tongs are currently being used with good results and have largely replaced the crutch field tongs. Gardner-Wells tongs are easy to apply and are less likely to dislodge than the crutch field tongs. The halo rings are often preferable to tongs because a rigid vest jacket can be applied that allows the patient to become ambulatory following successful traction and reduction of fracture dislocation.

Spinal Injury: Thoracolumbar Spine

Most thoracolumbar injuries are due to flexion-rotation forces. Stable fractures without cord injury are managed by kyphoplasty or conservatively. Patients with unstable fracture dislocation are managed with internal fixation to prevent further cord or nerve root damage.

Surgical Treatment

Historical Review

The timing of surgery has been under discussion for years. Most authors advocates early decompression, stabilization/fusion.[4,26] However, more recently in a retrospective analysis of 99 surgically treated patients with lower cervical spine injuries, Benzel and Larson (1987)[27] advocated delayed surgical intervention in patients after they are metabolically and neurologically stable. We are of the view that patients with cervical spine injuries requiring surgery should be operated upon 'early' giving the nervous tissue full chance to improve. This would also permit early mobilization and institution of rehabilitative process. Generally accepted techniques for reduction/fusion of traumatic fracture dislocation of cervical spine include posterior wire and bone fusion or anterior cervical fusion with dowel or wedge grafts.[28] The anterior approach is mainly used in injuries involving the anterior column of the spine, i.e. those concerning the vertebral bodies and intervertebral discs.

These include wedge compression fracture, burst compression of the vertebral bodies as well as the rupture of intervertebral discs and anterior longitudinal ligaments by hyperextension forces. Mann et al (1990)[29] reported their experience with 16 patients who underwent anterior decompression and bone grafting and plating. They achieved solid fusion in all cases. Casper et al (1989)[30] treated 60 cases of cervical trauma with Casper plating. All patients obtained fusion and stability were achieved immediately after surgery without external stabilization.

Locked facets, ruptured posterior ligaments, subluxation or dislocations generally need reduction and stabilization by the posterior approach (Staufer and Kelley 1977).[31] The various techniques available include Rogers technique, Forysyth technique, Robinson and Southwick technique (wire and bone), Daab plates and Roy-Camille plates.

The basic principles of treatment of cervical spine injuries are to reduce dislocation, to realign bony fragments, decompression of the spinal cord compression, stabilization procedures to maintain stability and rehabilitation (Flow chart 10.1). The goal of surgical treatment is manifold. In the acute stage the primary aim of surgical treatment is to furnish the spinal cord and nerve roots, the best possible environment for improvement and recovery. The salvaging of even a single nerve root may mean an enormous amount to a quadriplegic who will spend the rest of his life partially and/or wholly dependent on others.

The indication for surgery in cervical spine injury are:

i. Failure to achieve reduction/realignment with skull traction,
ii. Progressive neurological deficit with radiological evidence of cord compression,
iii. Incomplete spinal cord injury with impingement on cord by bone, disc and other material in neural canal,
iv. Unstable fracture of spine due to fracture of vertebral body, fracture dislocation, subluxation/dislocation,
v. Penetrating injury of the spinal cord, and
vi. Complete spinal cord injury with unstable spine.

Features suggestive of upper cervical spinal injury are:

- Predental space >3 mm.
- Overlap of C1 on C2 on AP X-ray film 6.9 mm.
- Dense type II fracture-dislocation >6 mm.
- C2-C3 axis translocation >3 mm.

Flow chart 10.1: Management of cervical spine injury

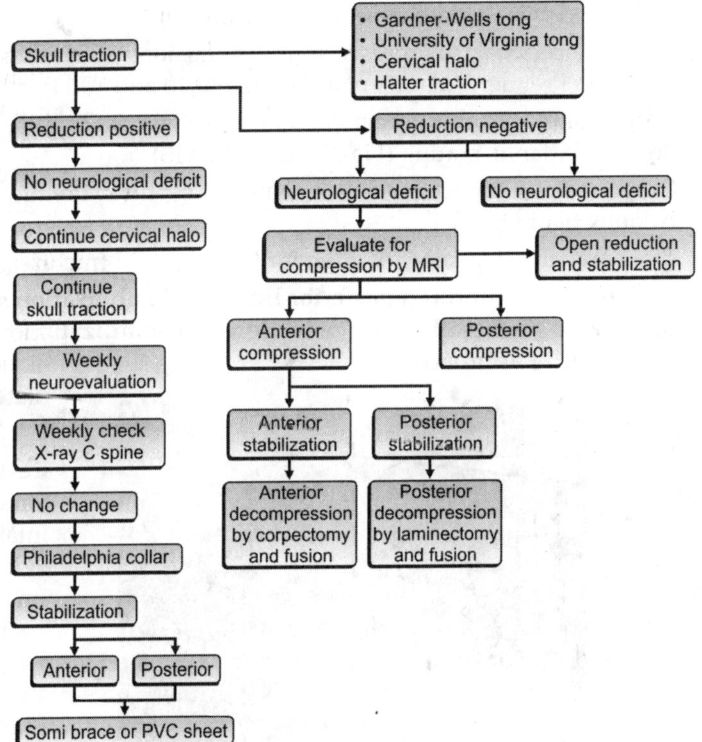

- Flexion-extension range >11 degrees (C1-C3).
- Fracture dislocation with more than 11 degrees angle between adjacent inferior surface of vertebral bodies.
- Loss of facet contact > 50%.
- Loss of facet parallelism.
- Interspinous widening.
- Rupture of transverse ligament on MRI.

The following cervical injuries are unstable on the basis of radiology:.

- Subluxation/dislocation/sagittal plane displacement of >3.5 mm.
- Fracture vertebral body with more than 40% reduction in the height of vertebral body.
- Fracture dislocation with more than 11 degrees angle between adjacent inferior surface of the vertebral body.

The Anterior Cervical Procedures Carried Out are:

Anterior cervical microdiscectomy and fusion.

Anterior cervical microdiscectomy + Fusion + Synthes/ Zephir's/Premier/Atlantis plating (Figs 10.10 and 10.11).

Corpectomy + Titanium cage placement + Synthes/Zephir's/ Premier/Atlantis plating (Figs 10.12 and 10.13).

Corpectomy + Bone grafting + Synthes/Zephir's/Premier/ Atlantis plating.

Transoral anterior screw fixation for the odontoid fractures.

Locked facets, ruptured posterior ligaments, subluxation or dislocations generally need reduction and stabilization by the posterior approach.

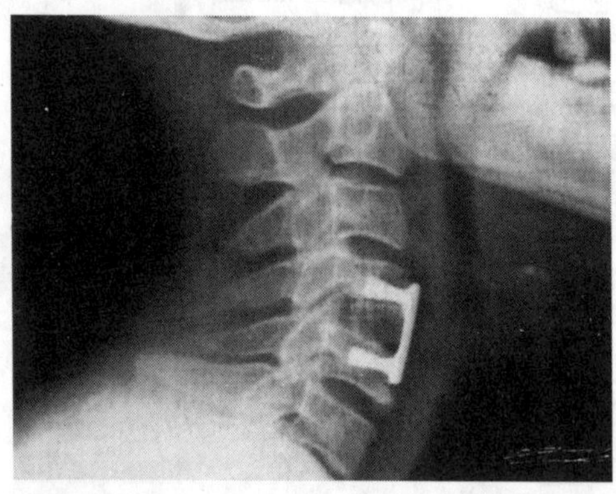

Fig. 10.10: C4-C5 fusion with bone grafting and plate + screw

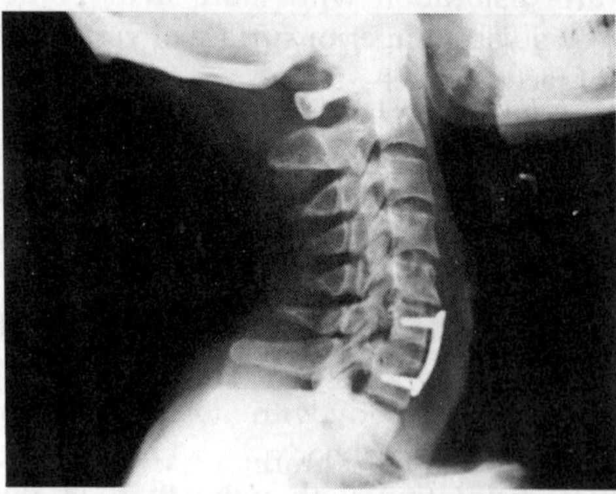

Fig. 10.11: C6-C7 fusion with bone grafting and plate + screw

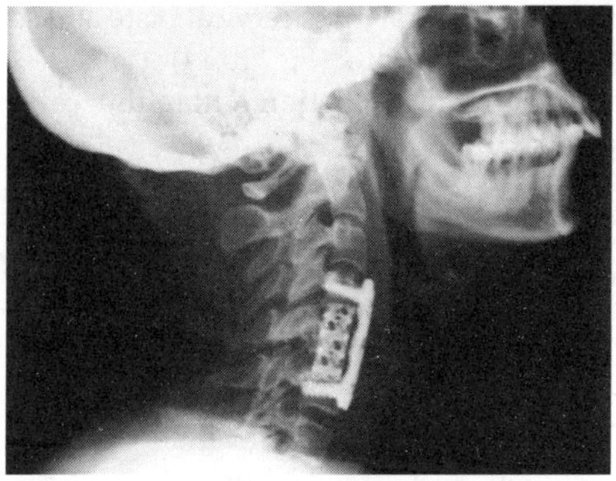

Fig. 10.12: C5 corpectomy + cage + plate

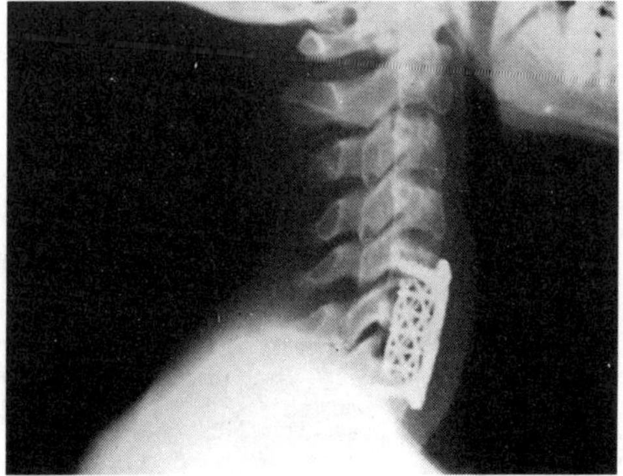

Fig. 10.13: C6 corpectomy + cage + plate

The Posterior Stabilization Procedures Available are:

- Pedicular screw and plate with bone graft.
- Pedicular screw and rod with bone graft.
- Sublaminar wiring and bone graft (post onlay graft).
- Interspinous wiring and bone grafting.

Hart Shill

- Rectangle and bone graft.
- Loops and bone graft.
- Sublaminar wire and bone graft.
- Lugue loop stabilization for the extensive cervical laminectomy.

- Magerl technique-lateral mass cervical plate and screw fixation.
- Posterior fusion by Apofix (Fig. 10.14)
- Posterior fusion by multistrand titanium cables and bone graft (Fig. 10.15).

Merits of Instrumentation

- The merits of instrumentation are strong fixation, easy patient nursing, decrease in patients pain, early mobilization, rehabilitation and no cervical halo vest required.

Complications

- Esophageal perforation by metallic implants.

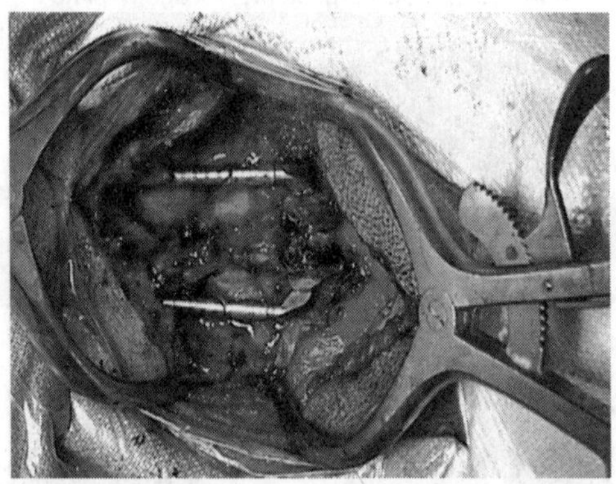

Fig. 10.14: Posterior cervical fusion by Apofix
(For color version, see Plate 3)

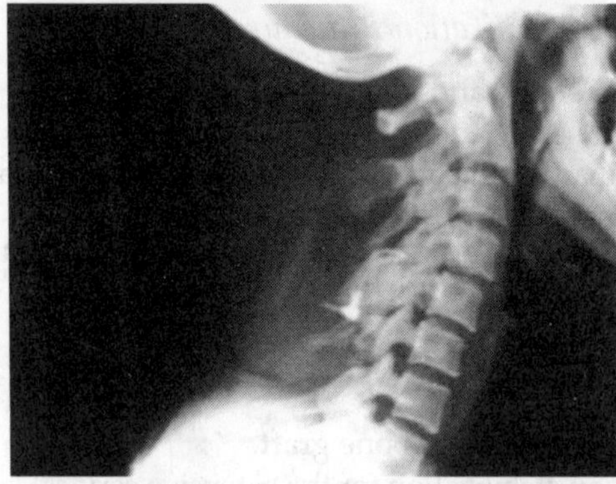

Fig. 10.15: Posterior cervical fusion with multistrand titanium cable

- Injury to vertebral artery.
- Graft displacement.
- Disc space infection.
- Meningitis due to damage to dura.

The indications for surgery for thoracolumbar spinal trauma remains same as cervical spine injury. The procedures carried outare as under.

Anterior Procedures

- Corpectomy and bone/cage (Fig. 10.16)
- Corpectomy and bone/cage + plating (Fig. 10.17)
- Corpectomy and bone/cage + rod fixation

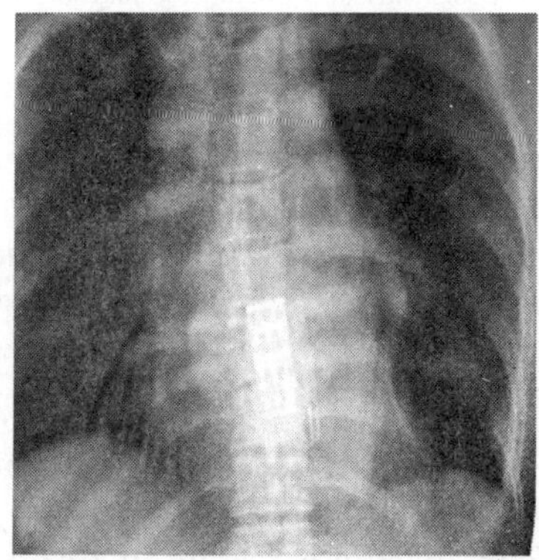

Fig. 10.16: Anterior thoracic titanium cage placement

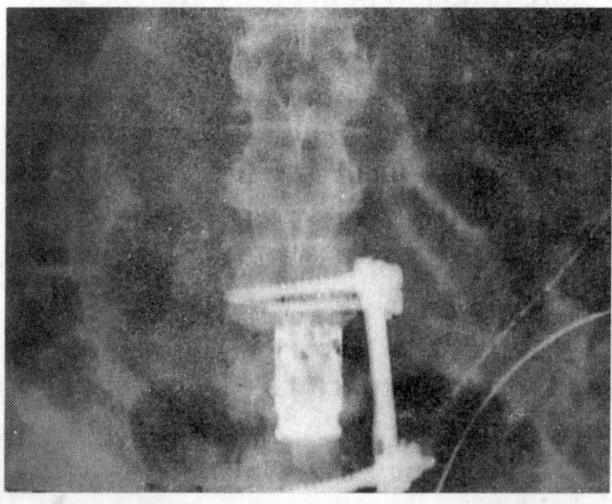

Fig. 10.17: L1 burst fracture anterior thoracic cage + plate and screw fixation

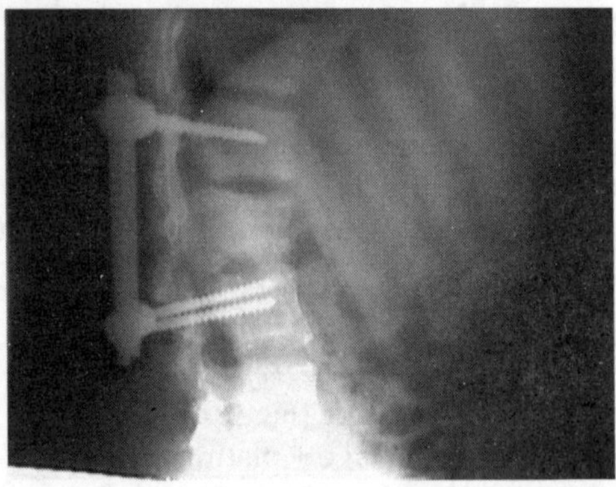

Fig. 10.18: D12 compression fracture posterior pedicular screw and rod fixation

Posterior Procedures

- Open pedicular screw and rod fixation (Fig. 10.18)
- Minimal access pedicular screw and rod fixation
- Percutaneous pedicular screw and rod fixation
- (Sextant system)

Both Anterior and Posterior

Rehabilitation: A major development in rehabilitation research has been the discovery of 'learned non-use' as a cause of neurological deficit. Inactivity results in turning off the neural circuits. By utilizing forced use 'rehabilitation' paradigm it is possible to restore function in people paralyzed for many years.

Prognosis

The outcome in spine injury depends on the initial degree of sparing from the trauma. The national Spinal Cord Injury Statistical Centre (NSCISC) database in 1991 confirmed this finding. The outcome is evaluated following acute care and rehabilitation as per Frankel classification from grade E to A.

The factors, which lead to poor prognosis in spinal cord injured patients, are chest infection, urinary infection, bedsore infection and pulmonary embolism. In terms of long-term outcome neurological recovery continues for some patients up to 18 months, after which further improvement is rare. However, the long-term outcome is poor if there is post-traumatic cord changes like myelomalacia, atrophy and syringomyelia.

CONCLUSION

The study of spine injury has evolved dramatically during the past several decades. A greater understanding of biomechanics and mechanism of injury has enabled a more accurate classification of these injuries. The understanding of pathophysiology has refined the protocol in medical management. The availability of CT and MRI scans has revolutionized the diagnostic evaluation, by delineating the exact level and extent of injury to the spine and spinal cord and guides for appropriate surgical approach.

The availability of varieties of internal devices (implants) for the stabilization of spine both anteriorly and posteriorly, high speed pneumatic drill, banked bones and addition of operating microscope has made a significant difference in the surgical management of these unfortunate individuals and have significantly improved the short-term and long-term outcome. Further development in the area of neural protection and axonal regeneration will undoubtedly provide the important key to the management puzzle of the spinal cord injured patients.

REFERENCES

1. Paradis GR, Janes JM. Post-traumatic atlanto axial instability: The fate of odontoid process fracture in 46 cases. Journal of Trauma 1993;13:359-67.
2. Ersmark H, Dalen N, Kalen R. Cervical spine injuries: A follow-up of 332 patients. Paraplegia 1990;28:25-40.
3. Stauffer ES. Clinical aspects of thoracic and lumbar spine and spinal cord injuries. Advances in Neurotraumatology. Vol 12, Springer, Vienna, 1987;P27-39.
4. White AA, Punjabi MM. The role of stabilisation in the treatment of cervical spine injuries. Spine 1984;12:522.
5. Denis F. The three column spine and its significance in the classification of acute thoracolumbar injuries. Spine 1983;8:817-31.
6. Huges JT. Pathology of the spinal cord. Lioyed Luke Medical Books. London, 1978.
7. Fawcett JW. Factors influencing the regeneration of axons in the central nervous system. Paraplegia 1991;29:287-93.
8. Schawb ME. Regeneration of lesioned CNS axons by neutralisation of neutrite growth inhibitors, a short review. Paralegia 1991;29:294.
9. Kakulas BA. The applied neurobiology of human spinal cord injury: A review. Paraplegia 1988;26:371-9.

10. Fehlings MG, Sekhon L. Cellular: Ionic and biomolecular mechanisms of the injury process. In: Benzel E, Tator CH, (Eds). Contemporary Management of Spinal Cord Injury: From Impact to Rehabilitation. Chicago. IL: AANS, 2000;33:112-6.
11. Tator CH, Fehlings MG. Review of the secondary injury theory of acute spinal cord trauma with emphasis on vascular mechanisms. J Neurosurg 1991;75:15-26.
12. Agrawal SK, Fehlings MG. Mechanisms of secondary injury to spinal cord axons in vitro: role of Na^{+}, $Na(^{+})$-$K(^{+})$-ATPase, the $Na(^{+})$-H^{+} exchanger, and the $Na(^{+})$-Ca^{2+} exchanger. J. Neurosci 1996;545-52.
13. Agrawal S, Nashmi R, Feblings MG. Role of L and N type calcium channels in the pathophysiology of traumatic spinal cord white matter injury. Neuroscience 2000;99:179-88.
14. Aki T, Toya S. Experimental study on changes of the spinal-evoked potential and circulatory dynamics following spinal cord compression and decompression. Spine 1984;9:800-9.
15. Allen AR. Surgery for experimental lesions of spinal cord equivalent to crush injury of fracture dislocation of spinal column: a preliminary report. JAMA 1991;57:878-80.
16. Burke DC, Berryman D. The place of closed manipulation in the management of flexion-rotation dislocations of the cervical spine. J Bone Joint Surg 1971;53(B):165-82.
17. Maynard FM, Reynolds GG, Fountain S, et al. Neurological prognosis after traumatic quadriplegia: three-year experience of California Regional Spinal Cord Injury Care System. J Neurosurg 1979;50:611-6.
18. Sonntag VK. Management of bilateral locked facets of the cervical spine. Neurosurgery 1981;8:150-52.
19. Katoh S, El Masry WS, Jaffray D, et al. Neurologic outcome in conservatively treated patients with incomplete closed traumatic cervical spinal cord injuries. Spine 1996;21:2345-51.
20. Kobrine AI, Evans DE, Rizzoli HV. Experimental acute balloon compression of the spinal cord: factors affecting disappearance and return of the spinal evoked response. J Neurosurg 1979;51:841-5.
21. Wiberg J, Hauge HN. Neurological outcome after surgery for thoracic and lumbar spine injuries. Acta Neurochir (Wien) 1988;91:106-12.
22. Frankel HC, Hancock DO, Hystop G, et al. The value of postural reduction in the initial management of closed injuries of the spine with paraplegia and tetraplegia. Paraplegia 1969;7:179-92.
23. Pang D, Wilerger JE. Cord injury with normal radiography. Journal of Neurosurgery 1982;57:114-29.
24. Donovan Post MJ, Green BA. The use of computed tomography in spinal trauma. Radiological Clinics of North America, 1983;21:327-75.

25. Bracken MB, Sheoard MJ, Collins WF, et al. A randomised controlled trial of methylpredisolone or naloxone in the treatment of acute spinal cord injury. New England Journal of Medicine 1990;332:1403-11.
26. Keim HA. Indications for spine fusions and techniques. Clinical Neurosurgery 1978;25:266-75.
27. Benzel EC, Larson SJ. Functional recovery after decompressive spine operation for the cervical spine fracture. Neurosurgery 1987;20:742-6.
28. Bohlman HH. Acute fracture and dislocations of the cervical spine: An analysis of three hundred hospitalised patients and review of literature. Journal of Bone and Joint Surgery 1979;61A:1191-42.
29. Mann DC, Burner BW, Keene JS, Levin AB. Anterior plating of unstable spine fractures. Paraplegia 1990;28:564-72.
30. Casper W, Barbier DD, Klara PM. Anterior cervical fusion and casper plate stabilisation for cervical trauma. Neurosurgery 1989;25:491-502.
31. Stauffer ES, Kelly EG. Fracture dislocation of the cervical spine. Journal of Bone & Joint Surg 1977;59A:45-48.

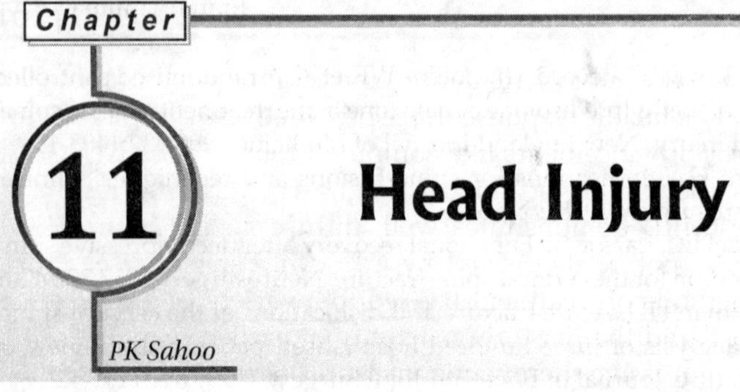

Head Injury

PK Sahoo

HISTORICAL REVIEW AND INTRODUCTION

Head injuries in the past were mostly due to falls, hunting's, accidents, tribal conflicts and war fare. In present days with rapid method of transport, increasing industrialization, regional conflicts fought with high-tech weapons, availability of accurate and deadly weapons in the society, the incidence and severity of head injury are increasing. Head injury is defined as a mechanical damage of cranium and intracranial contents (Meninges, brain, blood vessels and cranial nerves). Head injury is defined by WHO as equivalent to traumatic brain injury where following injury there is altered level of consciousness or post-traumatic amnesia (PTA), neurological signs or fracture of skull/intracranial lesions on radiology. Head injury is most serious traumatic brain injury which leads to morbidity, mortality and severe disability. It profoundly affects individual, family and society as a whole.

Head injury is not a single specific clinical or pathological entity but consists of a variety of lesions, ranging from scalp laceration or concussion to a gross brain damage and brainstem injury leading to instantaneous death. The clinical picture may be the admixture of concussion, compression due to intracranial hematoma, contusion, secondary brain edema, foraminal (Transtentorial and foramen magnum) herniation, which may all be seen in a single patient at different times. While managing such patients one must appreciate, that one is not dealing with a static but dynamic changing clinical picture resulting from traumatic force and natures attempt at resolution of the same. This has resulted in better understanding of the mechanism and pathophysiology of brain injury and evaluation of various primary and secondary brain injury following trauma.

Studies on cerebral circulation, intracranial pressure, biochemical and metabolic responses have provided with newer insights. Diagnostic advancements like computed tomography (CT) scans obviates the pitfalls of clinical diagnosis. Magnetic resonance imaging (MRI) demonstrates well, diffuse axonal injury (DAI) which may not be delineated by CT scan. Persistent search for better methods of treatment has led to a variety of management modalities and the masterly inactivity of earlier years has given place to aggressive therapeutic measures since the development of neurosurgery.

The outcome in a severely head injured patient can be adequately predicted within the first 24 hours. This is immensely important for management, as the expensive and limited intensive care resources of the hospital can be utilized meaningfully. Along with other symptomatic therapy, the treatment involves introduction of intracranial pressure (ICP) and judicious surgical intervention as and when necessary. Current research suggests that there is increase number of survivors and reduced number of complications. However, our mortality rate in severe head injury patients is still high in comparison to Western countries. There could be several factors for this. Our first aid facilities at the site of injury are extremely poor. The transportation is done by uneducated, nonmedical personnel, there is no facility for monitoring the conditions of the patient during transport and there is always a delay in transferring the patients from accident site to hospital due to medicolegal problems. First hour after accident is the GOLDEN HOUR for the victim, on the spot treatment, fast transportation, resuscitation in the transport can determine the fate of the victim. While it will be ideal for all severe head injured patients to be managed in neurosurgical center in Neuro ICU with ventilatory and monitoring facilities, this is neither possible nor practical under the present circumstances in our country. Head injuries are rapidly becoming a social problem. Unlike the disability caused by skeletal injuries, head injuries lead to loss of intellectual and other cognitive faculties with a resulting burden on the family and on society. Therefore, top priority should be provided in preventing, managing and rehabilitating such people.

Epidemiology

Incidence

Recent trends show that there is increase in road traffic accidents (RTAs), industrial mishaps, terrorist activities and natural calamities in India. By and large most common cause of head injury is RTA. 20% of the victims of RTA are drunk at the time of accident. Every year five lakhs accidents take place in our roads in which 10% of the vehicles get involved, resulting in 4 lakhs injury and one lakh death. Head injury is the most common cause of trauma death constituting 70% of deaths among trauma victims. Head injury not only heads the list for mortality but it claims a high place for causes of morbidity. 50% of the head injury deaths occur before reaching the hospital, i.e. at the site or during transport. 25% die due to primary and another 25% due to secondary brain injury in the hospital. Amongst the hospitalized patients cerebral concussion is the most frequent clinical form of head injury (70%). Cerebral contusion (15%) in the temporal or basifrontal region is the next common clinical form of head injury. Intracranial hematoma in the form of extradural hematoma (EDH), subdural hematoma (SDH) and intracerebral hematoma (ICH) constitutes 10% and diffuse axonal injury (DAI) constitutes 5% of all head injury patients.

Age Incidence

Road accidents kill mostly younger people who are in the prime of their life and who could have contributed to the progress of society. The most affected group is males aged 15 to 40 years.

Sex Incidence

Males predominantly affected by RTA in the proportion of M:F 2-4:1.

Causes

Indian statistics indicate that the incidence of road accidents is the highest in the world, in spite of total number of vehicles on the roads being less than in most developed countries. Hence, RTA continues to be the leading cause of head injury (60%) followed by fall from height (20%), terrorist activities and assaults constitutes 10%. Industrial mishaps, natural calamities and sports related activities including unhelmated boxing injuries constitute (10%) other causes of head injury.

Mechanism of Head Injury

Besides the direct impact of the injuring force, a variety of other mechanism plays a significant role in determining the type, extent and severity of damage to various structures. Multiple factors/ Mechanisms may affect in a single individual.

1. *Contact injuries*: A direct blow/contact/impact is necessary but head motion is not necessary. Contact injuries produces fracture of skull, extradural hematoma (EDH), intracerebral hematoma (ICH) and cerebral contusions.
2. *Acceleration injuries*: Direct blow to the vault is not necessary but head motion is necessary. In acceleration injuries surface strain produces acute subdural hematoma (SDH), center coup contusion and deep strains produces either concussion or diffuse axonal injuries (DAIs) and diffuse vascular injuries.
3. *Penetrating injuries*: The pathway taken by the bullet will depend on its type and velocity.
4. *Crush injuries*: In crush injuries usually the impact is bilateral. All the components like the scalp, skull bone, meninges, brain matter, cranial nerves and vessels may be involved.

Other Factors Responsible for Different Types of Traumatic Brain Injury

1. *The configuration of the interior of the skull*: The presence of bone edges like cristagalli, sphenoid ridge and petrous temporal bone in the interior of the skull produces basifrontal and temporal lobe contusion hematoma.
2. *Different mobility of various structure*: The density and elasticity of various structures, i.e. the scalp "skull" meninges and the brain being different, any force applied to the head results in variable mobility in relation to each other and results in shearing strains.

Pathophysiology of Head Injury

Primary brain injury: Primary brain injuries occur at the time of initial impact or injury. The injuries are concussion, DAI, intracerebral contusions and lesions due to associated injuries to the vessel like EDH, acute SDH, SAH, ICH. The primary injuries to the brain are preventable.

Secondary brain injury: The brain is neither completely fixed nor mobile in the rigid bony cranial cavity. It weighs 1,400 gm and approximately 2% of the total body weight. Seventy percent volume of intracranial cavity is occupied by glia and neuron and 10% each by CSF, blood and extracellular fluid. Increase in volume of any one of these components will raise the intracranial pressure (ICP). The normal ICP is 0 to 10 mm Hg. As the ICP rises the cerebral blood flow (CBF) or cerebral perfusion pressure (CPP) which is dependent on ICP reduces leading to hypoxia, ischemia and brain infarct and there is further increase in ICP.

The CBF or CPP = Mean arterial pressure (MAP) - ICP
The normal CBF is 50 ml/100 gm of brain tissue/per minute

The normal ICP is 0 to 10 mm Hg. When the ICP rises up to 25 mm Hg, it is dangerous but correctable and when the ICP is more than 40 mm Hg it is life-threatening. Facilities for monitoring of ICP are available in almost all the neurosurgical centers presently. The factors which increases ICP are hypoxia (PO_2 below 50 mm Hg), hypercarbia, brain swelling, edema, infarct, seizures, electrolyte imbalance, transfalcine, transtentorial or foramen magnum (Coning) herniation, hyperpyrexia, meningitis, brain abscess, halothane and nitrous oxide (NO_2).

The factors which reduces ICP are hyperoxia, hypocarbia, hypothermia, barbiturates, neuroleptanalgesia, osmotic diuretics.

Evaluation of Head Injured Patients

Clinical Evaluation

Aim

1. Simultaneous primary survey and resuscitation.
2. Prevent/limit secondary brain injury.
3. Recognize/stabilize associated injuries.

Evaluation and Management at the Site/ Primary Hospital Care–Management Plan

The management plan is based on:

1. Primary survey.
2. Resuscitation.

3. Secondary survey.
4. Definitive care.

Primary Survey

- A -Airway with cervical spine immobilization in neutral position until radiological examination excludes spinal injury.
- B - Breathing pattern and adequacy
- C - Circulation.
- D - Disability detection and documentation rapid neurological examination–A rapid examination based on AVPU scale is helpful (alert, responding to voice only, responding to pain only, unresponsive) check pupils.
- E - Exposure and evaluation as a whole completely expose the patient for an adequate examination but protect against hypothermia.
- F - Fluid administration.

Resuscitation

Prior to history taking and clinical evaluation in all polytrauma including head injury patients, proper management of airway, breathing and circulation is vital at the site of accident and in the casualty.

Airway

Proper management of airway is absolutely vital for good outcome. A trauma victim with loss of airway dies in three to four minutes. If however the airway is patent but the patient cannot breath, death ensues in 5-7 minutes (Untreated hypovolemic shock kills in 10-15 minutes). So the oral cavity has to be gently cleaned off all foreign bodies like food particles, broken teeth, blood, vomits, etc. to ensure patent airway.

Breathing and Oxygenation

The rate and type of respiration has to be observed. The simplest way to evaluate breathing is to observe the movements of the chest. The front and back of the chest has to be inspected. The best place to auscultate is the axilla since it is farthest from major airways. Ensure adequate ventilation. If the breathing is poor intubation/ mechanical ventilation/tracheostomy may be required urgently.

Circulation Support and Control of Hemorrhage

A loss of 10 to 15% circulating volume is tolerated. Clinical features of shock are seen when 25% circulating volume are lost and a loss of more than 50% proves fatal. All external bleedings should be arrested to prevent hypovolemic shock. In a head injury patient with shock spinal cord injury and abdominal injury should be excluded.

Documentation

A written record of the patients problems, treatment received and response to treatment should be documented. This information should include patient personal data, medical history, treatment initiated, the patients response to the treatment, laboratory and X-ray data. The names of referring and receiving surgeon should be included. If a patient is transferred, throughout transport, complete records of treatment given during transport should be mentioned.

Disability Detection

Boggy swelling on scalp (Scalp hematoma), wound on the scalp, fracture of the skull bone, compound head injury with brain matter/ CSF leak, facial injuries, bleeding ENT, periorbital ecchymosis (Racoon eyes), ecchymosis/swelling over the mastoid (Battle sign) and suboccipital ecchymosis should be noted.

Exposure and Evaluation of Extremity Injuries

After clearing airway, maintaining breathing and arresting any hemorrhage the whole body to be examined from head to toe and any injury has to be noted. Inspect and palpate the abdomen for any abdominal injury which should be managed at the earliest. Palpate/feel all the extremities to detect fractures of upper and lower limbs. Splint the fractures. Whole spine should be palpated without moving the patient to detect any cervical, thoracic or lumbosacral spinal injuries. Suspected spinal injury patients are to be moved by log rolling. Any flail chest, sucking wound of the chest, tension pneumothorax, massive hemothorax needs urgent attention. Chest compression test to find out fractures ribs, pelvic compression to find out fracture of the pelvic bones should be carried out.

Fluid Administration

In polytrauma patients with head injury IV line to be started at the site if possible. Fluid in the form of normal saline/Ringer's lactate solution to be given to maintain any fluid loss.

Evaluation of Head Injured Patients in Hospital (Secondary Survey)

History taking: The diagnosis of head injury is often obvious and the doctor examining the patient for the first time tends to neglect a complete history taking. A knowledge of the circumstances, mode of the accident and exact nature, extent and severity of injury is not only required for medicolegal purpose but also for proper and appropriate management of the patient.

a. The details of mode, the time and circumstances leading to injury should be recorded from eye witness, ambulance driver, police, relatives and any influence of alcohol also should be recorded.
b. The nature of accident, i.e. RTA, fall, assault or any other should be recorded.
c. Level of consciousness at the time of injury, during transport and at the time of examination is very significant to find out whether the patient is showing signs of improvement or deterioration.
d. History of convulsion modifies the clinical picture. Hence any convulsion at the time of accident or during transport should be inquired.
e. History of vomiting/ENT bleeds/CSF leaks should be inquired and recorded. Past history of epilepsy/DM/hypertension/IHD/renal disease/stroke/drug allergy should be asked for and recorded as these will have effect on the management and recovery. History of any treatment received at accident site and during transport like anticonvulsants, anticerebral edema measures, antibiotics, antidiabetic drugs and sedatives should be noted.

Neurological Evaluation

Level of consciousness: This is the most important single parameter which indicates the severity of injury and provides the most sensitive indicator for prognosis. Instead of terms like coma, semicoma or stupor, it is better to describe the best response that can be elicited from the patient with the least stimulus that elicits this response. The stimulus can be normal conversation, loud command, mild pain and deep pain. The response is described in terms of eye opening (E), best verbal response (V) and best motor response (M). It is necessary to check the level of consciousness frequently, more so when facilities for CT scan is not available as this is the most reliable indicator of a brain damage.

There are several classification scales available for recording the state of consciousness. The one which is most commonly used all over the world is the Glasgow coma scale (GCS) which provides a practical guidelines for initial and subsequent evaluation. The most important aspect of this score is to find out whether the patient is static, improving or deteriorating.

Glasgow coma scale (Jennett 1974)	Modified coma scale for infants
A. Eye opening (E)	*Eye opening (E)*
E 4. Spontaneously	E 4. Spontaneously
3. To speech	3. To speech
2. To pain	2. To pain
1. None	1. None
B. Best motor response (M)	
M 6. Obeys command	6. Spont movement
5. Localizes pain	5. Withdraws to touch
4. Normal flexion to pain	4. Withdraws to pain
3. Abnormal flexion to pain	3. Abnormal flexion
2. Extension to pain (Decerebrating)	2. Abnormal extension
1. None	1. None
C. Best verbal response (V)	
V 5. Oriented to time, place and person	5. Coos, babbles
4. Confused	4. Irritable
3. In appropriate words	3. Cries to pain
2. In comprehensible words (Groaning sounds)	2. Moans to pain
1. None	1. None

In a person who is fully conscious, alert and oriented, the Glasgow coma scale will be E4 M6 V5 (15/15) and the reduction in the score will be indicative of deterioration in the state of consciousness. The minimum score will be E1 M1 V1 (3/15) who has no eye opening (E1), no motor response (M1) and no verbal response (V1) to any kind of stimuli. While recording the Glasgow coma scale, it is the best response of that particular moment which is recorded. The best response is the motor response. By evaluating the GCS the severity of the head injury can be assessed clinically and also the prognosis can be predicted as follows:

GCS score	*Severity of head injury*	*0% cases*	*Fatality%*
13 to 15	Mild head injury	80%	10%
9 to 12	Moderately severe Head injury	10%	20%
3 to 8	Severe head injury	10%	70%

Limitation of GCS

1. Not applicable to children
2. Takes best motor response (M6), yet a patient could be monoplegic, hemiplegic or tetraplegic
3. Does not take into account pulse, BP, respiration and pupil size.
4. Can be impaired due to language problem, alcohol intoxication, intubation and tracheostomy.
5. Can be impaired with hypoxia due to blood loss and following seizures.
6. No check on cranial nerve function.
7. Eye opening and closing may be impaired by black eye and conjunctival chemosis.
8. Verbal response cannot be assessed in patients who are intubated/tracheostomized.

Post-traumatic or Antigrade Amnesia (PTA)

This is the duration of permanent loss of memory for events following injury till such time the patient regains full consciousness.

Very mild	> 5 minutes
Mild	> 1 Hour
Moderate	> 1 day
Severe	- 1 to 7 days
Very severe	- More than 7 days

Significance of PTA

- Post-traumatic amnesia is permanent. Hence PTA never recovers.
- Long PTA has poor prognosis.
- Medicolegal significance—Offence committed during PTA is not a cognigible offence.
- Some patients feel that they have not recovered unless the PTA recovers.

Retrograde Amnesia

It is the loss of memory to events prior to injury. The retrograde amnesia may be long extending over days/months/years. This period shrinks gradually leaving a permanent loss of memory for a fixed period prior to injury.

Examination of Pupil

The pupil should be observed in diffuse light before a focussed light is used to see the reaction. The size of the pupil should be recorded in mm rather than descriptive terms like constricted, small, dilated. The normal size of the pupil is 3 to 4 mm. Both direct and consensual responses need to be recorded. Pupillary response not only reflect the oculomotor pathways but also of visual pathways. Pupillary asymmetry is called anisocoria. One sided dilated pupil may suggest a developing hematoma on that side. However, pupillary dilatation may also occur due to injury to eyeball, injury to optic and oculomotor nerve which should be excluded. Besides diagnostic value dilated and fixed pupil has poor prognostic value. Once one pupil is dilated and fixed the mortality rate goes up to 50% and when both pupils are dilated and fixed the chances of recovery are bleak.

Corneal Reflex

Stimulation of the cornea with a soft wick of cotton results in contraction of orbicularis oculi. In the presence of facial nerve palsy a positive reflex elicits closure of the opposite eye and rolling up (Bell's phenomenon) of the ipsilateral eye. Corneal reflex has prognostic significance in an unconscious patient. It is one of the last reflexes to disappear and hence bilateral absence of corneal reflex is a Grave sign.

Oculocephalic Reflex

In a normal person sudden turning of head to one side results in the conjugate deviation of the eyes to opposite side, which readily corrects itself in few seconds. The absence of oculocephalic reflex indicate brainstem dysfunction or damage and is of grave prognostic significance. In an unconscious patient this should be carried out after excluding cervical spine injury.

Cold Caloric Test (Vestibulo-ocular Reflex)

The head is elevated to 30 degree. The resting position of the eye is observed. The external auditory canal is then irrigated with 20cc of ice cold water rapidly within 10 to 15 seconds. A record is made of the response of the eyeballs. After few minutes following the termination of response from one side the procedure is repeated on the other side.

Mechanism

Stimulation of the vestibular labyrinth with ice cold water results in a characteristic response of the eyeballs depending on the conscious state of the person and the integrety of the vestibulo-ocular pathway.

Interpretation: In normal subjects stimulation of the ear with cold water produces nystagmus with the eyes remaining in mid position. The slow component of the nystagmus is towards the side of the stimulation. In patients with impaired consciousness the response is modified. The eyes, instead of remaining in mid position deviate to the stimulated side. In lighter state of unconsciousness there may still be nystagmus with the eyes in deviated position. Conjugate deviation without nystagmus implies a deeper state of unconsciousness. With the hot water the response is reverse. Complete absence of reflex implies damage/ dysfunction to the brainstem is of grave prognostic significance.

Examination of fundus: Papilledema may develop quite rapidly in case of head injury. It has been recorded within 12 hours in some case.

Examination of other cranial nerves: If patient is conscious and cooperative all cranial nerve should be tested. Even in an unconscious patient seventh nerve can be easily assessed.

Gag reflex: Absence of Gag reflex implies damage/dysfunction of brainstem and is of grave prognostic significance.

Examination of Motor System

In an unconscious patient observation of the spontaneous posture and movement of limbs provides information regarding the motor system. With little practice it is always possible to discover even minor degree of weakness of a limb, be it an unconscious or an irritablc and uncooperative patient. Impairment of movement of a limb may frequently be due to an associated skeletal injury. The motor part in conscious and cooperative patients are recorded as per modified MRC classification (Medical Research Council) from 0 to 5. The abnormal motor responses are:

a. Decortication or abnormal flexor response when the upper limbs are in flexion and lower limbs are either in flexion or extension.
b. In decerebration or extensor response both the upper and lower limbs are in a state of extension. Both decortication and decerebration is suggestive of poor prognosis in head injured patients.
c. Diffuse flaccidity without any response can be found in: i. Severe intoxication state with alcohol, barbiturates or narcotic over dose; ii. In pontomedullary injury; iii. Traumatic myelopathy with flaccid quadriplegia.

Examination of the Sensory System

Except for response to pain examination of the sensory system is usually not possible in an unconscious and uncooperative patient. It seldom provides information of localizing value except in cases where associated spinal injury has been suspected.

Examination of Reflexes

Asymmetry of the deep tendon reflexes may be the only indication of the existence of a pyramidal tract lesion. Plantar reflex is even more important. However, bilateral extensor plantar response has little localizing value in an unconscious patient.

Clinical Grouping of Patients after Evaluation

Group I: Already conscious—A group of head injury patients who on arrival at casualty are found to be conscious. The GCS is E4 V5 M6 and no focal neurological deficit present. These patients can be observed for 24 hours and discharged with advice to report to casualty if there is intense headache, repeated vomiting, focal/ generalized convulsions, high fever or focal neurological deficit.

Group II: At admission itself or later while on observation deteriorates without period of improvement, i.e change in level of consciousness, focal neurological deficit, bradycardia or hypertension, intracranial hematoma has to be ruled out in these cases. Other conditions which may give rise to deterioration are:

a. Obstructed respiration with hypoxia or anoxia, hyperthermia, electrolyte imbalance, brain edema, convulsion and meningitis.

Group III: These group of patients show some neurological improvement at admission and then deteriorates during next few hours. In these patients EDH, SDH and ICH has to be excluded.

Group IV: All compound head injury patients with brain matter coming out and CSF leak needs hospitalization and management.

Group V: Alongwith head injury there is injury elsewhere in the body, i.e. flail chest, hemopneumothorax, sucking wound of chest, ruptured viscus, soft tissue injury and fractures. These patients require urgent attention.

Group VI: Brain death patients after head injury.

Clinical Diagnosis of Intracranial Hematoma (ICH)

1. Patients with head injury who continues to be unconscious after injury.
2. Patients with head injury who fails to show progressive uninterupted improvement is suspected to have an intracranial hematoma unless proved otherwise.
3. Patients with head injury after initial unconsciousness recovers and then become unconscious. ICH has to be ruled out (Table 11.1).
4. Focal neurological deficits in the form of monoparesis, hemiparesis, triparesis or guadriparesis, dysarthria, cerebellar signs.

5. Patients showing rising BP and bradycardia
6. Patients with pupillary abnormality (Anisocoria)
7. Head injured patients with evidence of raised ICT in the form of headache, repeated vomiting, VI paresis, papilledema.

Differential Diagnosis of Head Injury Patients

The following conditions has to be differentiated/excluded in head injured patients:

1. Alcoholic intoxication
2. Cerebrovascular accidents (CVAs)
3. Post ictal state
4. Poisoning
5. Subarachnoid hemorrhage due to burst aneurysms and arteriovenous malformation.
6. Hypoglycemia.

Conditions Leading to Deterioration in Head Injured Patients While Under Treatment

1. Respiratory inadequacy leading to hypoxia or anoxia
2. Delayed intracranial hematoma/contusion/mass effect
3. Cerebral edema and swelling
4. Brain ischemia and infarct
5. Seizures
6. Hyperpyrexia
7. Fluid and electrolyte imbalance
8. Dehydration
9. Hypoglycemia
10. Diffuse axonal injury (DAI)
11. Meningitis and brain abscess.

Definitive Care

This is the stage for comprehensive management in a neurosurgical center.

Criteria for Admission to Hospital with Head Injury

1. All moderate and severe head injury
2. Unconscious more than 10 minutes/confusion

3. Persisting altered level of consciousness
4. History of seizures and alcohol intake
5. Persistent severe headache/repeated vomiting
6. Open scalp wound/ENT bleed
7. Other associated injuries
8. Focal neurological deficits
9. Fracture skull and abnormal CT scan brain
10. Children and patients over 60 years of age
11. Responsible observation not available outside hospital/ No attendant.

Criteria for Neurological Consultation

1. Severe head injury cases (GCS< 8)
2. GCS 9 - 13, for more than 6 hr
3. Deterioration in GCS of two or more points
4. Focal neurological deficit
5. Compound H I
6. Penetrating injuries of brain
7. Suspected fracture base of skull
8. Depressed fracture of skull bone
9. Abnormal findings on CT scan
10. Persistent headache, vomiting, restlessness and confusion.

HEAD INJURY

Consultation information/transfer
What the neurosurgeon will need to know:

1. Name, age, address of patient
2. Mode and time of injury
3. Cardiorespiratory status
   - Blood pressure, pulse rate, respiration rate and type
4. GCS score
5. Pupillary response
6. Alteration in baseline observation
7. Associated injuries
8. Previous relevant medical conditions
9. Result of investigations.
10. Relevant previous medical condition, medications, allergies.

Table 11.1: Common causes of talk and die (Intracranial hematoma)

	EDH	*SDH*	*ICH*
Incidence	5%	50 to 70%	15%
MOI	RTA fall	Fall boxing	RTA
AGE	Any uncommon in elderly and up to 2 yr	Older age for chronic SDH	Any
Cause Vessels	Middle meningeal artery, meningeal and diploic vein	Bridging vein between cortex and dural sinus	Intrinsic cerebral
Time	48 hr	3 days acute SDH 3 weeks subacute SDH > 3 weeks chronic SDH	48 hr
Associated Brain Injury	Less	Very high	High
Associated Skull #	85%	Rare	Rare
Site	Temporal 70-80%	Whole hemisphere	Basifrontal Temporal
Shape	Lentiform	Crescent	Hyperdense lobe

Investigations

1. X-ray skull for alert neurologically intact patients. X-ray skull will reveal fractures–Linear, depressed, stellate, comminuted, compound, pneumocephalus and foreign body
2. X-Ray cervical spine to find out fractures, dislocations.
3. X-Ray chest PA view.

When CT scan facilities are not available, the following observations can be made when X-ray skull shows fractures of skull bones.

1. Fracture is associated with increased risk of intracranial hemorrhage.
2. Compound fractures and fracture base of skull are associated with increased risk of infection.
3. Depressed fracture skull with dural tear increases the risk of epilepsy.
4. Presence of intracranial air suggests fracture base of skull.

5. In progressive neurological deterioration the exploration should be carried out at the site of fracture in whom an extradural hematoma is suspected.

CT Scan Head

CT scan head is the basic investigation for head injured patients. However "no scan can replace the clinical judgment".

Indication of CT Scan

1. Unconsciousness for more than 30 minutes.
2. Altered level of consciousness.
3. Pupillary asymmetry.
4. Focal neurological deficit or hyperreflexia.
5. Depressed compound fracture/fracture skull bone known or suspected.
6. All penetrating injuries.
7. All severe/moderately severe head injury cases.
8. Persistent headache, vomiting.
9. Age-over 50 years of age.
10. Postoperative assessment.

Follow-up CT Scans

1. To detect delayed complications like hematoma, edema, infarct.
2. To find out communicating hydrocephalus, cerebral atrophy, encephalomalacia, porencephaly.

Finding on CT Scan

1. Fractures through bone windows (Fig. 11.1)
2. Hematoma EDH (Fig. 11.2), SDH (Figs 11.3 and 11.4), SAH (Fig. 11.5), ICH (Fig. 11.6).
3. Pneumocephalus
4. Foreign bodies (Fig. 11.7)
5. Secondary effects like cerebral edema, ischemia, infarct, midline shift, hydrocephalus, coning.

MRI Head

It is not a routine. However, diffuse axonal injury (DAI) (Fig. 11.8) may be missed in CT scan and can be detected by MRI scan. In

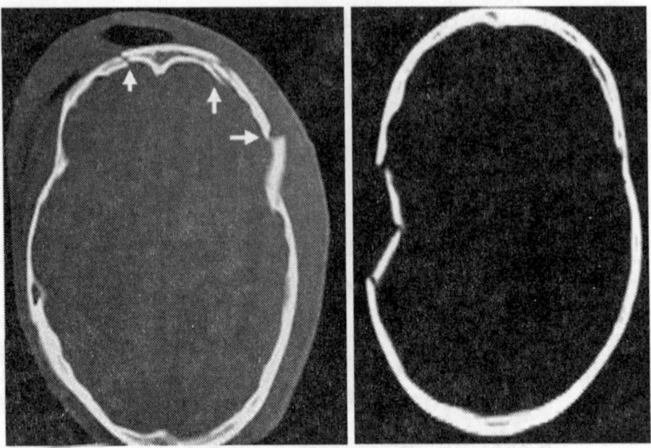

Fig. 11.1: Fracture skull on CT scan

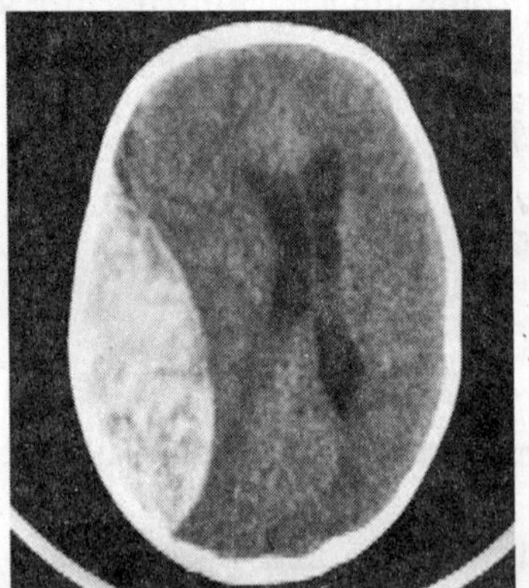

Fig. 11.2: Axial CT scan showing EDH

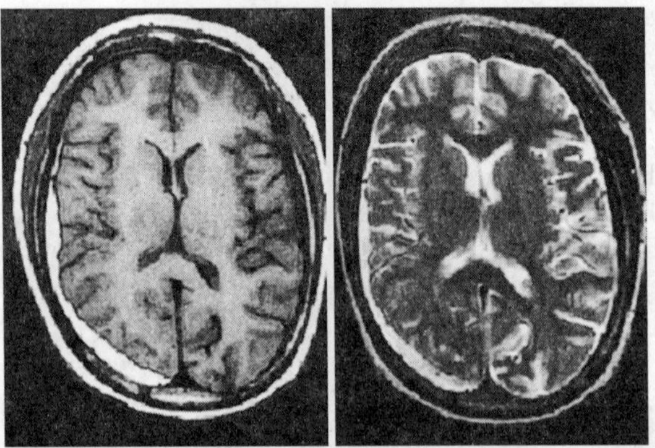

Fig. 11.3: Acute subdural hematoma

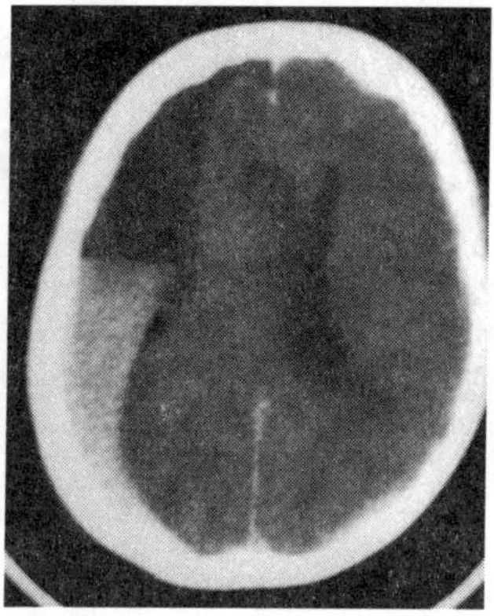

Fig. 11.4: Chronic subdural hematoma

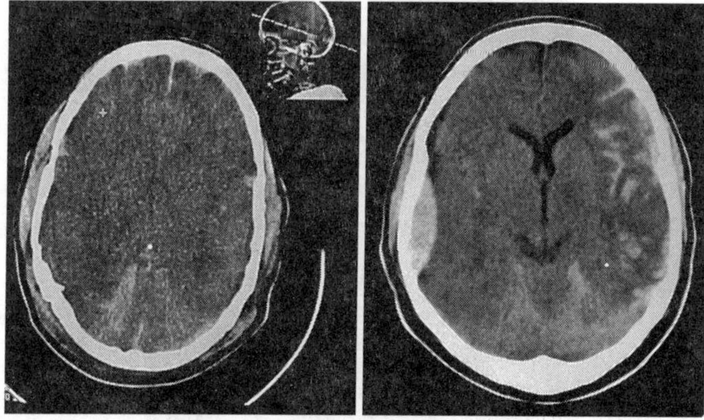

Fig. 11.5: Subarachnoid hemorrhage

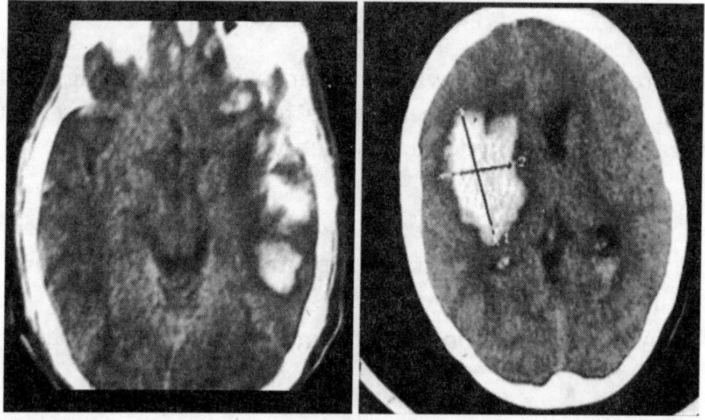

Fig. 11.6: Axial cranial CT showing intracerebral hematoma

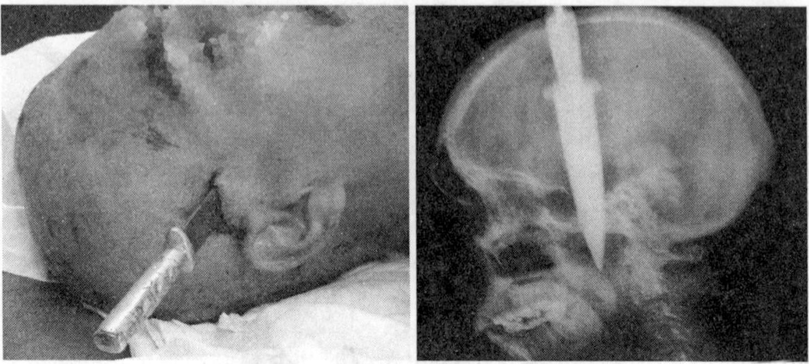

Fig. 11.7: Penetrating injury head with knife
(For color version, see Plate 3)

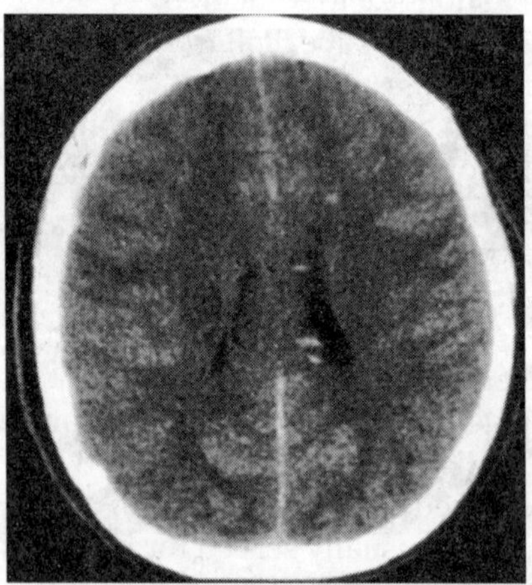

Fig. 11.8: Diffuse axonal

DAI there is damage in white matter axons connecting the two cerebral hemispheres. The lesion is found in corpus callosum, basal ganglia, corticomedullary junction and brainstem.

MR Angio/CT Angio

1. Detects vessel laceration, post-traumatic aneurysm, AV fistula, caroticocavernous fistula.
2. Arterial occlusions like thrombosis, embolism, spasm.

Management

It begins at the site of accident by emergency medical service (EMS) and the emergency medical team (EMT). The first hour after the accident is the GOLDEN HOUR for the victim. On the spot medical facilities, mode of transport and medical facilities in the ambulance can determine the fate of the victim.

Medical Management

At casualties and hospital "No head injury is trivial enough to ignore or serious enough to despair of" Hippocrates 4th century BC.

1. Record baseline parameters like pulse, BP, respiration
2. Head elevation–20 to 30 degrees
3. Put IV line, Ryle's tube, Folley's catheters.
4. Anticonvulsants.

Indication—known epileptics, history of convulsions, compound head injury with torn dura, depressed fracture of skull open or closed, prolonged unconsciousness, intracranial hematoma or intracranial infection.

Doses-5-20 mg/kg IV bolus in 10-15 mt followed by 5 mg/kg/24 hr.

5. H2 blockers—Ranitidine 50 mg IV 8 hourly.
6. IV Fluids—To mantain normovolemia and electrolyte balance. CVP at 8 to 10 cm of H_2O.
7. Anticerebral edema measures.
   a. Mannitol is usually served for life-threatening deterioration of the patients conditions. Dose should be 1-2 gm/kg/24 hr in 3-4 divided doses in a period of 20-30 minutes. Serum osmolality should be periodically measured to monitor dehydration.
   b. Furosemide - 1-2 mg/kg/24 hr in 2-3 divided doses.
   c. Oral glycerol - 1-2 oz 3 times daily.
8. *Antibiotics prophylaxis*—The antibiotics prophylaxis should be considered in the following situations. Patients on ventilator, GCS 8 or below, unconsciousness more than 24 hours, emergency surgery, CSF leak, compound head injury, suspicion of meningitis, patients below 5 years and above 60 years, known cases of DM, immunocompromised, severe anemia, hypoproteinemia, chest and urinary infection.

9. *Normothermia*—High temperature be brought down by tepid sponging, inj paracetamol 2cc IM.
10. *Restlessness*—The following can be the causes of restlessness in an unconscious head injured patients. Cerebral hypoxia, raised intracranial pressure, alcohol intoxication, full bladder. These causes should be ruled out before prescribing analgesics or tranquilizers. Haloperidol 2.5 mg IM should be given for restlessness.
11. Attention to nutrition by nasogastric tube feeding.
12. Care of eye, mouth, skin, bowel and bladder.
13. Continuous ICU monitoring—Pulse, BP, respiration, pupil size and GCS.

Protocol for Severe Head Injury

1. Head up 20-30 degrees neutral plane.
2. Endotracheal intubation and controlled ventilation with sedation and relaxation.

PaO_2 to be Mentained at 100 mm Hg and
$PaCO_2$ at 35–45 mm Hg

3. Mannitol 1 - 2 gm/kg/day in divided doses.
4. Fluid balance—Normovolemia CVP at 5 - 10 cm of H_2O.
5. Normothermia
6. Normal electrolyte and glucose level
7. Systolic BP 100-160 mm Hg
8. CT scan to find out surgical lesions. Evacuate mass lesions, ventricular drainage for hydrocephalus.
9. ICP monitoring if no surgical lesions on CT scan. ICP to be mentained at 5 - 10 mm Hg.

Dos for Head Injury Patients

- Watch for respiration—normal breathing—if breathing is not normal first attend to the respiration
- Suctioning of mouth, nose and tracheostomy tube
- If patient is drowsy Ryle's tube should be inserted and stomach contents empites to prevent aspiration
- Remove all tight fitting clothes.
- Make a recording of the pulse rate and blood pressures
- Suture/bandage all obvious external bleeding wounds

- Look for spine, chest, abdominal pelvic and extremity injuries and splint all fractures
- Neurological evaluation by GCS and record pupillary reaction.
- Start IV line for IV fluids and antibiotics.
- Take blood samples for basic hematological parameters, grouping and crossmatching
- Catheterize if the patient has a distended bladder.

Don'ts for Head Injury Patients

- No oral fluids
- No sedations
- Not to pack the bleeding ear, nose or mouth
- Not to keep the foot end elevated
- Not to apply tight bandage of head and neck together
- Not to explore the cranial wound with a finger or instrument
- No steroids
- Not to restrain a restless patient
- No lumbar puncture
- Don't transport the patient in an unstable condition

Indications for Controlled Ventilation

1. Inadequate spontaneous respiration
2. Poor neurological status GCS 8 or below
3. Spontaneous extension posturing
4. Repeated generalized convulsions
5. Spontaneous hyperventilation
6. ICP over 25 with no remediable cause
7. Associated chest injury
8. Postoperative – All the patients with tense brain at the end of surgery.

Indications for Tracheostomy

Most valuable in our settings where proper ICU with ventilatory facilities are not available.

1. Prolonged unconsciousness
2. GCS below 8

3. Maxillofacial and chest injury care of the tracheostomy is very important.

ICP Monitoring

Indications

1. All patients operated for head injury and electively ventilated.
2. All patients with mass lesion on CT scan but not operated because of good GCS.
3. All patients with GCS 8 or below but has no mass lesion on CT scan.

Methods

1. Ventricular catheter
2. Subarachnoid bolt
3. Epidural monitor
4. Parenchymatous monitor. Duration—24 to 48 hr.

Indications for Surgery

1. Severe head injury (GCS 8 or below) lesion in 3 or more cuts of CT scan with midline shift more than 2 mm or obliteration of the basal cisterns.
2. Mild to moderate head injury. Lesion in 5 or more cuts of CT scan with midline shift of more than 5 m
3. Large intracranial hematoma producing mass effect and raised ICP.
   a. Patient is deteriorating
   b. Patient is not improving
   c. Patient having shown improvement, then deteriorates.
4. Surgery for putting subarachnoid bolt and ICP monitoring or intraventricular catheter.
5. Compound head injury with brain matter coming out.

Surgery for Head Injury

1. Under GA craniotomy or burr hole craniectomy (better in a center).
2. Remove hematoma, necrotic brain, FB, comminuted depressed fragments and dural closure or duroplasty (Table 11.2).

Table 11.2: Surgical procedures

EDH	*SDH*	*ICH*
Craniotomy	Large craniotomy	Craniotomy
Evacuation	Evacuation	Evacuation of contusion hematoma
Control of bleeder	Control of bleeder	Control of bleeder
Hitching of dura	Duroplasty/dura closure	Dura closure/duroplasty

3. Avoid craniotomy/burr hole near sagittal/transverse sinus.
4. Emergency bitemporal craniectomy in morribund patients where CT scan is not available.

The Myth of Six Burr Holes (Three on Each Side)

Before the advent of CT scan all the concepts of head injury were not clear. When a head injury patient use to deteriorate, the surgeon did not know what to do. Three burr holes were put on one side starting from the temporal, then frontal and parietal regions. If no hematoma was found then three burr holes use to be put on the opposite side. Most of the times the burr holes use to be negative on the opposite side. Now we know these cases are DAI and any number of burr holes would prove negative and do not help to decrease the raised ICP. EDH, SDH, ICH will give some indication for localization and a craniotomy can be made at the site of localization. In the absence of localization an unilateral or bilateral decompression will have some beneficial effects to reduce the ICP rather than making 6 burr holes on both sides.

Surgery in Chronic Head Injury

- Chronic SDH
- Subdural effusion
- Post-traumatic hydrocephalus
- CSF fistula
- Cranial defects
- Growing skull fracture

Poor Prognostic Factors in Head Injury

1. GCS 8 or less.
2. Bilaterally dilated and fixed pupil.

3. Extremes of age.
4. CT scan shows DAI, acute SDH, multiple ICH and contusion.
6. ICP more than 30.

Outcome in Head Injury Patients (Glasgow Outcome Scale)

Grade 1: Good recovery–Resumption of normal lifestyle but may have minor sequelae.

Grade 2: Moderate disability–Disabled but independant.

Grade 3: Severe disability–Conscious but dependant.

Grade 4: Persistent vegetative state–Unresponsive and speechless (Sleep/wake but not sentiment)

Grade 5: Death

Prevention of Head Injury

Primary Prevention

1. Improve road condition and vehicle design.
2. Use helmets, seat belts and airbags.
3. On the spot treatment by emergency medical team.

Secondary Prevention

1. ABC of trauma by emergency medical team.
2. Case monitoring and appropriate medical therapy.
3. Appropriate surgical therapy where indicated.

Tertiary Prevention

Physical, vocational and psychological rehabilitation.

CONCLUSION

1. Nearly 70-75% of head injury patients do not require surgical intervention as they have cerebral concussion or minor head injury.
2. Detailed history taking and repeated neurological evaluation is essential to detect surgically correctable lesions where CT scan facilities are not available readily.
3. CT scan of the head is the GOLD STANDARD for confirming clinically suspected intracranial hematoma and surgically correctable lesion.

4. Prompt and appropriate management with good ventilation and tracheostomy when necessary and early evacuation to neurological center reduces morbidity and mortality in severe and moderately severe head injury patients.
5. Death due to secondary brain injury is preventable.
6. Advances in neuro ICU with controlled ventilation, ICP monitoring and newer neurosurgical instruments and techniques reduces morbidity and mortality in severe head injured patients.

Thoracic Trauma: General Consideration

SK Kochar

INCIDENCE

The incidence of chest trauma varies from 12 to 25% depending on whether the series have predominant blunt trauma or penetrating trauma. Similarly, it also shows variation if the reporting is from metropolis or rural areas. It accounts for approximately 25% of trauma related deaths.[1] For those patients who survive thoracic injury, nearly one half have a significant degree of long-term disability.[2] Thoracic trauma may be as a result of vehicle accident, crush injury, stab wounds, gunshot wounds or fall from hills or industrial accident, and blast injury following bomb explosions. Injury may vary from simple rib fracture to extensive pulmonary contusion. Associated injuries are present in 80% of patients. Most common being extremity injury and head injury.[3] The American College of Surgeons Committee on Trauma has divided these injuries into two groups.[4]

Immediately Life-threatening

- Airway obstruction
- Tension pneumothorax
- Open pneumothorax
- Massive hemothorax
- Flail chest
- Cardiac tamponade

Potentially Life-threatening

- Pulmonary contusion
- Myocardial contusion

Table 12.1: Specific type of injury

Injuries	*Percentage*
Chest wall	45
Pulmonary	26
Hemothorax	25
Pneumothorax	20
Heart	9
Diaphragm	7
Aorta and great vessels	4
Esophagus	0.5
Miscellaneous	21

- Aortic disruption
- Traumatic diaphragmatic hernia
- Tracheobronchial disruption
- Esophageal disruption

Occurrence of specific type of injury is shown in Table 12.1.[5]

Mechanism of Injury

Chest injuries occur by three principal mechanisms. The most common is body acceleration and deceleration, where organ inertia lags behind skeletal acceleration or deceleration. It mostly happens in vehicle accidents. The next most common type is body compression, where the force exceeds the ultimate strength of the skeleton, such as crush injuries or falls. The third type is high speed impact, where the violence exceeds viscus (organ) tolerance. It is localized, caused by a projectile such as bullet or sharpnel.

Different mechanisms produce basically two types of injury, e.g. blunt and penetrating.

Classification

Chest injury may be classified according to anatomical location and by the injuring agent as shown in Table 12.2.

Initial Evaluation and Management

Prehospital Care

Conditions which are influenced by prehospital care are: compromised airway, potential fracture of the cervical and thoracic spine, flail chest, pulmonary contusion, sucking chest wound,

Table 12.2: Classification of chest injuries

Anatomical site	*Injuring agent*	*Physiological impact*
• Chest wall	Penetrating	Stable
• Pleura and lungs	Blunt	Unstable
• Heart		
• Great vessels		
• Mediastinal viscera		
– Trachea		
– Bronchi		
– Esophagus		

tension pneumothorax, and pericardial tamponade. Patient with sucking chest wound should have the wounds covered with vaseline gauge and be sealed on three sides thus avoiding potential tension pneumothorax. If confidently diagnosed tension pneumothorax should be treated by pushing 16-gauge needle covered with holed finger stall at other end into second space. A patient with multiple ribs fracture if feasible, should lie on that side to decrease the flail or should have sand bags placed at the side of the chest wall to decrease its movement. Fluid administration in the prehospital phase is very vital in chest trauma as overload is easy and harmful in cases of pulmonary contusion and flail chest while in the patient with pericardial tamponade, the addition of fluids to increase the right heart filling pressures will improve the hemodynamics temporarily.

Hospital Care

Evaluation of thoracic trauma forms the initial ABC's of any polytrauma management as airway and breathing may be immediately life-threatening. After securing, the airway attention is focussed on breathing and circulation. Chest trauma may present as a respiratory distress or circulatory collapse.

Respiratory distress may be due to:

- Sucking (Open) chest wound
- Tension pneumothorax
- Flail chest
- Pulmonary contusion
- Hemothorax

Circulatory collapse/instability may be due to:

- Massive hemothorax, and
- Cardiac tamponade.

All these conditions can be diagnosed clinically though some include chest X-ray as a fundamental examination in thoracic injuries.[6] Position of trachea, movements of chest wall on respiration, surgical emphysema, dullness or tympanic percussion notes, diminished breath sounds on auscultation and muffled heart sounds are important clinical signs which clinches the diagnosis.

Resuscitation

It begins by securing and maintenance of airway and oxygenation by using supplemental oxygen and intravascular volume expansion via 16-gauge intracaths intravenous lines. Initial choice of fluid is isotonic saline/Ringer's lactate followed by matched blood transfusion. Although most patients may be managed by endotracheal intubation, some have anatomical injury or distortion of the upper airway. Patients with subcutaneous emphysema extending into neck may have laryngotracheal injury, and acute airway obstruction can occur during intubation. Fiberoptic laryngoscope is useful in assessment of the airway just before intubation. Such patients should not be sedated and paralyzed because the combination of acute airway obstruction and anatomical distortion of the airway will lead to severe hypoxia. The endotracheal tube should be of sufficient size to permit suctioning and flexible endoscopy. This requires a minimum size of 8F in adults. Decompression of hemothorax and pneumothorax should be considered part and parcel of airway management in patients with chest injuries. Emergency department thoracotomy (EDT) (Flow chart 12.1) has been suggested as a life saving intervention in selected patients with chest injuries.

Current Indications and Contraindications for EDT[7]

Indications

- Salvageable postinjury cardiac arrest.
- Patients sustaining witnessed penetrating trauma with <15 minutes of prehospital CPR.
- Patients sustaining witnessed blunt trauma with < 5 minutes of prehospital CPR.
- Persistent severe postinjury hypotension (SBP ≤ 60 mm Hg) due to:

Flow chart 12.1: Emergency department thoracotomy

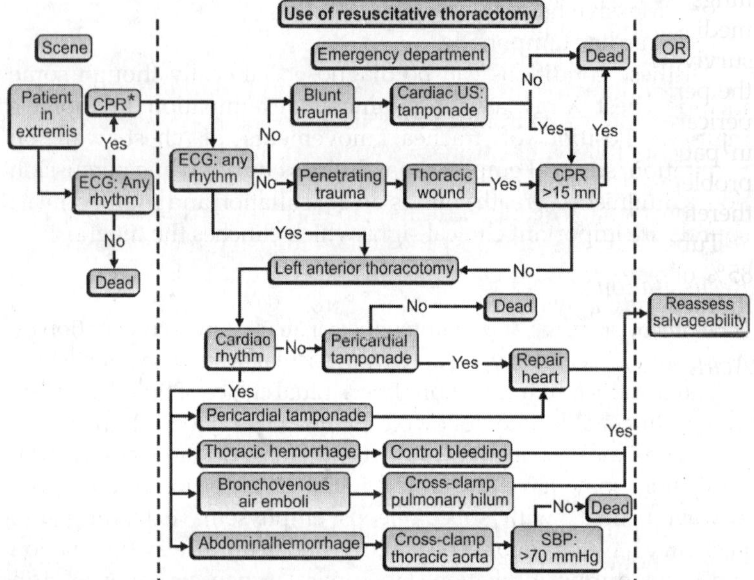

- Cardiac tamponade
- Hemorrhage–intrathoracic, intra-abdominal, extremity, cervical
- Air embolism.

Contraindications

Penetrating trauma: CPR>15 minutes and no signs of life pupillary response, respiratory effort, or motor activity.

Blunt trauma: CPR > 5 minutes and no signs of life or asystole.

The primary objectives of EDT are to: (a) release pericardial tamponade; (b) control cardiac hemorrhage; (c) control intrathoracic bleeding; (d) evacuate massive air embolism; (e) perform open cardiac massage; and (f) temporarily occlude the descending thoracic aorta. Combined, these objectives attempt to address the primary issue of cardiovascular collapse from mechanical sources or extreme hypovolemia.

Complications of EDT

Technical complications of EDT involve virtually every intrathoracic structure. The list of such misadventures included lacerations of the heart, coronary arteries, aorta, phrenic nerves, esophagus, and lungs, as well as avulsion of aortic branches to components of the mediastinum. Additional postoperative morbidity among ultimate survivors of EDT includes recurrent chest bleeding, infection of the pericardium, pleural spaces, sternum, and chest wall, and post-pericardiotomy syndrome. Previous thoracotomy, typically seen in patients following coronary bypass, virtually assures technical problems from the presence of dense pleural adhesions and is therefore a relative contraindication to EDT.

Tube thoracostomy is the only invasive procedure that 85% of patients with chest trauma may require. Indications for thoracotomy may be acute or nonacute.

Acute indications for thoracotomy are:

- Cardiac tamponade
- Initial thoracotomy loss >1000 ml, or continuing loss > 200 ml/hr for 4 hr
- Acute deterioration: Cardiac arrest in the emergency department with penetrating truncal trauma, resuscitative thoracotomy
- Massive air leak from chest tube
- Traumatic thoracotomy
- Vascular injury at the thoracic outlet
- Endoscopic or radiographic demonstration of tracheal or bronchial injury
- Endoscopic or radiographic evidence of esophageal injury
- Radiographic evidence of great vessel injury.

Indications for thoracotomy after trauma but in the nonacute setting include:

- Unevacuated clotted hemothorax
- Chronic traumatic diaphragmatic hernia
- Chronic (or neglected) post-traumatic empyema
- Infected intrapulmonary hematoma
- Tracheoesophageal fistula
- Missed tracheobronchial injury.

Algorithm for initial resuscitation of patients with chest trauma is shown in Flow chart 12.2.

Tube Thoracostomy Technique

The skin of the involved hemithorax is prepared with an antiseptic solution. The interspace at the level of the nipple is identified. This

Flow chart 12.2: Initial resuscitation of patients with chest trauma

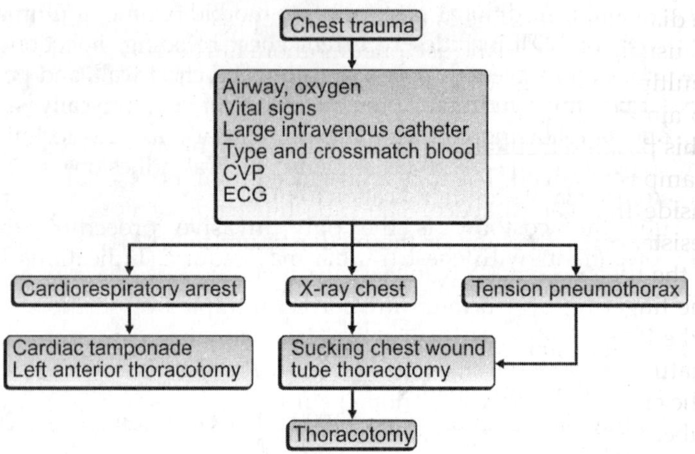

is usually the fifth or the sixth interspace. If the patient is conscious, the skin in the interspace in the midaxillary line is anesthetized by local infiltration. The needle is directed superiorly, and a tract is infiltrated up to and over the upper edge of the immediately superior rib and into the pleural space. The periosteum of the rib should be infiltrated because the tube will lie on the superior edge of the rib. A 3 cm transverse skin incision is made at the site of skin infiltration. A curved artery forcep is inserted and by spreading, a track in the subcutaneous tissue is created, passing superiorly and slightly posteriorly. The top of the rib above the skin incision is felt with the tip of the clamp, and the clamp is slipped vertically into the interspace. The clamp is kept in close approximation to the superior aspect of the rib so as to avoid the neurovascular bundle that courses along the inferior edge of the next superior rib. The intercostal muscles are divided transversely by blunt dissection with the forcep, and the forcep is passed into the pleural space. This can be painful because the pleura is difficult to anesthetize. The clamp is then withdrawn and the right index finger is passed with a sweeping motion along the tract made by the forcep and inserted into the pleural space. The tract is thus enlarged. The inside of the chest wall should be palpated to ensure an intrapleural location and to check for adhesions between the lung and the chest wall. The finger is withdrawn and a curved artery forcep with a large chest tube is inserted through the tract. The end of the tube is clamped. Although a small tube may be adequate for relief of pneumothorax, a tube of 32 F to 36 F in diameter is indicated in cases of trauma as hemopneumothorax is usual, rather than just pneumothorax. The tube, which has multiple holes, is advanced into the thorax. The clamp is used to aim the tube in a superior and a slightly posterior direction. This position facilitates dependent drainage blood and fluid. The clamp is removed. The tube is advanced until the last hole is well inside the pleural space. The tube must not be forced against resistance, or the lung or the mediastinum might be perforated. If the tube does not advance easily, it should be withdrawn and the finger reinserted to ensure correct intrapleural position. The tube is then reinserted using the clamp for direction. A vertical mattress suture of 0 silk is used to close the skin around the tube. The ends of this suture or another suture can be used to secure the tube. The end is firmly and securely fixed to the skin at the site of insertion with a heavy suture, such as 0 silk, that is passed several times around the tube. An occlusive dressing of gauze with petroleum jelly may be placed on the wound and the tube. The tube is attached to a continuous water seal drainage system with a suction of 20 cm of water. A chest radiograph is immediately obtained to ensure correct positioning of the tube and successful results of its insertion in terms of lung expansion and evacuation of hemopneumothorax and pneumothorax.

Incisions

The incisions used for a patient requiring operation for a chest injury is dictated by the diagnosis and anticipated injuries. The basic incisions are:

Anterolateral Thoracotomy

Indications: Resuscitative thoracotomy, injuries to heart, injuries to left lung.

Technique: The left arm is abducted to allow access to the left hemithorax. The skin is incised in the fifth intercostal space, from the edge of the sternum to the posterior axillary line. Underlying tissue is rapidly divided just superior to the upper border of the sixth rib. A self-retaining chest wall retractor is inserted, and the wound opened to expose the heart and left lung. A wound to the heart posteriorly or a concomitant right thoracic injury may require extension of the incision across the sternum. The internal mammary arteries will be transected when this incision is made. Therefore, these vessels must be identified and securely ligated.

Left Posterolateral Thoracotomy

It provides excellent exposure of the left lung, lower esophagus, descending aorta, proximal left subclavion artery and some excess to the proximal left common carotid artery.[8]

Right Posterolateral Thoracotomy

It provides good exposure for managing pulmonary, tracheal and proximal esophageal, superior and inferior vena cava injuries.

Book Thoracotomy

The "book" or "trap door" incision is an en block left third -interspace anterolateral thoracotomy and partial upper sternotomy with a supraclavicular extension. This incision is useful for left sided arterial injuries, especially in the area of the clavicle. At times, the clavicle is removed to increase exposure.

REFERENCES

1. LoCicero J, Mattox KL. Epidemiology of chest trauma. Surg Clin North Am 1989;69:15.
2. Landercasper J, Cogbill T, Lindsmith L. Long-term disability after flail chest injury. J Trauma 1984;24:410-4.
3. Beeson A, Saegesser F. Colour atlas of chest trauma and associated injuries. Oradell, medical economics book, 1983.
4. Thal ER, Ramenofsky ML, et al. Advanced trauma life support course for physicians. Subcommittee trauma, 1987-88. Chicago, III. American College of Surgeons, 1988.
5. Kemmerer WT, Eckert WG, Gathright JB, et al. Pattern of thoracic injuries in fatal traffic accidents. J Trauma 1961;1:595.
6. Wiot JF. The radiological manifestation of blunt chest trauma. JAMA 1975;231:500.
7. C Clay Cothren, Ernest E Moore. Emergency department thoracotomy for the critically injured patient: Objectives, indications, and outcomes World Journal of Emergency Surgery 2006;1:4
8. Schaff HV, Brawley RK. The operative management of penetrating vascular injuries of the thoracic outlet. Surgery. 1977;82(2):182-91.

Injuries of Chest Wall

SK Kochar

Chest wall injuries are the most common injury sustained in the thoracic trauma. Its incidence varies from 35 to 45 percent[1] among the specific type of thoracic injuries. Injury to the chest wall may follow blunt trauma or penetrating injury. The incident is higher in blunt trauma than penetrating injuries. In blunt trauma, the mechanism is crushing injury or a fall from height. Vehicle accident is the most common cause for blunt trauma. In India stab wounds are more common than gunshot wounds. Chest wall injuries range from relatively trivial, such as a simple isolated rib fracture, to fatal flail chest or huge defects.

Pathophysiology

Trauma to the chest wall may result in fracture rib or ribs and injury to pleura, intercostal nerves and intercostal vessels. The injury results in severe pain which increases on inspiration and thus it interferes with ventilatory effort. It results in shallow breathing, tachypnea, and hypoventilation; and results in a relative increase in dead space, decreased cough effectiveness, and retained secretions. These abnormalities may progress to hypercarbia, hypoxia, and later, infection and septicemia. Thus, control of pain is of vital importance in chest wall trauma.

A number of ribs may get fractured at two places and the intervening segment may move in and out with respiratory effort. Occasionally, there may be bilateral rib fractures or a larger segment involvement on one side giving rise to significant flailing. When there is significant flailing, the mediastinum swings with breathing, producing hypoventilation of both lungs. The loss of normal levels of negative intrathoracic pressure contributes to hypoventilation.

Atelectasis occurs, tidal volume decreases, arteriovenous shunt appears, the alveolar-arterial oxygen gradient increases, and hypoxia supervenes.[2] Associated pulmonary contusion which often is present, adds loss of compliance, increased airway resistance, and decreased gas diffusion. Retained secretions, pulmonary edema, arteriovenous shunting, and the work of breathing all increase over the first 2 or 3 days.[3]

An opening in the chest wall allows atmospheric air to enter the pleura, permitting the intrapleural pressure to rise and producing pneumothorax and collapse of the lungs. This results in sucking chest wound. The air entering the hemithorax during inspiration, depending upon the size of the hole and not allowing the lung to expand and exiting during expiration. Ventilation is compromised and it may proceed to respiratory distress when the size of the defect approaches or exceeds the cross-sectional area of the trachea. The wound may produce an valve like effect, resulting in tension pneumothorax.

Classification

- Single rib fracture
- Multiple rib fractures
- Flail segment, chest
- Clavicular, scapular, sternal fractures
- Chest wall defects: Penetrating injuries
  - Sucking chest wound
  - Chest wall hemorrhage
- Traumatic asphyxia

Diagnosis

The clinical spectrum of simple fracture rib/ribs may range from only pain and restricted chest wall movement to major physiological derangements. Conscious patient often points out at the site of pain and the fracture. In doubtful cases compression of the chest wall at a site little away from the fracture produces pain. There may be crepitus or discontinuity at the fracture site, and occasionally, surgical emphysema may be a predominant feature on physical examination. A flail segment, chest may be evident on physical examination. It is important to assess the associated pneumothorax, hemothorax and pulmonary contusion (Figs 13.1 and 13.2). In alert patients without evidence of chest wall tenderness, reduced air-entry or abnormal respiratory effort, selective use of CT chest scanning as a screening tool could be adopted (Fig. 13.3). This is supported by the fact that most chest injuries can be treated with simple observation. Intubated

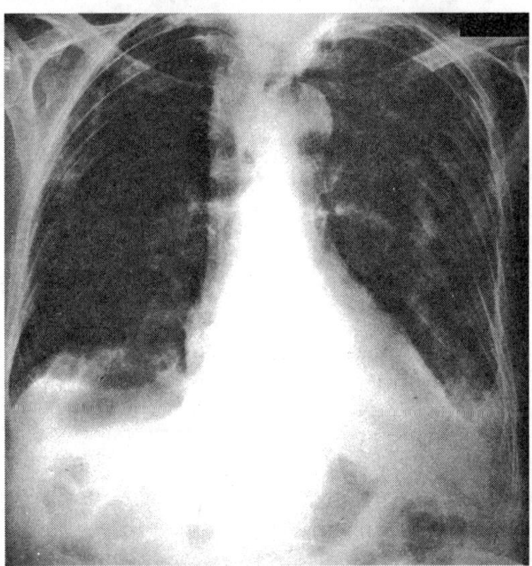

Fig. 13.1: Multiple left rib fractures, pulmonary contusion and hemothorax

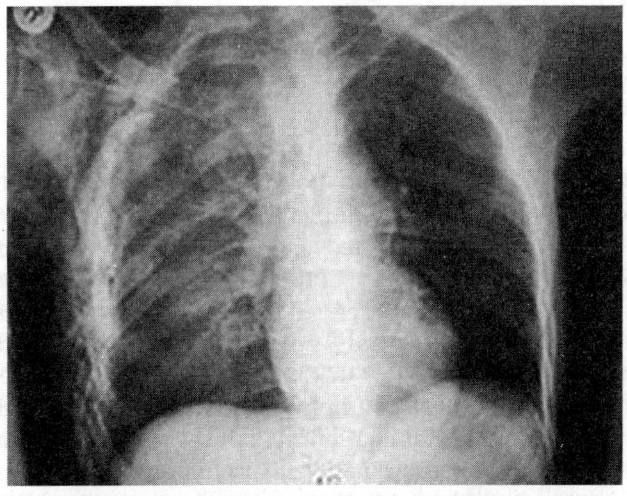

Fig. 13.2: Multiple rib fractures, pulmonary contusion surgical emphysema and flail segment

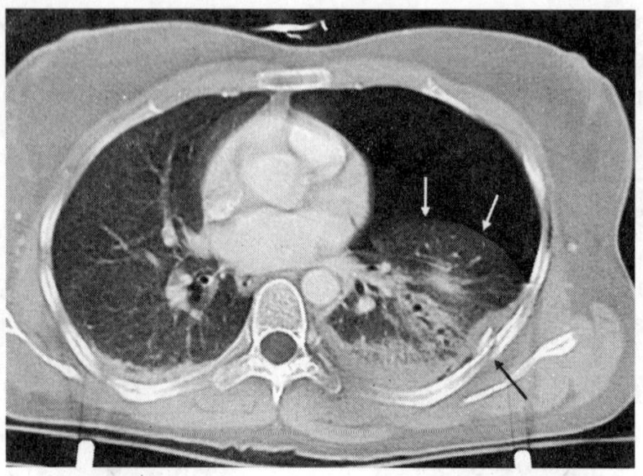

Fig. 13.3: Flail segment with pulmonary contusion and collapse

patients, in most instances, should receive a routine CT chest scan in their first assessment.[4]

Pulmonary complication may take 24-48 hours to appear, thus re-evaluation is desirable in all fracture rib patients. When the first or second ribs are fractured, one should be specially alert to injuries of adjacent nervous and vascular structures because of the narrow thoracic inlet and the magnitude of the trauma necessarily involved.[4a] Routine arteriograms on detection of first rib fracture is no more indicated.[5] Indications of arteriography are:

- Abnormality in pulse or circulation to the upper limb
- Brachial plexus injuries
- Large hematoma at the base of the neck or the upper chest
- Extrapleural and mediastinum hematomas on the chest films
- Marked displacement of the first rib segment.

When sternal fracture or costochondral dislocation are present, cardiac injury should be ruled out. Fracture of lower ribs on the right side should make one alert about the injury to the liver and similarly when there is fracture of lower ribs on the left side, spleen is in the danger of getting injured. In severe crush injury a patient may suffer from traumatic asphyxia. Clinical features of this rare syndrome are, craniofacial cyanosis, facial edema, petechiae, subconjunctival hemorrhage and occasional neurological symptoms. Neurological symptoms may be, loss of consciousness, seizures, confusion, and temporary or permanent blindness.[6,7] Hematuria, hemoptysis, epistaxis are occasionally present.

In penetrating injuries the defect may be a simple perforation or may be huge defect. Laceration of intercostal vessel may produce bleeding which at times may necessitate thoracotomy.

Management

The aim of treatment is to detect/prevent pulmonary complications. Rib's fracture produces pain which results in respiratory splinting, inhibition of cough, retention of secretions, atelectasis, hypoxia, pneumonia, lung abscess and may even result in death. Pain relief is most important in management of fracture ribs. Around the clock analgesics, deep breathing exercises are often that is all required to be done. Strapping is discouraged and if analgesics are not adequate, pain relief by intercostal nerve block is the treatment of choice. The nerve of the fractured ribs should be blocked, as well as one above and one below the involved ribs. It is generally more advantageous to block these nerves well posteriorly, near the rib angle. A long acting anesthetic is preferred. Blocks may be repeated once or twice at the interval of 12-24 hours. Table 13.1 illustrates the changes in several indices of ventilation and respiratory mechanics resulting from intercostal nerve blockade in a patient with multiple rib fractures and pulmonary contusion.[8]

Where facilities/expertise is available and the pain relief with nerve block is not adequate, epidural catheter placement and anesthesia give excellent pain relief. Other modalities of pain relief used for patients of fracture ribs are intrapleural injection of long acting anesthetic and transcutaneous electrical nerve stimulator.[9,10] In Indian subcontinent due to high incidence of pulmonary tuberculosis, intrapleural catheter or injection is not a safe proposition and it should be avoided. Table 13.2 compares the changes in arterial oxygen pressure that occurs following different types of pain relief modalities for fracture ribs.[8]

Table 13.1: Changes in ventilation variables before and after intercostal nerve block

Variables	*Before*	*After*
Tidal volume	380 ml	700 ml
Negative inspiratory force	–22 cm H_2O	–30 cm H_2O
Minimum volume	6.6 l/min	9.26 l/min

Table 13.2: Comparison of pain relief modalities for rib fracture patients

Modality	*Expected change in PaO_2 (mm Hg)*
Systemic analgesic	–4
Transcutaneous electrical nerve stimulator	+7
Intercostal block	+40
Intrapleural catheter	+70

Surgical fixation of unstable or multiple ribs have been controversial. However if thoracotomy is being resorted to for one or the other indication the advantage should be taken and the ribs be fixed with plates or wire sutures. There are significant advantages to fixation, including earlier ambulation, better tracheobronchial toilet, and less long-term deformity.[11] When multiple lower ribs are fractured it is useful adjuvant to resort to nasogastric aspiration as it will avoid gastric distention and further complications.

Management of penetrating wounds includes closure of any open wound and insertion of a chest tube for control of pneumothorax and hemothorax. After the initial management and evaluation the wound is definitely debrided and closed in an operation theater. Though one chest tube placed in 5th intercostal space in midaxillary line is enough, some advocate two tubes, one placed along the anterior and one along the posterior pleural space.[11] When the wound is grossly contaminated the skin is left open after the underlying intercostal muscles have been closed with interrupted sutures. When the wound has become clean and the patient's condition allows, secondary closure is done. When the defect is large, closure may be difficult. It may be accomplished with the help from reconstructive colleague as these patient will need raising of musculocutaneous flaps. When the wound is parasternal, the internal mammary vessels may be injured. Bleeding from the intercostal or internal mammary arteries, being under systemic pressure, does not tamponade and hemothorax and usually continues until shock or frank pulmonary insufficiency occurs. Surgical ligation is usually required.

FLAIL CHEST

Unstable segment of chest wall, following thoracic trauma, moving paradoxically to the rest of chest wall has been termed as flail chest. It may be classified as sternal, anterior, lateral, or posterior depending on the location of this segment. In anterior segment there is separation of the sternum from costochondral junctions on either sides or adjacent ribs are fractured on both sides. In other cases multiple ribs are fractured at two places giving rise to flail segment. This may be placed laterally or posteriorly. The incidence of flail chest varies from 5 to 13%.[1] Flail chest mostly results from direct impact. Common mechanism includes high speed contact with steering columns, autopedestrian trauma, motorcycle accidents, and falls. Flail chest may result from severe compression injury resulting from vehicle, industrial accidents.

Pathophysiology

The force which gives rise to compression and multiple ribs fracture does manage to contuse the underlying lungs. Hemothorax occurs in approximately half the patients and many develops pneumothorax. Flail chest injury results in abnormality of ventilation, oxygenation and compliance. The relative contribution of the unstable chest wall vs concomitant pulmonary contusion and parenchymal injury is not well established. Large flail segments may disrupt the normal bellow action of the thorax. Pain and muscular splinting restrict chest wall expansion leading to abnormal respiratory mechanics. However, most of the pulmonary dysfunction observed in flail chest is probably secondary to underlying pulmonary contusion[12,13] and not due to concept of Pendelluft.[14] Excessive fluid resuscitation during prehospital phase or during anesthesia may precipitate respiratory distress syndrome in these patients.

Diagnosis

Diagnosis of flail segment/chest is primarily clinical. Physical examination of chest wall anteriorly, posteriorly and laterally will demonstrate the flail segment during respiratory excursion. Occasionally the flail may not appear immediately after trauma due to muscular splinting of the chest. Shackford et al documented delay in diagnosis in 14% of their patients from 18-75 hours after hospitalization.[15] X-ray chest may demonstrate fracture of multiple ribs at two sites and these are the patients who should be observed for paradoxical movements of the chest wall. Any airway obstruction, such as mandibular fracture or aspiration, increases inspiratory intrathoracic negative pressure and thus may increase or may even produce inspiratory flailing; expiratory obstruction, especially groaning and grunting, increases expiratory pressure and the resultant outward displacement of the flail segment of the chest wall.

Sagittal and coronal reformats of a thoracic MSCT scan also identifies rib fractures quite well. Because many of these patients sustain concomitant internal thoracic injury, thoracic CT scanning images may be available for reasons other than rib fracture identification (i.e. evaluation of an abnormal mediastinal contour). Three-dimensional (3-D) reconstruction of helical CT images is also possible though not widely available.

Management

The aim of management is to: i. restore the normal movement of the chest wall, ii. decrease the work of breathing, iii. restore the oxygenation to near normal, iv. decrease the progressive pulmonary damage, and v. prevent complications.

Adequate airway: As mentioned earlier any airway obstruction will increase the flailing. An adequate airway is essential. Tracheobronchial toilet, humidification, effective suction of bronchi, relief of bronchospasm if any, limited bronchial irrigation, bronchoscopy or even tracheostomy may be required to achieve good airway.

Relief of pain: Multiple rib fractures need pain management as described earlier in fracture ribs. In fact pain relief becomes the cornerstone of the management. Around the clock analgesia, epidural blocks preferably with epidural catheter so that it can be topped up 8-12 hourly, intercostal nerve blocks are some of the ways of achieving this. Adequate analgesia certainly improves pulmonary function and toilet.

Judicious fluid administration: During resuscitation, anesthesia, every effort must be made to avoid fluid overload. A central venous catheter may be used for monitoring. Crystalloids should be replaced by the blood at the earliest and red cell mass be maintained near normal to maximize oxygen transport. Diuretics may be used after resuscitation to maintain central venous pressure and osmolality near normal limits.

Antibiotics: Broad spectrum antibiotics are indicated for prevention of infection and further complications.

Stability of Chest Wall

External stabilization with towel clips, wires, pins or pack were routinely used till 1970's. In the late 50's it was realized that the same can be achieved with "internal" splinting by endotracheal intubation and forced volume ventilator.[16] This became the standard treatment till Tinkle and associates[17] introduced the concept of selective management in the 1970s by demonstrating that many patients do not require "internal pneumatic stabilization. The major therapeutic question is: in which patients, and when, should endotracheal intubation and controlled breathing be used?

Indications for Ventilation in a Flail Chest Patients

1. Respiratory failure is manifested by one or more of the following criteria;

Respiratory rate	> 35 or <8
CO_2 tension	>50 torr
Vital capacity	< 10-15 ml /kg
Maximum inspiratory force	< -25 cm H_2O
Alveolar to arterial oxygen tension difference (FiO_2=1.0)	>350 torr
Shunt	>15%
Dead space to tidal volume ratio	>0.6
Static compliance	<30 ml/cm H_2O

2. Clinical evidence of sever shock
3. Associated severe head injury with lack of airway control or need to hyperventilate.
4. Severe associated injury requiring surgery.
5. Airway obstruction.
6. Significant pre-existing chronic pulmonary disease.
7. Injuries of more than seven ribs.
8. Bilateral multiple injuries.

When the decision is made to intubate and ventilate the patient, one should completely re-evaluate both pleural spaces. If there is significant evidence of pulmonary injury, even without pneumothorax, thoracostomy tubes are indicated. A small or even potential pulmonary air leak can be converted to tension pneumothorax by the ventilator. Controlled ventilation should be used. Intermittent mandatory ventilation does not stabilize the chest wall effectively and may lead to the fatigue of the patient.[18]

Not all patients require intubation. Flail chest patients without respiratory impairment generally do well without ventilatory assistance. More attention to management of basic physiologic derangements and close nursing and medical care improve clinical results and decrease costs. The best way to avoid ventilators is early aggressive attention to correction of these derangements before the need for artificial ventilator arises.

Elements of Treatment of Flail Chest without Mechanical Ventilation

- Chest physiotherapy
- Supplemental oxygen therapy
- Humidification of inspired air
- Incentive spirometry
- Tracheobronchial toilet
- Effective analgesia
- Intermittent positive pressure breathing
- Nebulized bronchodilator administration
- Therapeutic fiberoptic bronchoscopy
- Continuous reassessment
  - Physical examination
  - Serial chest X-ray
  - Serial arterial blood gas determinations
  - Oximetric monitoring
  - Serial spirometric testing
  - Surveillance for pulmonary morbidity.

Outcome and Complications

Pulmonary complications are common following flail chest. These are hospital acquired pneumonia, major atelectasis, pleural effusion, tracheobronchitis, bronchopneumonia's, barotrauma, tracheal injury, and tracheoesophageal fistula. Most of these complications are due the use of ventilators and management of these patients in ICU. About one half of critically ill patients in an intensive care unit becomes colonized with gram-negative flora within three days and nasocomial pneumonia may occur in one-fourth of colonized patients.[19] The overall incidence of barotrauma has been reported to be less than 5%[20] but the risk has been found to be as high as 40% in patients on continuous positive pressure.[21] Prolonged endotracheal intubation may result in tracheal stenosis, vocal cord ulcers, and vocal cord paralysis.[15]

Mortality in patients with flail chest remains high despite advances in the management. Factors which influence the mortality are:

- Thoracic factors
  - Pulmonary contusion,
  - Number of fractured ribs.
- Extrathoracic factors
  - Presence of shock at admission,
  - Head injury,
  - Hepatic and/splenic trauma.

Mortality was 34% in 60s and 29.6% in 70s and up to 16% in 80s.[12,15,22]

Long-term Sequelae

The long-term sequelae of flail chest injury are not well documented. However, pulmonary function test (PFT) may remain impaired for a very long time as shown in Table 13.3.[23]

Role of Surgery

In general, operative fixation is most commonly performed in patients requiring a thoracotomy for other reasons or in cases of gross chest wall deformity. Flail chest from multiple myeloma, sternal absence, or total sternectomy more frequently responds well to surgical fixation. Underlying pulmonary injury with respiratory insufficiency resulting from changes in tidal volume and minute ventilation in these patients is rare.

Table 13.3: Pulmonary function test in long-term follow-up of flail chest survivors

PFT	*Abnormal(%)*	*Normal(%)*
Chest tightness	25	75
Chest wall pain	49	51
Subjective dyspnea	63	37
Chest expansion	46	54
Chest X-ray	100	0
Spirometry	57	43
Diffusion testing	10	90
Dyspnea tread mill testing	70	30

Sternal Fracture

These injuries most commonly occur in vehicular accidents and from direct impact to the anterior chest. The classic injury mechanism remains direct impact of the sternum against the steering column of an automobile involved in a deceleration crash. Severe flexion injuries of the vertebrae may also produce sternal fractures. Sternal injuries are commonly associated with costochondral dislocations of multiple ribs, and therefore, with flail chest. The majority of sternal fractures involve the upper or mid portion of the body. Comminuted fracture are rare. Sternal fractures are associated with other significant injuries in 50-60% of patients.[24] These includc rib fractures, long bone fractures and head injury. With sternal injuries, one should always suspect rupture of a bronchus, rupture of major arteries, and especially, myocardial injury, because the heart is compressed between the sternum and the vertebrae.[25]

The clinical manifestations of sternal fracture include anterior chest pain, tenderness, ecchymosis, swelling, and palpable deformity. The diagnosis is made primarily by physical examination as sternum is subcutaneous, it is easily palpated, and the fracture or step-off can usually be felt.

Treatment

The initial focus should be on the management of associated injuries followed by careful reduction of claviculosternal dislocations that may be compromising the trachea or vascular or nervous structures at the thoracic inlet. Cardiac monitoring in an intensive care unit should be considered for any multiply injured patient with a sternal fracture. Myocardial injury must be investigated with serial electrocardiograms, cardiac enzyme determinations and echocardiography, as indicated. Analgesia and local infiltration may be all that is needed for fracture sternum. However, many patients are best managed by early fixation of the sternum by direct wiring.

REFERENCES

1. Lo Cicero J, Mattox KL. Epidemiology of chest trauma. Surg Clin North Am 1989;69;15.
2. Trunkey DD. In Blaisdell FW, Trunkey DD. Trauma Management, Vol III. Cervicothoracic Trauma. New York, Thieme, 1986.

3. Richardson JD, Polk HC Jr, Flint LM. Trauma: Clinical Care and Pathophysiology, Chicago, year Book Medical Publishers, 1987.
4. Traub M, Stevenson M, McEvoy S, Briggs G, Lo SK, Leibman S, Joseph T. The use of chest computed tomography versus chest X-ray in patients with major blunt trauma. Injury 2007;38(1):43-7.
4a. Philips EH, Rogers WF, Gasper MR. First rib fracture: Incidence of vascular injury and indication for angiography. Surgery 1981;89:42-47.
5. Lazrove S, Harley DP, et al. Should all patients with first rib fracture undergo arteriography? J Thorac Cardiovas Surg 1982;83:532-7.
6. Purdy RH, Cogbill TH, Landercasper J, Ryan DK. Temporary blindness associated with traumatic asphyxia. J Emerg Med 1988;6:373.
7. Landercasper J, Cogbill TH. Long-term follow-up after traumatic asphyxia. J Trauma 1985;25:838.
8. Flint LM. An integrated approach to thoracic injury. In Najarian JS Delany JP. Progress in Trauma and Critical Care Surgery (eds) St Loius, Mosby Year Book, 1992.
9. Mackersie R, Shackford S, Hoyt D, et al. Continuous epidural fantanyl analgesia. Ventilatory function improvement with routine use in treatment of blunt chest injury. J Trauma 1987;27:1207-12.
10. Sloan J, Muwanga C, Waters E, et al. Multiple rib fractures. Transcutaneous nerve stimulation verses conventional analgesia. J Trauma 1986;1120-22.
11. Pate JW. Chest wall injuries. Surg Clin North Amer 1989;69:59-70.
12. Richardson JD, Adams L, Flint LM. Selective management of flail chest and pulmonary contusion. Ann Surg 1982;196:481.
13. Shackford Sr, Smith De, Zarins CK, et al. The management of flail chest: A comparison of ventilatory and nonventilatory treatment. Am J Surg 1976;132:759.
14. Malony JV, Schmutzer KJ, Raschke E. Paradoxical respiration and "Pendelluft". J Thorac Cardiovasc Surg 1061;41:291.
15. Shackford SR, Virgilio RW, Peters RM. Selective use of ventilatory therapy in flail chest injury. J Thorac Cardiovasc Surg 1981;81:194.
16. Avery EE, Morch ET, Benson DW. Critically crushed chests: A new method of treatment with continuous mechanical hyperventilation to produce alkalotic apnea and internal pneumatic stabilisation. J Thorac Surg 1956;32:291.
17. Trinkle JK, Richardson JD, Franz JL, et al. Management of flail chest without mechanical ventilation. Ann Thorac Surg 1975;19:355.
18. Hood RM (Ed). Management of thoracic injuries. Springfield, Charles C Thomas, 1969.
19. Northey D, Adess ML, Hartsuck JM, et al. Microbial surveillance in a surgical intensive care unit. Surg Gynecol Obster 1974;139:321.

20. Cullen DJ, Caldera DL. The incidence of ventilator induced pulmonary barotrauma in critically ill patients. Anesthesiology 1979;50:185.
21. Bone RC, Francis PB, Pierce AK. Pulmonary barotrauma complicating positive end expiratory pressure. Am Rev Respir Dis 1975;111:921.
22. Clark GC, Schecter WP, Trunkey DD. Variables affecting outcome in blunt chest trauma: Flail chest vs pulmonary contusion. J Trauma 1988;28:298.
23. Landercasper J, Cogbill Th, Lindesmith LA. Long-term disability after flail chest injury. J Trauma 1984;24:410.
24. Wojcik JB, Morgan AS. Sternal fractures: The natural history. Ann Emerg Med 1988;17:912.
25. Snow N, richardson JD, Flint LM Jr. Myocardial contusion: implication for patients with multiple traumatic injuries. Surgery 1982;92:744-50.

Injuries of Lungs and Pleura

SK Kochar

Injuries to lungs and pleura are second in incidence to injuries to chest wall. In a study of 1500 patients done at Switzerland the incidence of pneumothorax 20%, hemothorax was 21%, and pulmonary contusion 21%.[1] In another study from 60 hospitals and 15,047 patients of chest trauma, incidence of pneumothorax 20%, hemothorax 25% and pulmonary contusion was 26%.[2] Injuries to lungs and pleura can be classified as immediately life-threatening and potentially life-threatening. Mechanism of injuries may be direct impact, compression/crushing, acceleration/deceleration and high speed impact. It may be blunt or penetrating. Causes of these injuries are vehicle accidents, stab injuries, gunshot wounds and fall from heights. Vehicle accidents being the most common and blunt trauma being more common than penetrating.

PLEURA

Whatever may be the cause, air entering the pleura disrupts the normal intrapleural pressure resulting in pneumothorax. The lung collapses to various extent depending on the quantity of air, the rate of air entering the pleural space and the status of adhesion of the pleura to the wall. The pneumothorax may be open, tension or uncomplicated pneumothorax. Injury to the lungs, intercostal vessels and intrathoracic vessels may result in hemothorax. This may be mild to massive. Both parietal and visceral pleural surfaces are highly vascularized, which facilitate delivery of inflammatory mediators and removal of toxic products of infection. Thus, when an infected fluid collection is completely evacuated from the pleural space and the lung fully re-expanded, primary healing occurs. Pleural responses to blunt and penetrating trauma are similar, representing the nonspecific responses of the pleura to disruption, infection, and inflammation.

PULMONARY PARENCHYMA

Wounds following stab wounds and low velocity gunshots result in laceration of the pulmonary parenchyma without much devitalization. It may result in hemothorax, pneumohemothorax or pneumothorax. Complete evacuation of the pleural space and re-expansion of the lungs are usually adequate to control bleeding from the relatively low pressure pulmonary vessels.[3] High velocity gunshot wounds are associated with a large amount of tissue destruction due to cavitation and blast injury. This result in a large area of injured or devitalized pulmonary parenchyma that may predispose to infection. Thus, the incidence of empyema following these injuries is higher than after low velocity injuries.

Classically blunt injuries to the lungs have been grouped into: lacerations, hematomas, contusions. In fact as is evident on CT scan studies, these lesions represent various spectrum of the same injury and these can coexist. Pulmonary lacerations may be the result of direct puncture by the fractured rib or tearing due to the compressive/crushing/shearing force. Lacerations due to shearing forces tends to be associated with pulmonary contusion.

Pulmonary hematoma present soon after the injury and since not accompanied by hemo/pneumothorax usually have little effect on gas exchange or pulmonary function. These get absorbed slowly and resolve over a number of days without any active treatment. However, pulmonary hematoma may get become infected secondarily and form abscess cavities.[4]

In pulmonary contusion there is extensive interstitial hemorrhage with alveolar collapse and alveolar flooding with blood and proteins. This leads to atelectasis and consolidation in adjacent areas of uninjured lung tissue, or shunting, and results in hypoxia that is relatively refractory to enhanced inspiratory oxygen concentration.[5,6] Pulmonary contusions are usually localized and there is loss of the normal selective permeability of the injured capillary membrane.[7]

Pneumothorax

Open Pneumothorax

Following penetrating injuries or as result of loss of chest wall in severe blunt injuries there is a defect in chest wall through which air passes in and out during respiration resulting in sucking chest wound. As the size of the defect approaches two third of the size of the tracheal diameter, air passes preferentially through the lower resistance injury tract rather than through the normal airways.[8] This severely compromises oxygenation and ventilation and is immediately life-threatening. Diagnosis is obvious and the treatment is urgent. In the prehospital settings and in the emergency room till the definitive treatment can be offered, the wound should be covered with sterile occlusive dressing and taped securely on three sides. In those patients who are offered endotracheal intubation and ventilator for associated injuries the wound should not be closed as it may result in tension pneumothorax. Subsequently, the patient is taken to operation theater and wound debridement and closure is done. Tube thoracostomy is performed at the remote selected site, preferably 5th intercostal space midaxillary line to drain the pneumothorax and hemothorax, if any.

Tension Pneumothorax

Tension pneumothorax develops following pneumothorax when the air cannot exit. Following pneumothorax the injured lung collapses and the further escape of air into the pleura stops. When the air continues to enter pleura during inspiration but does not exit during expiration the tension pneumothorax results. Similarly, in penetrating injuries if the air enters during inspiration and does not escape during expiration due to valve like injury or the chest wall wound have been sealed but the air from injured lung continues to escape it results in tension pneumothorax. The consequence of this condition is progressively increasing intrathoracic pressure in the affected hemithorax resulting in impaired venous return and mediastinum shift. Tachypnea, tachycardia, hypotension are invariably present. The classic picture of tracheal deviation, respiratory distress, unilateral diminished breath sounds, distended neck veins and hyperresonance is often absent.[9] Needle thoracocentesis not only confirm the diagnosis but it will also relieve the emergent situation if connected to under water seal. The definitive treatment is tube thoracostomy. If the lung does not expand, further evaluation by bronchoscopy is required.

Uncomplicated Pneumothorax

Pneumothorax may be suspected when the patient has got rib fractures or complains of chest pain, and on clinical examination, there is tympanic note on percussion of the involved hemithorax and the breath sounds are diminished on auscultation. X-ray chest confirm the diagnosis (Fig. 14.1) and the treatment is tube thoracotomy. Pneumothorax may take almost 24 hours to develop and thus the need to evaluate chest trauma patient repeatedly. Occasionally though suspected, it may not be evident on X-ray chest. These patients should be observed with serial X-ray and repeated clinical examination and prophylactic chest tube should be reserved for the following conditions:

1. Prior to transfer to other hospital,
2. Prior to administration of general anesthesia, and
3. Prior to ventilatory support.

HEMOTHORAX

The incidence of hemothorax is 20 to 25% among chest trauma patients. It may follow blunt or penetrating injuries. It may develop acutely or it may take anything from 24-48 hours to accumulate and be clinically evident. Up to 300 ml may not be detected clinically or by X-ray chest (Fig. 14.2), and if suspected, small hemothorax can be detected with ultrasonography. Bleeding from chest injuries may arise from pulmonary lacerations, intercostal vessels, pulmonary or bronchial vessels. In penetrating injuries hemothorax may result from injuries to liver and spleen when the diaphragm has been transgressed.

Diagnosis

Patient may have features of hypovolemic shock and massive collection may further decrease the venous return. Respiratory compromise is usually present if hemothorax is massive. Attention should be paid to correct the blood volume. Bleeding often stops as the pulmonary vessels are low pressure system and there is high concentration of tissue thromboplastin. However, when the bleeding is arterial and from hilar vessels it usually requires aggressive surgical treatment.

Management

Initial management is to achieve hemodynamic stability with intravenous fluid therapy supplemented by blood transfusion. Thoracocentesis as a form of treatment for hemothorax is not a acceptable modality as it fails to evacuate the hemothorax completely and may even hasten the clotting. The aim is not only to evacuate the hemothorax completely and allow the lungs to expand but also to evacuate rapidly for assessment of rate of bleeding and decrease the chances of clotting and adhesion formations. Tube thoracotomy preferably using size 36 F is the treatment of choice. The color of blood, quantity is noted down as it may indicate the need of thoracotomy.

Indication for thoracotomy are:

i. Initial loss more than 1000 ml,
ii. Continuous loss > 200 ml/hr for 4 hr,
iii. Bright red color blood.

Occasionally, one have to use two tubes, one anteriorly to the lungs and the other posteriorly to drain hemothorax well. 5-15% of the patients treated with tube thoracotomy will develop clotted hemothorax or go onto develop fibrothorax.[10] Smaller clotted hematoma may absorb and treated conservatively. The generally accepted indications for surgical evacuation of clotted hemothorax are:

1. Clotted hemothorax large enough to produce loss of 25% of lung volume on chest X-ray.
2. The presence of air fluid level within the residual hemothorax suggesting infection.
3. Fever or leukocytosis.

Ideal time to operate the clotted hemothorax is first week post injury and as the time elapses the adhesion develops and gradually get converted into avascular fibrotic process. Thus, the surgery become more and more hazardous and fraught with complications. It is better to prevent clotted hemothorax by draining acute hemothorax well and adequately.

POST-TRAUMATIC EMPYEMA

Not every hemothorax resolves completely and not all the penetrating wounds chest heal by primary union. The exact incidence of post-traumatic empyema is not known but incidence is higher in penetrating injuries than blunt injuries.

Etiopathogenesis consist of:

1. Penetrating injuries,
2. Infected residual hematoma,
3. Contamination of pleural space in thoraces—abdominal injuries,

4. Ascending infection through chest tubes placed for pneumo/hemothorax,
5. Secondary to pneumonia in flail chest/pulmonary contusion.

Diagnosis

Fever, leukocytosis, fluid collection on X-ray chest are cardinal signs of post-traumatic empyema. Aspiration of purulent/turbid material on thoracocentesis or in the chest tube drainage confirms the diagnosis. The material should be subjected to culture and sensitivity tests. Organisms encountered are *Staphylococcus* or *Streptococcus* in penetrating injuries and gram-negative in cases of thoracoabdominal injuries. When associated with nasocomial pneumonia organisms are mostly the same as are isolated in the sputum.

Management

In some cases of empyema, tube thoracotomy often provides adequate treatment.[11] Response to treatment means that follow-up films show complete drainage of pleural fluid, fever settling down and leukocytosis resolving. If fever and leukocytosis persist and X-ray chest shows minimal changes further evaluation with CT scan chest is desirable.[12] If CT scan demonstrates a residual fluid collection, surgical intervention is indicated. Ideally, surgical intervention early in the course of the disease is easier, response is good and complications are less. Posterolateral thoracotomy is ideal approach. Infected debris removed, all loculations are broken up and the lung is expanded. Chest is drained with three tubes placed in the anterior, posterior and inferior positions. These are removed within 6-7 days. Quite often the assessment and decision-making get delayed due to reliance on tube thoracotomy for a longer period and in these situations resection of the rib, drainage of the loculated pus followed by healing by secondary intention is the treatment of choice.

PULMONARY CONTUSION

Pulmonary contusion classically has been defined as damage to the lung parenchyma that results in edema and hemorrhage without accompanying pulmonary laceration. Recently studies based on CT scan concluded that "pulmonary contusion" is in fact a pulmonary laceration surrounded by intra-alveolar hemorrhage without significant interstitial injury.[13] When one studies the etiopathogenesis and relates it to pathophysiology, it is not difficult to conclude that classical pulmonary contusion, pulmonary laceration, and pulmonary hematoma may be representing spectrum of the same disorder which results due to varying degree of compressive/decompressive injury to pulmonary parenchyma.

Pathophysiology

The degree of distribution of pathologic changes in pulmonary contusion may vary widely, depending on the severity of the injury. In the patients with less severe damage, there are usually focal areas of intra-alveolar hemorrhage with only minimal evidence of interstitial and intra-alveolar edema. There is minimum, if any, alteration in the physiologic function of the lung. With more severe injury, the intra-alveolar extravasation of blood occurs which may be focal, segmental, or lobar in distribution. Alveolar hemorrhage with rupture of alveolar walls and small blood vessels and transudation of fluid into alveolar, and interstitial spaces can be seen microscopically. If there is loss of integrity of the larger pulmonary vessels with the pulmonary injury, hemorrhage may not occur into the alveoli but may dissect along the soft tissues surrounding the vessels and bronchi. In the most severe pulmonary contusions, there is widespread damage to the lungs, and at post-mortem examination the lungs are heavy, edematous, and consolidate. The combination of blood, fluid and cellular debris leads to atelectasis by obstruction of the bronchioles and alveoli. The resultant atelectasis removes these areas as effective units of ventilation and produces alterations in ventilation/perfusion ratio with systemic hypoxia. The elasticity of lungs is reduced and work of respiration is increased which result in an oxygen deficit leading to additional hypoxia and respiratory acidosis. This may result in increased cardiac output to satisfy increased oxygen demand which if carries on for prolonged period may result in cardiac decompensation. Myocardial decompensation will result in inadequate tissue perfusion with accumulation of lactic acid. Thus, metabolic acidosis will be superimposed on the already established respiratory acidosis. Unless it can be corrected, the combination may prove fatal.

Diagnosis

Clinical findings of chest pain, difficulty in breathing, varying grades of hypoxia, diminished breath sounds without any accompaniments, in blunt injury chest patient with or without clinical evidence of fracture ribs should suggest pulmonary contusion. Dyspnea, tachypnea, and weak cough may be the only clinical features. In the early stages (10 to 12 hr) the radiological features may be absent and one may have to rely entirely on history and clinical features to institute the treatment. The radiological diagnosis has been based on the classic findings of a pulmonary infiltrate seen within hours of trauma (Fig. 14.1). The infiltrate may be irregular, coarse nodular densities that are discrete or confluent; homogeneous consolidation; a combination of changes of irregular and homogeneous; or diffuse, often patchy, infiltration of the lung that diminishes and usually disappears completely within a few days.[14-16]

Management

Studies have demonstrated that contused areas of the lungs are sensitive to fluid overload and more so to crystalloids and large volume of unfiltered blood. Thus in prehospital setting and in emergency department fluid should be administered judiciously in cases of patients with thoracic trauma and if the need be central

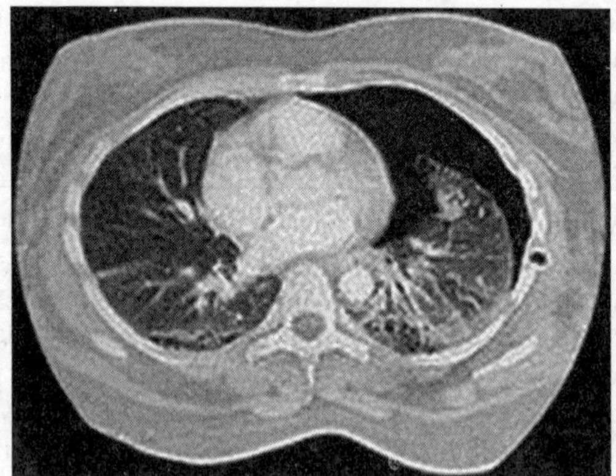

Fig. 14.1: CT scan showing rib fracture, pneumothorax and pulmonary contusion

venous pressure monitoring should be done. Beginning with clinical studies of Avery et al[17] the volume controlled ventilator has been the cornerstone of treatment for chest injuries causing hypoxia for more than 30 years till Trinkle et al[18] proposed a selective approach based on the level of derangement in pulmonary function.

Management consist of aggressive pulmonary care with chest physical therapy, turning of the patient in bed, ambulation, endotracheal suctioning, and bronchoscopy. Pain relief with local intercostal block or epidural analgesia, intravenous fluid administration with CVP monitoring and systemic antibiotics. Indications for intubation are:

- Respiratory distress
- Head injury
- Need for general anesthesia
- Shock
- Airway obstruction.

Many patients never require intubation or may be extubated in less than 72 hr. Most of the patients will respond to the treatment but severe cases will need endotracheal intubation and control of respiration with volume cycled respirator for achieving adequate oxygenation. Indications for ventilator therapy are:

Respiratory rate	>35
Vital capacity (ml/kg body weight)	<15
FEW 1(ml/kg body wt)	<10
Inspiratory force (cm H_2O)	<-25
PaO_2 (mm Hg)	<70 (supplemental O_2)
A-aDO_2 (mm Hg)	>450 (on 100% O_2)
$PaCO_2$ (mm Hg)	>55
VD/Vt	0.60

[FEV1=Volume of gas expired during a forced, rapid expiration from a maximum inspiration in 1 second; A-aDO_2=Alveolar-arterial gradient; Vd/Vt= dead space to tidal volume ratio]

Patients may be divided into three groups depending on severity of the disease (Figs 14.2 to 14.5).

Group 1 patients: These patients may have minimal symptoms and have radiological evidence of pulmonary contusion. Clinical findings of tachypnea, tachycardia, and loose rales may be present. Relief of pain, chest physiotherapy, tracheobronchial lavage, bron-

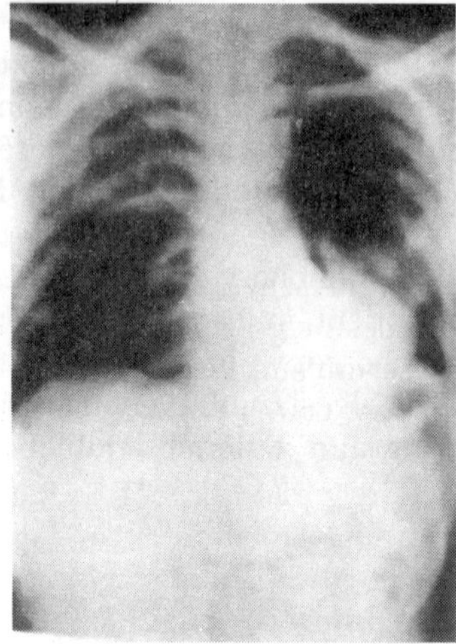

Fig. 14.2: X-ray chest demonstrating multiple ribs fractures and pulmonary contusion on right side and pneumothorax on left side

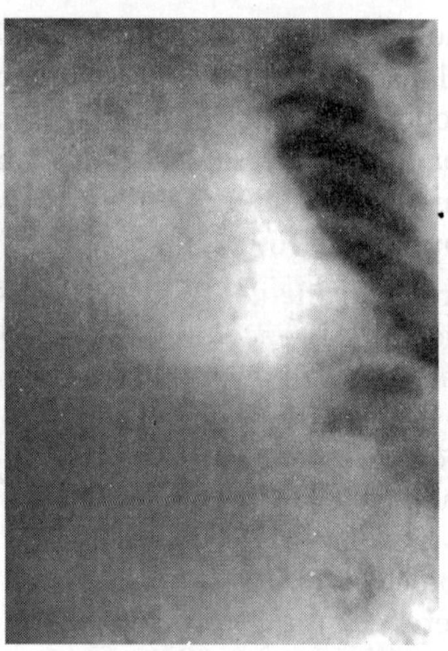

Fig. 14.3: Massive hemothorax right side following GSW chest right

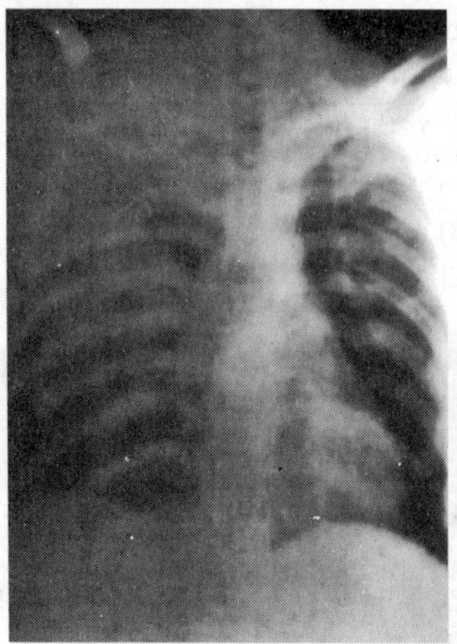

Fig. 14.4: GSW chest. Multiple rib fractures, hemothorax and pulmonary contusion

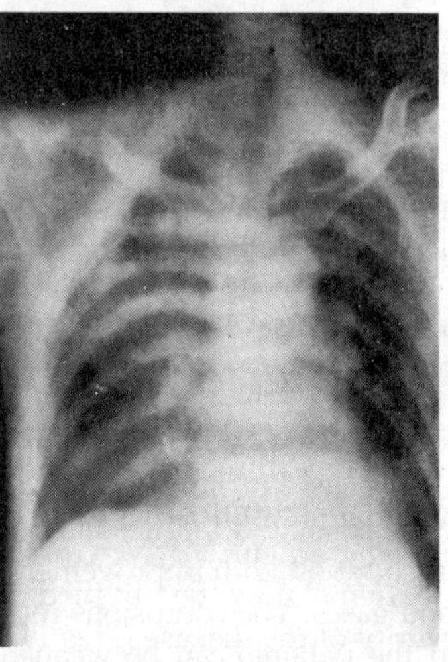

Fig. 14.5: GSW chest showing bullet tract, surgical emphysema, fracture ribs and contusion lung right

chodilators and broad spectrum antibiotics often result in successful management. Intravenous fluids if required, ideally plasma or blood should replace crystalloids as soon as these are available. For blood fine screen filters should be used. The resolution of parenchymal abnormality takes 72-96 hours and survival rates approaches 100%.

Group 2 patients: Initial clinical features are tachypnea, tachycardia and the presence of scattered loose rales heard on auscultation. There is copious amount of mucous, serum and then frank blood in the tracheobronchial tree. The patient cough incessantly and becomes restless, apprehensive and develops labored respiration. The pattern is one of progressive respiratory insufficiency. If facilities are available blood gas analysis should be done. Coincident with the deterioration with the patient's condition there is a progressive fall in PaO_2 and pH, an increase in the $PaCO_2$ and a widening of the alveolar-arterial oxygen gradient. Besides the management as described for group 1 patients, these patients will be benefited with respiratory support. Indications have been already mentioned (vide supra).

Important aspects are:

- Use lowest FiO_2 possible to maintain PaO_2 at 60 mm Hg.
- Use positive end-expiratory pressure if unable to maintain PaO_2 of at least 60 mm Hg on an FiO_2 of 0.6.
- Maintain hematocrit between 40 and 45%.
- Maintain pH between 7.35 and 7.45.
- Limit crystalloid solution to 50 ml/hr.
- Use bronchodilators for bronchospasm.
- Use nasogastric suction.
- Correct metabolic acidosis with intravenous infusion of soda bicarb.
- Make frequent cultures of tracheobronchial secretions.

The course of illness in the majority of group 2 patients is characterized by gradual resolution of the parenchymal abnormalities in association with improvement in clinical condition and in arterial blood gases. The contusions resolve radiologically in 10 to 14 days and the patients can be weaned successfully from the respirator. Mortality rate inspite of optimum therapy is 15%.

Group 3 patients: These patients have sustained a severe pulmonary contusion and show early signs of respiratory failure. Despite the early use of an endotracheal tube, respiratory support, 100%

oxygen, PEEP, maintenance of normal hematocrit and careful regulation of intravenous fluids, the course of disease is one of the rapid, progressive respiratory insufficiency and death occurs from hypoxia within 72-96 hours of injury. The new modes of ventilatory support, viz. high frequency jet ventilation, simultaneous independent lung ventilation, extracorporeal membrane oxygenation have been reported to be successful in isolated cases but it has not improved the survival rate. The important aspect is that in these patients multiple organ failure is so overwhelming that it is doubtful that mere support of oxygenation will be enough to reverse it. Extracorporeal membrane oxygenation may well be used to treat such patients, but it will be successful only as part of a concerted attack on multiple organ failure.

Most of the current practice in treatment of PC-FC derives from a modest quantity of Class II and III work, extrapolation of animal research and "local custom". There is currently no credible human evidence that "fluid restriction" improves outcome though it has been shown to improve oxygenation in animal models. Respiratory dysfunction after contusion may ultimately be shown to relate more to direct traumatic and indirect biochemical effects of the injury rather than amounts of fluid administered. In terms of ventilatory management, the bulk of current evidence favors selective use of mechanical ventilation with analgesia and chest physiotherapy being the preferred initial strategy. When support is required, no specific mode has been shown to be superior to others though there is reasonable evidence that addition of PEEP or CPAP is helpful in improving oxygenation. While the literature supporting the use of independent lung ventilation in severe unilateral. Pulmonary contusion is largely observational, the majority of work supports the opinion that it may be beneficial in select patients. Finally, surgical fixation of flail chest has not been credibly compared to modern selective management, but may also be a valuable addition to the armamentarium in appropriate circumstances.[19]

PULMONARY LACERATION

Pulmonary laceration may follow blunt or penetrating injuries. Penetrating injuries may be due to stab wounds or gunshot wounds. There is extensive damage when gunshot wound is following high velocity weapons (Figs 14.6A and B). Pulmonary

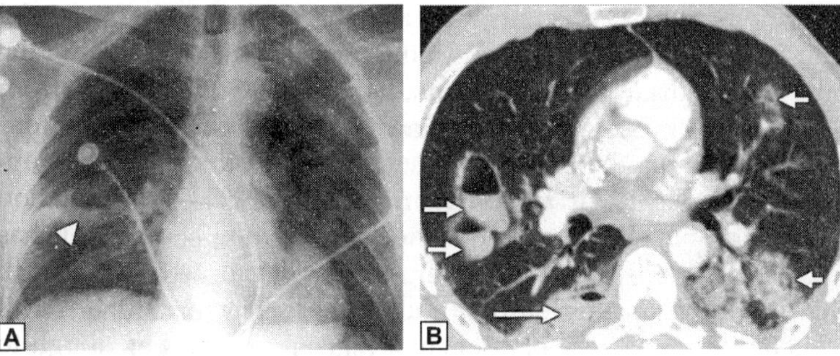

Figs 14.6A and B: Pulmonary lacerations: (A) Chest radiograph shows multifocal patchy airspace opacities in both lungs with an air-fluid level in the midportion of the right lung (arrowhead), findings that represent pulmonary contusions and a laceration, respectively, (B) CT scan reveals multiple pulmonary lacerations (large arrows) in the central portion of the right upper lobe (compression rupture injury) and in the paraspinal portion of the right lower lobe (compression shear injury). Small arrows indicate pulmonary contusions in the left lung. (Radiographics 2008;28:1555-70)

laceration following blunt injuries may be due to the puncture by the fractured rib or may be due to shearing forces. In the later case it is accompanied with pulmonary contusion. Pulmonary laceration has been classified into four types on the basis of CT scan (*see* Fig. 14.1).[19a]

Type 1: Laceration is usually seen as an air filled area or an air fluid interface in an intraparenchymal cavity. Occasionally, the laceration ruptures through the visceral pleura, producing a pneumothorax.

Type 2: Lacerations appear on CT as an air-containing cavity or intraparenchymal air-fluid interface within the paravertebral lung.

Type 3: Lacerations appear as small peripheral cavities or peripheral linear radiolucencies that are always in proximity to the chest wall where a rib has been fractured. Pneumothoraces are often associated with this type of lacerations which are in reality penetrating injuries. A severe form of this will be seen in stab/ gunshot wounds wherein addition hemothorax is also present.

Type 4: Lacerations result from previously formed, firm pleuro-pulmonary adhesions that tear the lung when the overlying chest wall is suddenly compressed or fractured.

Pulmonary lacerations following blunt injury is managed on the lines of management of pulmonary contusions as outlined above after draining the pneumo/hemothorax.

Pulmonary lacerations following stab injuries/gunshot wounds result in hemothorax and/or pneumothorax. Most of these injuries are easily managed with tube thoracotomy. Patients with continued bleeding or large air leaks require open thoracotomy and simple closure of the laceration using absorbable sutures. Limited pulmonary resection must be reserved for patients with concomitant vascular or bronchial injuries. A major resection is rarely necessary for adequate treatment.[20] In cases of massive bleeding, clamping the hilum of the lung may be necessary for temporary control while the site of bleeding is identified and individual vessels are repaired.[21] Principles of management of gunshot wounds of the lung are: prompt and appropriate resort to tube thoracotomy, thoracotomy when evidence of retained blood or blood clot follows tube thoracotomy, resection of contused parenchyma in the face of severe hypoxemia, and prophylactic antibiotics.

Complications

Complications are not common but include infection, pulmonary abscess, and bronchopleural fistula (a fistula between the pleural space and the bronchial tree). A bronchopleural fistula results when there is a communication between the laceration, a bronchiole, and the pleura; it can cause air to leak into the pleural space despite the placement of a chest tube. The laceration can also enlarge, as may occur when the injury creates a valve that allows air to enter the laceration, progressively expanding it.[22] One complication, air embolism, in which air enters the bloodstream, is potentially fatal, especially when it occurs on the left side of the heart. Air can enter the circulatory system through a damaged vein in the injured chest and can travel to any organ; it is especially deadly in the heart or brain. Positive pressure ventilation can cause pulmonary embolism by forcing air out of injured lungs and into blood vessels.[23]

REFERENCES

1. Beeson A, Saegesser F. Colour atlas of chest trauma and associated injuries. Oradell. Medical Economics Book. 1983.
2. LoCicero J III, Mattox KL. Epidemiology of chest trauma. Surg Clin North Am 1989;69:15.
3. Beall AC, Crawford HW, DeBakey ME. Considerations in the management of acute traumatic haemothorax. J Thoracic Cardiovasc Surg 1966;52:351.
4. Hankings J, Attar S, Turney S, et al. Differential diagnosis of pulmonary parenchymal changes in thoracic trauma. Am Surg 1973;39:309.
5. Carrico CJ, Hudson LD. Post injury acute pulmonary failure. In Shires GT (Ed): Principles of Trauma Surgey, third ed. NewYork, McGraw-Hill, 1984.
6. Moore FD. Post-traumatic pulmonary insufficiency. Philadelphia, Saunders, 1969.
7. Brigham KL, Harris TR, Bowers RE, et al. Lung vascular permeability. Inferences from measurments of plasma to lung lymph protein transport. Lymphology 1979;12:177.
8. Daughtry DC, Daughtry JD. The initial management of thoracic trauma. In Daughtry Dc (Ed): Thoracic Trauma Boston, Little, Brown, 1980.
9. Eddy AC, Carrico CJ, Rusch VW. Injury to lung and pleura. In Moore EE, Mattox KL, Feliciano DV (Eds): Trauma, second ed. California, Appleton and Lange, 1991;357-71.
10. Kish G, Kozloff L, Joseph WL, et al. Indications for early thoracotomy for management of chest trauma. Ann Thorac Surg 1976;22:23.
11. Thomas DF, Glass JL, Bisch BF. Management of streptococcal empyema. Ann Thorac Surg 1966;2:658.
12. Stark DD, Federle MP, Goodman PC. CT and radiographic assessment of tube thoracostomy. AJR 1983;141;163.
13. Wagner RB, Jamieson PM. Pulmonary contusion: Evaluation and classification by computed tomography. Surg Clin North Am 1989;69:31-40.
14. Crawford WO Jr. Pulmonary injury in thoracic and nonthoracic trauma. Radiol Clin North Am 1973;11:527.
15. Stevens E, Templeton AW. Traumatic nonpenetrating lung contusion. Radiology 1965;85:247.
16. Williams JR, Bonte FJ. Roentgenological aspect of nonpenetrating chest injuries. Springfield, Charles C Thomas, 1961;36.

17. Avery E, Morch E, Benson D. Critically crushed chests. A new method of treatment with continuous mechanical hyperventilation to produce alkalotic apnoea and internal pneumatic stabilisation. J Thorac Surg 1956;32:291-311.
18. Trinkle K, Richardson J, Franz J, et al. Management of flail chest without mechanical ventilation. Ann Thorac Surg 1975;19:355-63.
19. Bruce Simon, James Ebert, Faran Bokhari, Jeanette Capella, Timothy Emhoff, Thomas Hayward III, Aurelio Rodriguez, Lou Smith. Practice Management Guideline for "Pulmonary Contusion-Flail Chest" June 2006 EAST Practice Management Workgroup for Pulmonary Contusion-Flail Chest
19a. Wagner RB, Crawford WO Jr, Schimpf PP. Classification of parenchymal injuries of the lungs. Radiology 1988;167:77.
20. Kirsh MM, Sloan H (eds). Management of pulmonary contusion and related injuries. In Blunt chest Trauma. Boston, Little Brown, 1977, p19.
21. Moghissi K. Laceration of the lung following blunt trauma. Thorax 1971;26:223
22. Miller LA . "Chest wall, lung, and pleural space trauma". Radiologic Clinics of North America 2006;44 (2): 213–24.
23. Matthay RA, George RB, Light RJ, Matthay MA, (Us). "Thoracic trauma, surgery, and perioperative management". Chest Medicine: Essentials of Pulmonary and Critical Care Medicine. Hagerstown, MD: Lippincott Williams & Wilkins 2005;pp. 580.

Injuries of Diaphragm

SK Kochar

Incidence of diaphragm injury is 4.5%[1] if all cases of polytrauma are taken into account. When only penetrating injuries to chest are considered the incidence rises to almost 15% and when the wound of entry is located anteriorly and below nipple the incidence is more than 30%.[2] Thus in all wounds in the lower chest the diaphragmatic injury must be suspected and looked for. Due to its intimate relation with abdominal organ, associated intra-abdominal injury may go up to 45% in gunshot wounds[3] though the incidence is lower for stab wounds. When considering diaphragmatic injury one must keep in mind that anteriorly the diaphragm rises to 4th space on right side and 5th space on left side.

Mechanism of Injury

The injury to the diaphragm may follow penetrating wound or due to blunt trauma. Penetrating injuries are due to gunshot wounds or stab wounds while blunt injury is commonly encountered in vehicle accidents/compression due to house collapse/fall from heights or direct forceful impact as in lathi blow or fall against lap seat belt. In penetrating injuries stab which are directed downward and below nipple line to lower chest are more likely to injuries to the diaphragm than the one in the right hypocondrium. Any gunshot wounds to the lower chest, where entry is below nipple line one must assume that the diaphragmatic injury has occurred till not proved otherwise. In penetrating injury the incidence of right and left diaphragm are equal in frequency[4] but in blunt injury the rupture on left side is five to six times more common.[5] This could be due to the fact that the liver dissipates the force generated by blunt trauma broadly over the right hemidiaphragm more adequately and protects it from rupture. Penetrating injuries are rents in diaphragm of size of 1-2 cm but shot gun wounds from close range may give rise to disruption of a larger area of diaphragm. Blunt injuries are larger and irregular tears and these usually radiate posterolaterally from the central tendinous portion of the left, and less from the right hemidiaphragm. Bilateral diaphragmatic tears and complex unilateral rents extending into the pericardial surface are also reported.[6]

Diagnosis

Sign, symptoms of associated injuries overshadow the diaphragmatic tear. Tear of right side may be detected at thoracotomy when dealing with the chest injury or at laparotomy when dealing with intra-abdominal injuries. As it often happens most of the penetrating injuries of chest are treated with thoracotomy without further investigation and the diaphragmatic injury is missed. Similarly, in blunt injury patient may not be subjected to laparotomy as the indications may not exist and the injury to diaphragm may be missed. Strong suspicion of diaphragmatic injury in all cases of penetrating injury to chest below nipple line and to investigate to rule it out, will definitely decrease the missed injuries.

Blunt trauma produces no external signs that are pathognomic of diaphragmatic injury. The patient with multiple displaced ribs and/or sternal fractures has clearly sustained severe trauma and requires meticulous attention directed to the possibility of a diaphragmatic injury. Physical examination is helpful in those patients who have acute herniation of abdominal contents into left chest following injury of left dome of diaphragm. The physical signs are: (i) prominence and immobility of the left chest, (ii) displacement of the area of cardiac dullness to the right, (iii) absence of breath sounds over the left thorax, (iv) auscultation of bowel sounds over the left thorax, and (v) tympany to percussion over the left thorax.

X-ray chest may demonstrate pneumothorax/hemothorax or lower lobe pulmonary contusion on the involved side in 50% of the cases of penetrating injury.[7] In blunt trauma the relevant dome of the diaphragm may be raised on the right side while on left stomach or colonic gas shadow may be visualized (Fig. 15.1). Fluoroscopy which has gone out of vogue is often helpful but in polytrauma it may not be practical to perform. USG has been found to be fairly accurate in the evaluation of diaphragmatic rupture.[8] In fact we perform USG in all cases where diaphragmatic rupture is suspected after the patient has been adequately resuscitated. Being dynamic it not only demonstrates the tear but it also defines the movement of the diaphragm and assesses the pleural cavity, liver and the spleen which are commonly associated injured organs.

Multidetector CT with coronal and sagittal reformation can show even a small diaphragmatic discontinuity and help identify any herniated viscera (Figs 15.2 and 15.3). Other CT signs of diaphragmatic injury include the "collar" sign, the "dependent viscera" sign, diaphrag matic thickening, and peridiaphragmatic contrast material extravasation. The collar sign is produced by a waiste-like constriction of herniated viscera at the site of herniation. The dependent viscera sign results from the abdominal viscera falling dependently against the posterior chest wall through the diaphragmatic tear. Injuries to the diaphragm are commonly accompanied by hemothorax and hemoperitoneum. Blood on both sides of the diaphragm without obvious intra-abdominal injury should raise suspicion for possible diaphragmatic injury. CT has an overall sensitivity in the diagnosis of blunt diaphragmatic rupture of 70–100%, with a greater sensitivity for left-sided injuries, and a specificity of 75–100%.[9]

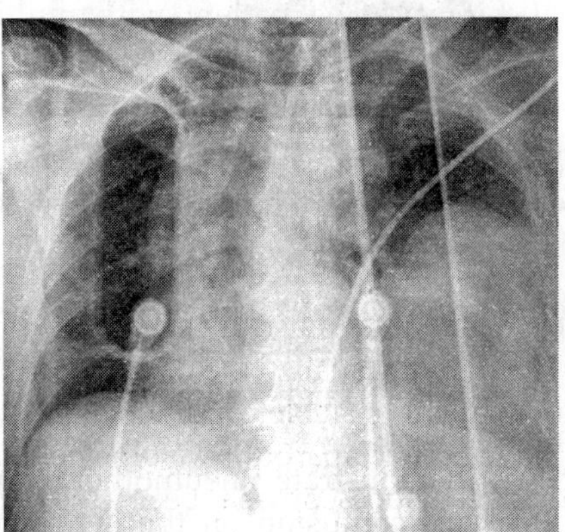

Fig. 15.1: Diaphragmatic injury. Chest radiograph shows marked elevation of the left hemidiaphragm

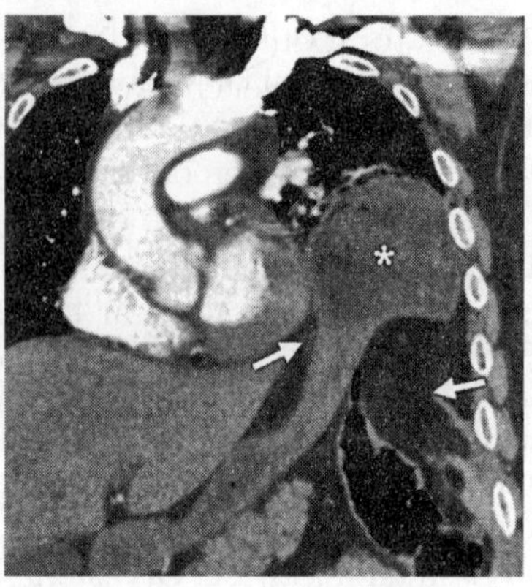

Fig. 15.2: Diaphragmatic injury. Coronal reformatted CT images reveal a large left diaphragmatic defect (arrows) with herniation of the stomach (asterisk) into the thorax

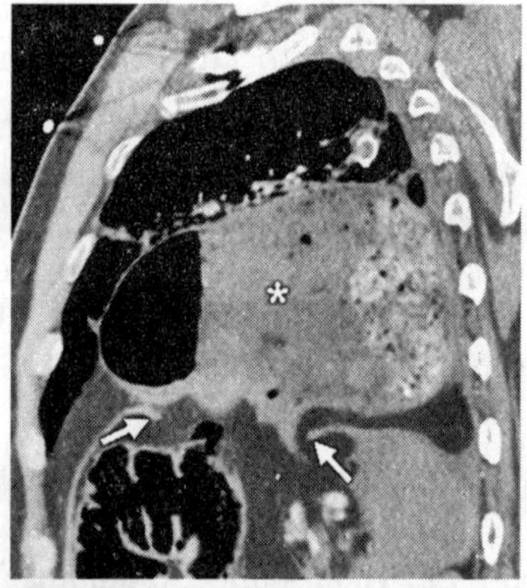

Fig. 15.3: Diaphragmatic injury. Sagittal reformatted CT images reveal a large left diaphragmatic defect (arrows) with herniation of the stomach (asterisk) into the thorax

Magnetic resonance imaging (MRI) may aid in the diagnosis because it can accurately visualize the diaphragm's anatomy. MRI may be used in a patient in stable condition who has an equivocal diagnosis and no need for laparotomy (some penetrating injuries) or for late diagnosis. Thoracoscopy has been used to better visualize the diaphragm when the diagnosis is unconfirmed and laparotomy is not required. The best way to diagnose diaphragmatic injury is to suspect it and to look for it during laparotomy/thoracotomy in case of penetrating injuries to lower chest and in blunt polytrauma.

Management

The abdominal approach to repair is most useful in the acutely injured patients because it allows thorough exploration of the abdomen. The thoracic approach is preferred for chronic hernia because the sac of the hernia must be excised to achieve a satisfactory repair. The repair is done in two layers. The first layer is formed from mattress sutures of 0 suture, the second layer is of 2-0 suture. Nonabsorbable material is used. Repair must be done for all tears however small it may be. Occasionally, one may have to use prosthesis to close the defect. Polypropylene patches seem to be favored by most surgeons.

Laparoscopy is an excellent diagnostic and therapeutic tool in hemodynamically stable patients. Left-sided diaphragm injury can be successfully treated with laparoscopic repair. However, right-sided diaphragm may be better with thoracoscopic repair[10] Large traumatic diaphragmatic injuries adjacent to or including the esophageal hiatus are best approached via laparotomy.[11]

REFERENCES

1. Rodkey GV. The management of abdominal injuries. Surg Clin North Am 1966;46:627.
2. Robison PD, Harman PK, Grover FL, et al. The management of penetrating lung injuries in civilian practice. J Thorac Cardiovasc Surg 1988;95:184.
3. Moore JB, Moore EE, Thomson JS. Abdominal injuries associated with penetrating trauma in the lower chest. Am J Surg 1980;140:724.
4. Schneider CF. Traumatic diaphragmatic hernia. Am J Surg 1956;91:290.
5. Brooks JW. Blunt traumatic rupture of the diaphragm. Ann Thorac Surg 1978;26:199.
6. Bernatz PE, Burnside AF Jr, Clagett OT. Problem of the ruptured diaphragm. JAMA 1958;168:877.
7. Miller OL, Bennet EV, Root HD, et al. Management of penetrating and blunt diaphragmatic injury. J Trauma 1984;24:403.
8. Ammann A, Brewer WH, Maull KI, et al. Traumatic rupture of the diaphragm. Real time sonographic diagnosis. Am J Radiol 1988;140:915.

9. Mirvis SE, Shanmuganathan K. Imaging hemidiaphragmatic injury. Eur Radiol 2007;17:1411-21.
10. Opasanon S, Akaraviputh T, Keorochana K, Somcharit L. The role of laparoscopic management in suspected traumatic diaphragmatic injury patients: a tertiary care center experience. J Med Assoc Thai. 2009 Jul;92(7):903-8.
11. Matthews BD, Bui H, Harold KL, Kercher KW, Adrales G, Park A, Sing RF, Heniford BT. Laparoscopic repair of traumatic diaphragmatic injuries. Surg Endosc. 2003;17(2):254-8.

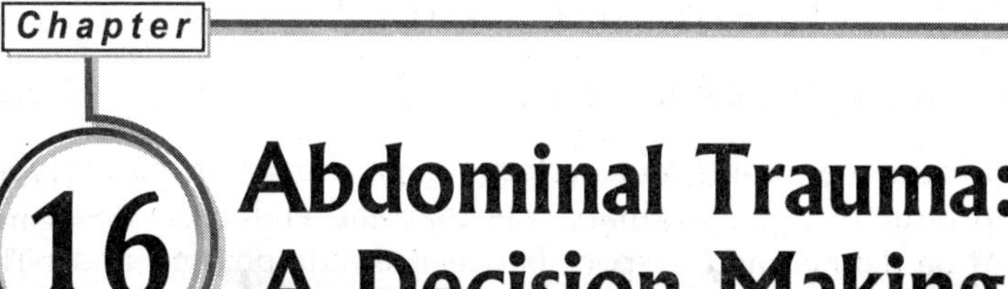

Chapter 16 Abdominal Trauma: A Decision Making

Gurjit Singh, B Easwaran

Abdominal trauma makes a sizeable portion of all trauma cases across the globe. Blunt and penetrating abdominal trauma are major causes of morbidity and mortality particularly because it can be very difficult to recognize clear symptoms early. Blunt trauma is often a diagnostic challenge while penetrating trauma is difficult to evaluate. Morbidity and mortality of delayed diagnosis is very high while the outcome of timely treatment is very rewarding.

In blunt abdominal trauma, the spleen and liver are the most commonly injured organs with a mortality rate of roughly 8.5%.[1] Nearly three quarters of all blunt abdominal trauma injuries involve vehicle.[2] Almost two-thirds of injuries occur in males with a peak incidence in patients between ages 14 and 30.

Penetrating abdominal trauma has a slightly higher mortality rate, depending on the mechanism of injury. It ranges up to about 12% and is responsible for more than a third of urban trauma center admissions and 12% of rural trauma center admissions. Gunshot and stab wounds combine to cause 95% of penetrating abdominal injuries. Penetrating abdominal injuries have a significantly higher morbidity rate than blunt trauma, with the most serious morbidities arising from wound site infection and development of intra-abdominal abscesses.

Pediatric patients warrant special mention because their abdominal anatomy differs from adults. Fewer than 10% of pediatric injuries are considered abdominal trauma in nature, however more than 80% of pediatric abdominal injuries are caused by blunt force trauma.[1] Pediatric abdominal injuries may be caused by abuse and organ injury rates differ from adults due to unique pediatric anatomy.

Anatomical Considerations

The abdomen holds and protects major organs of the digestive, reproductive, genitourinary, vascular and endocrine systems. It can be defined as the space between the diaphragm and pelvic bony structures on the superior and inferior aspects respectively; the flanks along the lateral walls; the abdominal muscles anteriorly; and the vertebrae and back muscles along the posterior cavity wall.

Four regions divide the abdominal cavity. Firstly the intra-thoracic region which runs from the base of the 12th ribs to the diaphragm includes spleen, stomach, diaphragm and a portion of liver. The ribs make complete assessment of the cavity difficult but not impossible. Second region beginning at the superior aspects of the iliac crests and called pelvic abdominal region. It is the space within the pelvic bones and contains the bladder, rectum, small intestine and female reproductive system. Third is retroperitoneal region which gets separated by connective tissue. It contains the kidneys, ureters, pancreas, aorta and inferior vena cava. Finally, the remaining space is the true abdominal region which contains the large and small intestines, part of the liver, a gravid uterus and distended stomach. The peritoneum is the connective tissue membrane holding in the contents of the true abdominal region. Traditionally, the true abdominal region is divided into four quadrants: right upper, right lower, left upper and left lower.

Organs are defined as either solid or hollow. Solid organ generally bleed when injured whereas hollow organs spill their contents into the abdominal cavity causing peritonitis.

Pediatric patients have many unique abdominal anatomical differences worth mentioning. There is significantly less protection as the muscle walls are thinner and there is less fat. Ribs protecting the thoracic abdomen have an increased flexibility compared to adult ribs and while this protects the rib from damage, it more easily allows injury to the abdominal organs. Solid organs within the pediatric abdomen have a larger surface area relative to adult organs, thus a greater area is exposed for potential injury. The organ attachments are also more elastic which increase the chances of tearing and shearing injuries. In the pediatric patient the bladder also extends to the umbilicus increasing its chance for injury.

Abdominal trauma can be caused by vehicle accidents, stabs wounds, gunshot wounds, bomb/explosive blasts, compression/ crushing injuries, direct blow or impact and seat belt injuries.

Classifications

Blunt injuries
- Acceleration/deceleration injuries
- Direct blow/impact
- Compression injuries
- Crushing injuries

Penetrating injuries
- Gunshot injuries
  - Low velocity
  - High velocity
- Shot gun injuries
- Stab injuries
- Bomb/explosive blasts.

Pathophysiology

Vehicular trauma is by far the leading cause of blunt abdominal trauma in the civilian population. Auto to auto and auto to pedestrian collisions have been cited as causes in 50-75% of cases. Rare causes of blunt abdominal injuries include iatrogenic trauma during cardiopulmonary resuscitation, manual thrusts to clear an airway, and the Heimlich maneuver.

Intra-abdominal injuries secondary to blunt force are attributed to collision between the injured person and the external environment and to acceleration or deceleration forces acting on the persons internal organs. Blunt force injuries to the abdomen can generally be explained by three mechanisms.

The first is when rapid deceleration causes differential movement among adjacent structures. As a result, shear forces are created and cause hollow, solid, visceral organs and vascular pedicles to tear, especially at relatively fixed points, of attachment. For example, rupture occurring between mobile aortic arch portion and distal aorta, at renal pedicles, at duodenojejunal junction or retrohepatic vena cava.

The second is when intra-abdominal contents are crushed between the anterior abdominal wall and the vertebral column or posterior thoracic age. This produces a crushing effect to which solid viscera (e.g. spleen, liver, kidneys) are specially vulnerable.

The third is external compression forces that result in a sudden and dramatic rise in intra-abdominal pressure and culminate in rupture of a hollow viscus organ thereby spilling their contents into the abdominal cavity.

Penetrating trauma occurs when an object enters through the skin and wall of the abdominal cavity. The most common mechanism for penetrating trauma is gunfire followed by stabbing and blast of explosive devices. Other causes include impalement and animal bites. As the object enters the abdominal cavity, it injuries the organs in two ways. First, the object physically damages organ tissues as it penetrates. Second, while passing through organ tissue, the object sends a wave of pressure in all directions, stretching the organs, which can injury adjacent organs and not just the impacted organ. Organs stretch because of their elastic nature and can cause both a temporary and permanent cavity. The greater the speed of a penetrating object, the more kinetic energy is transmitted to the organs, increasing the chance for ricochet off bony objects and for fragmentation.

Pattern of organ involved in a large series[3] shows relative incidence of spleen 46%, liver 33%, mesentery 09% involvement in that order. However in penetrating injuries small intestines is most commonly injured organ followed by liver, colon and stomach.[4]

Assessment

During the care of any trauma patient, begin an initial assessment following the ABCDE mnemonic.

An abdominal assessment becomes a key component of the secondary assessment and requires adequate time to complete thoroughly.

However, it is imperative not to develop tunnel vision, looking for abdominal trauma findings and ignoring the remainder of the assessment. While evaluating abdomen as part of the entire body, prioritize injuries in order of importance and severity.

The initial assessment of a trauma patient begins at the scene of the injury, with information provided by the patient, family, bystanders, or paramedics. Important factors relevant to the care of a patient with blunt abdominal trauma, specifically those involving motor vehicles, include the following:

- The extent of vehicular damage.
- Whether prolonged extrication was required.

- Whether passenger space was intruded.
- Whether a passenger died.
- Whether the person was ejected from the vehicle.
- The role of safety devices such as seat belts and airbags.
- The presence of alcohol or drug use.
- The presence of head or spinal cord injury.
- Whether psychiatric problems were evident.

When evaluating penetrating trauma, determine the object, distance it traveled to the patient, speed, on scene external blood loss and time of injury. The distance the object traveled to the patient is actually important as the chance for serious injury decreases if the distance exceeds 10 feet (3 meters).[5]

Resuscitation is performed concomitantly and continues while physical examination is performed and completed. The secondary survey is the identification of all injuries via a head-to-toe examination.

It is imperative for all personal involved in the direct care of a trauma patient to exercise universal precautions against body fluid exposure.

The evaluation of a patient with blunt abdominal trauma must be accomplished with the entire patient in mind, with all injuries prioritized accordingly. This implies that injuries involving the head, the respiratory system or the cardiovascular system may take precedence over an abdominal injury. The abdomen should neither be ignored nor be the sole focus of the treating clinician and surgeon.

The initial clinical assessment of patients with blunt abdominal trauma is often difficult and notably inaccurate. Associated injuries often cause tenderness and spasms in the abdominal wall and make diagnosis difficult. Its general accuracy increases if the patient is examined repeatedly and at frequent intervals.

However repeated examinations may not be feasible in patients who need general anesthesia and surgery for other injuries. The greatest compromise of the physical examination occurs in the setting of neuralgic dysfunction, which may be caused by head injury or substance abuse.

When there are indicators of abdominal trauma (Table 16.1) repeat an abdominal examination as time permits to look for the most reliable signs of internal injuries: The most reliable sign of an intra-abdominal injury is shock without an otherwise identifiable cause.[6]

Table 16.1: Indicators of abdominal trauma
• Mechanism of injury consistent with abdominal compression
• Bent steering wheel
• Safety belt impressions
• Shock without a obvious cause
• Soft tissue injury to the lower thorax, back, flank or abdomen
• Significant tenderness on palpation on coughing
• Involuntary guarding

The physician evaluating the abdomen should answer two questions: (a) Is there an intra-abdominal injury and (b) does this injury require operative repair? While addressing these issue, two principles should not be violated: (a) the ABCs should be adequately assessed before focusing on the abdomen and (b) clinical examination should be the most important element of the evaluation.

Despite the technological advances, which undoubtedly add greatly to the ability to evaluate the abdomen, clinical examination remains of paramount importance. Clinical examination can determine the need for emergent exploration following abdominal trauma by the presence of one or both of two signs: (a) peritonitis and (b) hemodynamic instability. In the absence of these two signs, there is time for more detailed investigations.

Hemodynamic stability (or instability) is a term, which is widely used but insufficiently understood. At the initial stage, the hemodynamic status is usually assessed by crude methods, such as heart rate, blood pressure and urine output monitoring, serum hemoglobin measurement and evaluation of the skin and capillary refill. Although such information is very important, one needs to remember the limitations of using these measurements to assess hemodynamic instability. Hypotension may be occurring in the presence of spinal cord injury without blood loss. Hypertension may occur even in the presence of blood loss due to increased intracranial pressure and as Cushing's reflex. A blood pressure of 110 mm Hg may be normal for a 25-year-old man, abnormally high for a six-month-old baby and profusely low for a 70 years old hypertensive woman. The heart rate can be high for cause unrelated to bleeding such as pain or anxiety, on the other hand a normal or low heart rate cannot exclude bleeding particularly in patients, with high spinal cord injuries, chronic cocaine intoxications or beta-blocker medication. Paradoxical bradycardia occurs in up to 29% of hypotensive trauma patients.[7] For this reason a more precise description of the hemodynamic status of the patient is highly desirable. Pulmonary artery catheterization is not logistically feasible in most acute trauma areas. Now non-invasive technology allows continuous monitoring of the cardiac output, stroke volume, and transcutaneous oxygen tension.[8] In summary hemodynamic instability is a valid reason for laparotomy as long as the physician recognizes the limitations of vital signs and incorporates additional elements in the decision making to increase its accuracy.

Physical Examination

Begin an abdominal examination by exposing the entire abdomen from the nipple line to the groin. The standard sequence for an abdominal assessment is: inspection, palpation, percussion and auscultation.

On inspection there may be tell-tale evidence of the injury to the abdomen. Ecchymosis, contusions, lacerations, abrasions will point out to the involvement of the abdomen and could be taken, as a pointer to internal hemorrhage in case of patient in shock. Lap belt impression is a strong, indicator of injury. Two bruising pattern, i.e. Cullen's sign around umbilicus and Grey-Turner's sign in the flanks are indicative of blunt force hemorrhage, aortic leak, pancreas or kidney bleeds but appear late. One must look for abdominal distention. Expose genitalia to look for swellings, bruising and blood accumulation. Identify any impaled object or entrance wound from a penetrating object. Do not routinely remove impaled objects from the abdomen at preliminary examination.

Palpate abdomen for masses, tenderness, rigidity guarding and deformity systematically in each quadrant. Palpate inferior ribs for any tenderness which may suggest fracture and possible injury to underlying organ like liver or spleen. Renal angles and spine should be examined for any tenderness. The iliac crest and symphysis pubis should be compressed to establish possibility of a pelvic fracture.

Abdomen is examined for free fluid. Auscultation of chest will suggest rupture of diaphragm when bowel sounds are heard in thoracic cavity.

Bowel sounds will be absent following hollow viscus injury or a bruit may be heard over renal artery area in case of injury to the vessel.

A rectal examination should be performed to search for evidence of bony penetration from a pelvic fracture and the stool should be evaluated for gross or occult blood. The evaluation of rectal tone is important for determining the patient's neurological status and palpation of high riding prostate suggest urethral injury.

Pediatric patient are assessed and treated at least initially as adults with respect to the primary and secondary surveys. However, obvious anatomical and clinical differences exist and these must be kept in mind. The child's physiologic response to injury is different, communication is not always possible, hence physical examination findings become more important. The pediatric patient's blood volume is less, predisposing them to rapid exsanguination; technical procedures tend to be more time consuming and challenging and a child's relatively large body surface area contributes to rapid heat loss. Perhaps the most significant difference between pediatric and adult blunt trauma is that for the most part, pediatric patient can be resuscitated and treated nonoperatively.[9]

Concept of tertiary examination was first introduced by Enderson et al to assist in the diagnosis of any injuries that may have been missed during the primary and secondary surveys.[10] The tertiary survey involves a repetition of the primary and secondary surveys and a revision of all laboratory and radiographic studies. In one study a tertiary trauma survey detected 56% of injuries, missed during the initial assessment within 24 hours of admission.

Laboratory Investigations

There are no specific investigations which can point out to organ injury but many investigations directly or indirectly indicate intra-abdominal injury. Fall of hemoglobin, hematocrit indicate internal hemorrhage though it may take sometime to fall and besides that it depends on the quantum and the rate of bleeding. Pretrauma hemoglobin level is not known for assessing the fall but it is important to be part of baseline investigation. Valuable blood studies in the initial evaluation of a patient with abdominal trauma vary by institution but should include a CBC count, coagulation studies, blood type and blood crossmatch, urine analysis and urine pregnancy test in females of appropriate age. Serum electrolyte values, creatinine level and glucose value are often obtained for reference but typically they have little or no value in the initial management period. The serum lipase or amylase level is neither sensitive nor specific as a marker for major pancreatic or enteric injury. Normal levels do not exclude a major pancreatic injury. Elevated levels may be caused by injuries to the head and face or by an assortment of nontraumatic causes (e.g. alcohol, narcotics, various other drugs). Amylase or lipase levels may be elevated because of pancreatic ischemia caused by the systemic hypotension that accompanies trauma. However persistent hyperamylasemia or hyperlipasemia should raise the suggestion of significant intra-abdominal injury and is an indication for aggressive radiographic and surgical intervention.

Although the overall value of plain films in the evaluation of patients, with blunt abdominal trauma is limited they can demonstrate numerous findings.

Chest radiograph may aid in diagnosis of abdominal injuries such as ruptured hemidiaphragm (e.g. a nasogastric tube seen in the chest) or pneumopertioneum (Figs 16.1 and 16.2).

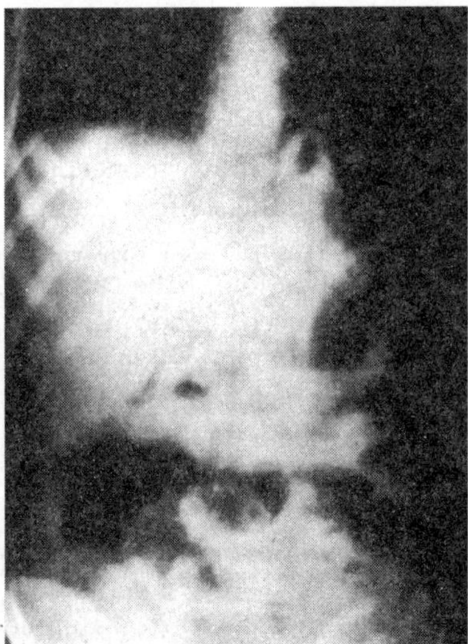

Fig. 16.1: Across the table view demonstrating air behind the parietes in case of perforated hollow viscus

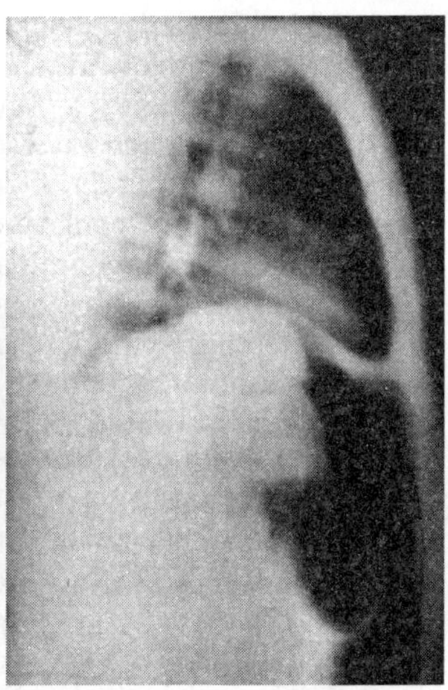

Fig. 16.2: Plain X-ray abdomen (standing) showing air under the dome of diaphragm

A search should be made for rib, pelvic, vertebral body and transverse spinous process fractures as these may indicate nearby visceral damage. There may be loss of renal or psoas shadow in case of retroperitoneal hemorrhage. Displacement of gastric air bubble and any soft tissue mass in liver or splenic area will indicate presence of a hematoma. Trapped retroperitoneal air from duodenal perforation may be seen.

As part of emergency department's assessment, the physician is likely to select one or more of the following three tests to look for the blood in the abdomen. Viz diagnostic peritoneal lavage (DPL), focused assessment with sonography for trauma (FAST) and computed tomography (CT).

Diagnostic Peritoneal Lavage

Diagnostic peritoneal lavage (DPL) was developed by Root et al in 1965.[11] It is rapid inexpensive, accurate and relatively safe. Subsequent studies have confirmed the efficacy of DPL in diagnosing abdominal hemorrhage as well as its superiority over physical examination alone.[12]

DPL is indicated in blunt trauma in: (1) Patients, with a spinal cord injury, (2) those with multiple injuries and unexplained shock, (3) obtunded patients with possible abdominal injury, (4) intoxicated patients in whom abdominal injury is suggested, and (5) patients with potential intra-abdominal injury who will undergo prolonged anesthesia for another procedure. The only absolute contraindication to DPL is the obvious need for laparotomy. Relative contraindications, include morbid obesity, a history of multiple abdominal surgeries and pregnancy.

Whatever may be the method of introduction of the catheter, 1l of 0.9% sodium chloride solution is infused. If permitted by clinical condition, the patient is rolled from side-to-side or time is given for infused fluid to mix with peritoneal contents. Fluid is then drained out by gravity by lowering the bottle to the floor.

The fluid is sent to laboratory for RBC count, WBC count, amylase and alkaline phosphatase levels and the presence of bile, bacteria. The criteria for positive DPL[13,14] is shown in Table 16.2.

The accuracy DPL has been reported between 92% and 98%.[15] The high sensitivity of DPL is due to the significant false positive rate of the technique.[16] Several authors have highlighted the importance of interpreting DPL results in the context of the overall

Table 16.2: The criteria for positive DPL

Index	*Positive*	*Equivocal*
Aspirate		
Blood	>10 ml	>5 ml
Fluid	Enteric contents	–
Lavage		
Red blood cells	>100,000/mm^3	>50,000/mm^3
White blood cells	>500/ mm^3	>200 /mm^3
Enzymes	Amylase >20 IU/L	–
Alkaline phosphatase	>3 ml	
Bile	Confirmed biochemically	

clinical condition of the patient. A positive DPL does not necessarily mandate immediate laparotomy in the hemodynamically stable patient[17] DPL has been shown to be more efficient than CT scan in identifying patients that require surgical exploration.[18]

The complication rate associated with DPL is quite low.[19] The incidence of complication is lower for open DPL compared to with the closed technique. The false positive rate for DPL is increased in patients with pelvic fracture.[20] In order to avoid sampling the retroperitoneal hematoma, a supraumbilical approach has been recommended, theoretically reducing the chances of false positive result.[21]

The advantages of DPL for detection of hollow visceral injuries have been clearly demonstrated.[22] Two studies which advocate analysis of DPL fluid for amylase and alkaline phosphatase consistent with enteric injuries have been disputed.[23] Similarly, the utility of DPL white blood cell (WBC) count has been questioned.[24] DPL is sensitive for mesenteric injury and, infact has been shown be superior to CT for the diagnosis of this injury.[25]

DPL has been shown in some studies to have diagnostic accuracy of 98-100%, sensitivity of 98-100% and specificity of 90-96%. It has some advantages, including high sensitivity, rapidity, and immediate, interpretation. Its limitations include iatrogenic abdominal injury and its high sensitivity which can lead to non-therapeutic laparotomies.

However because the technique is invasive and fails to identify the source of bleeding and the need for operative repair, DPL is used with decreasing frequency over the years. Therefore, DPL in today's health care environment is used predominantly when CT or FAST are not available, if there is insufficient expertise to make decision based on the FAST result or if the FAST results are negative but there is no other source to account for the hemodynamic instability.[26]

Ultrasound

It is an excellent modality for solid organ injury and also for assessment of retroperitoneal structures. However, it has not been of much help in hollow viscus injury. It is noninvasive, may be easily performed and can be done concurrently with resuscitation (Fig. 16.3).

In addition, the technology is portable and may be easily reported if necessary. In most cases procedures may be completed within 3 to 4 minutes. The test is specialty useful for detecting intra-abdominal hemorrhage in the multiply injured or pregnant patient.[27]

In recent years, focused assessment sonography for trauma (FAST) has emerged as a useful diagnostic test in the evaluations of blunt abdominal trauma.

In 1996, the examination was first termed focused abdominal sonography for trauma. However, in 1997 the FAST consensus conference committee concluded that the acronym should stand for focused assessment with sonography for trauma.

The FAST examination is based on the assumption that all clinically significant abdominal injuries are associated with

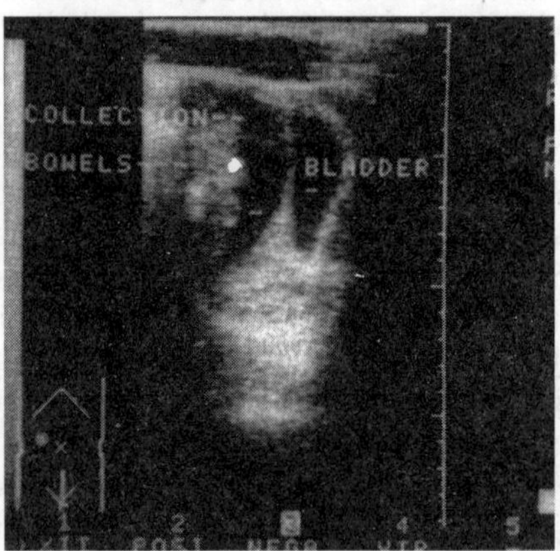

Fig. 16.3: USG abdomen showing free fluid in the abdomen as collection around the loops of intestines following traumatic intestinal perforation

hemoperitoneum. However, the detection of free intraperitoneal fluid is based on the factors such as the body habitus, injury locations, presence of clotted blood, position of the patient, the amount of free fluid present.

The minimum threshold for detecting hemoperitoneum is unknown and remains a subject of interest. Kawaguchi and colleagues found that 70 ml of blood could be detected.[28] While Tiling et al found that 30 ml is the minimum requirement for detection with ultrasound.[29] They also concluded that a small anechoic shape in the Morison pouch represents approximately 250 ml of fluid, while 0.5 cm and 1 cm stripes represent approximately 500 ml and 1 l of free fluid, respectively. In the hands of most operators ultrasound will detect a minimum of 200 ml of fluid[30] although another report claims that 400 to 600 ml of fluid are needed in the trauma setting.[31]

The current examination protocol consists of 4 acoustic windows with the patient supine. These windows are pericardiac, perihepatic, perisplenic and pelvic (known as the 4 Ps).

A noted drawback to the FAST examination is the fact that a positive examination relies on the presence of free intraperitoneal fluid. Injuries not associated with hemoperitoneum may not be detected by this modality.[32] Thus, ultrasound is not a reliable method for excluding hollow visceral injury.[32] In addition the FAST examination cannot be used to reliably grade solid organ injuries.

Ultrasound is not a good modality for further imaging (in contrast to as a screening proceeding) because it misses up to 25% of liver and spleen injuries, most renal injuries and virtually all pancreatic, mesenteric and gut injuries.[31] It also misses a high proportion of retroperitoneal hemorrhage and bladder rupture. Combining the results for ultrasound in 1535 abdominal trauma patients from eight published series, an average sensitivity for hemoperitoneum was 88% and that for organ injury of 74%.[31] Unfortunately a negative ultrasound (absence of hemo-peritoneum) does not rule out significant organ or viscus injury that might require surgery or observation. Almost regardless of volume an ultrasound diagnosis of free fluid alone does not predict that surgery is needed or that surgery will be therapeutic. In addition, in best hands, there is at least a 15% false negative rate for detecting hemoperitoneum with ultrasound.[35] Ultrasound poorly identifies active hemorrhage and also does not accurately predict the need for surgery in splenic injury. Ultrasound is also insensitive to perforation of gut and to pancreatic injury.

Rozyeki et al studied 154 patients and reported that ultrasound was the most sensitive and specific modality for the evaluation of hypotensive patients with blunt abdominal trauma (sensitivity and specificity 100%).[31] However, taking every patient with positive FAST to the operating room may result in an unacceptably high negative laparotomy rate.

Hemodynamically stable patients, with negative FAST results require close observations, serial abdominal examination and a follow-up FAST examination. However, strongly consider performing CT scan especially if the patients is intoxicated or has other associate injuries.

Hemodynamically unstable patients with negative FAST results are a diagnostic challenge. Options include DPL, exploratory laparotomy or possibly a CT scan after aggressive resuscitation.

Overall FAST has a sensitivity between 73% and 88% a specificity between 98% and 100% and is 96 to 98% accurate.[33] This level of accuracy is independent of the practitioner performing the study. Surgeons, emergency medicine physicians, ultrasound technicians and radiologists give equivalent result.[34]

CT Scan

Abdominal CT is becoming the test of preference for evaluating the abdomen of patients with blunt abdominal trauma who are hemodynamically stable and complain of abdominal tenderness or are unevaluable. CT detects hepatic laceration that is either segmental or lobar (Fig. 16.4).

It allows estimation of the amount of intra-abdominal fluid and accurate imaging of solid parenchymal injuries in most patients.[35] Abdominal CT plays a major role in the decision to manage the injured spleen, liver or kidney nonoperatively. It can also reveal other associated injuries, notably vertebral and pelvic fractures, and injuries in the thoracic cavity. It has the capability to determine the source of hemorrhage. It can detect retroperitoneal injuries and provides excellent imaging of the pancreas, duodenum and genitourinary system (Figs 16.5 and 16.6).

Indications for CT scan are:[36]

- Severe blunt trauma with multiple injuries
- Unexplained but stable hypotension

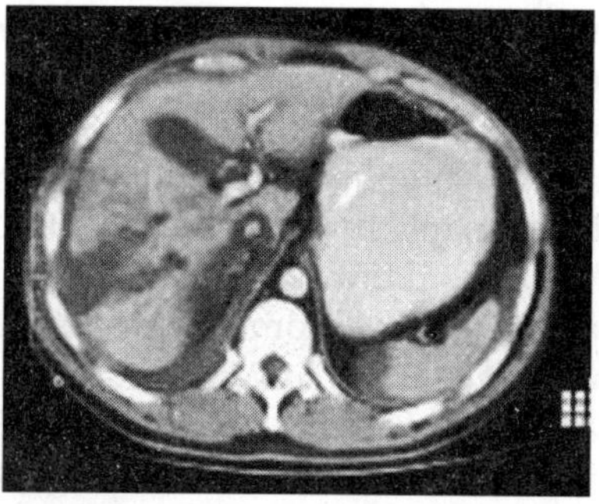

Fig. 16.4: CT scan showing grade IV injury of liver

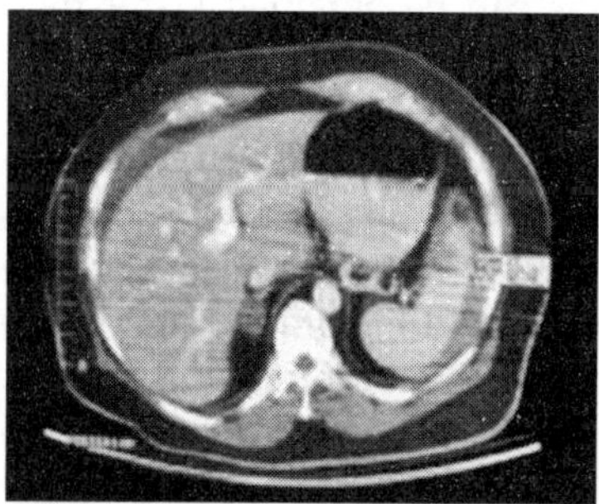

Fig. 16.5: CT scan showing perihepatic and perisplenic collection

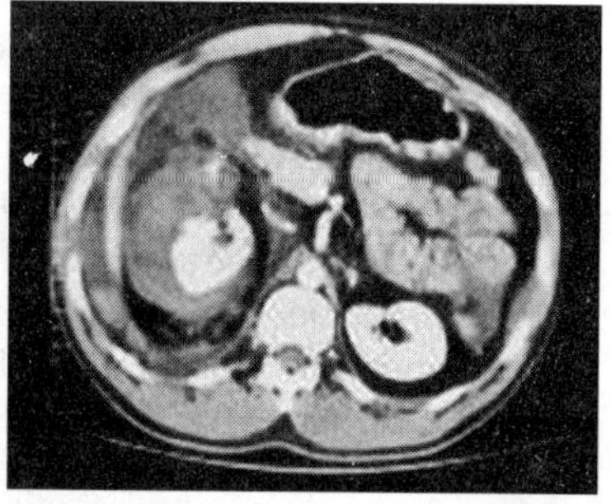

Fig. 16.6: CT scan showing perinephric hemorrhage and disruption of renal parenchyma

- Positive abdominal findings
- Unreliable clinical examination
  - Altered sensorium
  - Spinal injury
  - Unreliable DPL
  - Abnormal X-ray of the lower chest and abdomen
  - Falling hematocrit
  - Microscopic hematuria with shock
  - Gross hematuria from a suspected renal cause.
  - Serum hyperamylasemia
  - Abnormal quantitative peritoneal lavage.

Computed tomography has proved more accurate than excretory urography in evaluating the extent of renal parenchymal injury, perirenal hemorrhage, and the presence or absence of extravasated urine.[37]

Limitations of CT scan include marginal sensitivity for diagnosing diaphragmatic, pancreatic, hollow viscus and mesenteric injuries.[38] It has been suggested that in children the presence of unexplained fluid on abdominal CT should not always be an indication for laparotomy because the incidence of significant intra-abdominal injuries is only 3%.[39]

It is an accurate modality for deciding if patient needs a period of close observation. The trend towards placing helical computed tomography scanners close to or in emergency department has substantially diminished the delay in getting patient to the CT scanner and has decreased adult scan time to less than 40 seconds.

In most circumstances, results from a helical computed tomography of the abdomen and pelvis can be obtained faster than results from a detailed ultrasound examination that includes evaluation of abdominal organs and gut.

If multidetector computed tomography with rapid image display capability is available in or next to an emergency department, abdominal CT can be performed in about 2 minutes excluding time needed for patient transport to computed tomography scan setup and archiving of images. Including all time requirements, patient turn around with rapid-process multidetector CT can be less than 10 minutes for a trauma patient. For single slice incremental CT turn around time is some what longer, usually 20 minutes. Scanning multiple body regions increases these times variably. An experienced radiologist should carefully examine images on film, picture archiving and communication system (PACS) or at the CT console, where images can be altered to seek bone injury, pneumoperitoneum, or subtle organ injury.

It should be noted that various schemes for using CT to grade liver or spleen lacerations are not helpful in deciding whether a patient needs surgery. The decision must be based on the clinical status of the patient in combination with the image findings.

If evidence of extensive hemorrhage is discovered on CT exams, the patient may be taken to the operating room or under arteriography plus embolization to control the hemorrhage.

Abdominal CT is done with administration of intravenous and oral contrast to optimize the visualization of the organs. However oral contrast is time consuming and potentially dangerous.

Role of abdominal CT has been recently expanded in the evaluation of patients with abdominal gunshot wounds, selected for no operative mangement.[40] The CT scan may show the direction of a bullet tract and thus help in selecting patients who may be managed nonoperatively.

It may be reasonable to use CT, in conjunctions with the clinical information, to decide whether to observe patient in the hospital for a day or send them home promptly at the completion of their investigations in the emergency department. The high sensitivity of CT in detecting injuries that require observation in the hospital means that negative CT may be adequate to release the patient to home in selected cases. However with a negative ultrasound, it is not adequate to safely release the patient to home wherein a period of 12 to 48 hours is used to observe the patient as reflected in the design of many outcome based investigations.[41]

As abdominal CT is used more and more frequently, it becomes essential to monitor the possibly inappropriate use of technology. CT scanners at the front door of emergency rooms and portable CT scanner are being introduced.[42] Some remain skeptical about the ever diminishing value of clinical examination and the training of a whole new generation of surgeons who are depended on CT to diagnose abdominal pathology. On the other hand there is no doubt that diagnostic accuracy and avoidance of unnecessary operation is related to the ability to image the abdomen accurately. Whether we like it or not abdominal CT has become an indispensable tool in the evaluation of abdominal trauma.

DIAGNOSTIC LAPAROSCOPY

Role of diagnostic laparoscopy (DL) in trauma is still evolving. The acuity of most trauma patients requiring an operation does not allow the time required to set up and use of laparoscopic equipment.

Similarly patient who do not need an operation can be followed clinically or imaged by CT without the need for interventional diagnostic procedure.

However, one of the potential benefits postulated is the reduction of nontherapeutic laparotomies.

With modification of the technique to include smaller instruments, portable equipment and local anesthesia, bedside laparoscopy with or without gas insufflations has been proposed as a convenient screening tool at the emergency department or intensive care unit.

The major limitations of DL in trauma are related to the inability to "run" the bowel, diagnose retroperitoneal injuries expose adequately deep lying organs and estimate accurately the quantity of hemoperitoneum.[43] Studies have shown that close to half to the existing injuries can be missed by laparoscopy.[43] At the same time DL has an excellent sensitivity and specificity (>95%) when used as a screening tool to establish the presence of peritoneal violation, hemoperitoneum, or enteric content spillage.[43]

At this point there is only one clear cut indication for DL which relates to penetrating left thoracoabdominal trauma. In 42% of patients with such injuries, the diaphragm is involved (50% for gunshot wounds, 32% stab wounds). Many of such patients do not have other injuries requiring laparotomy. Additionally imaging tests are inaccurate in diagnosing; small, uncomplicated diaphragmatic penetrations. Direct visualization of diaphragm by laparoscopy remains the only reliable method to identify these injuries. In a prospective study, Murray et al[44] evaluated 110 patients, laparoscopically who had left thoracoabdominal, penetrating injuries and no indication for laparotomy and found an incidence of 24% of occult diaphragmatic injuries. The conclusion of study was that all patients with penetrating trauma to the left lower chest and without an indication for laparotomy should undergo laparoscopic evaluation of the left hemidiaphragms to exclude an occult injury regardless of the presence or absence of associated clinical or radiographic findings. Incidence of occult injuries will be similar to the right hemidiaphragms, the "buttressing effect" of the liver masking clinical findings.

Rigid Sigmoidoscopy

The value of rigid sigmoidoscopy is significant when it comes to evaluating the extraperitoneal rectum. Injuries to this part of the intestinal tract may not produce symptoms initially and escape diagnosis until septic complications prompt their investigation sigmoidoscopy may reveal intraluminal blood or the exact injury. It may not be possible to identify the precise site of injury. Therefore, if blood is found in the rectum by sigmoidoscopy the patient should be treated as if an injury exists. Patients with pelvic gunshot wounds who are taken to the operation room can be placed in mild lithotomy position and procedure could be done before or during the operation, if there are doubts about extra-peritoneal rectal injuries.

DECISION MAKING

The trauma patient often presents a diagnostic puzzle. Delaying laparotomy is associated with serious morbidity on the other hand, negative laparotomies are not without significant consequences for the patients.[45] The full appreciation of patient's picture, taking into account all available information provided by clinical examination, radiographic findings, and laboratory tests is more useful than the adherence to rigid protocols that prevent individualization (Figs 16.7 and 16.8).

The advent of trauma ultrasonography, increasing use of CT and successful application of nonoperative techniques have drastically changed the therapeutic algorithms over the last years, including the indications for operation. However, the two signs which remain absolute indications for laparotomy following blunt or penetrating trauma are peritonitis and hemodynamic instability. In the presence of either of these two, patient should be taken to operation theater without delay. A third indication relates

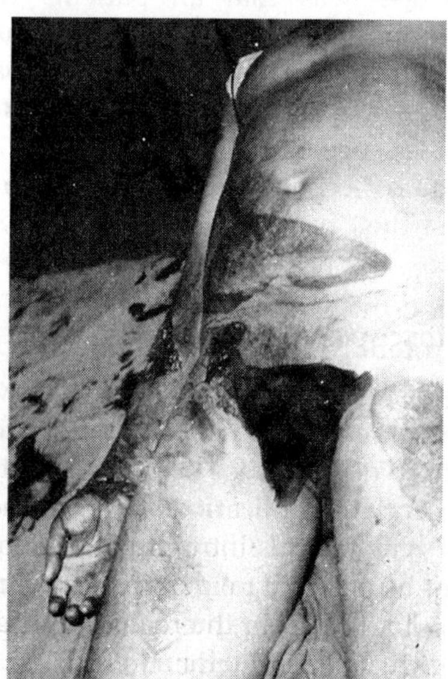

Fig. 16.7: Road traffic accident. Tell tale abrasions on the abdominal wall *(For color version, see Plate 4)*

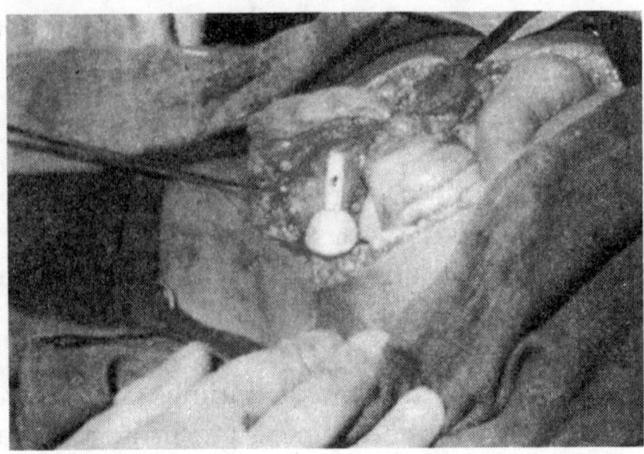

Fig. 16.8: Blunt injury abdomen, transection of sigmoid colon and bladder rupture *(For color version, see Plate 4)*

to the inability to examine the patient reliably after penetrating injury due to associated head injury, spinal cord injuries, severe intoxication or other injuries requiring emergent operation.

EVALUATION OF BLUNT TRAUMA

Besides clinical examination, plain films, and routine laboratory tests, immediate use of FAST and DPL should be made in the emergency room. In view of increasing experience gamed by FAST, DPL is becoming less frequently used investigation. Positive ultrasonography for intra-abdominal fluid in the presence of hemodynamic instability equals emergent laparotomy negative ultrasonography in the presence of hemodynamic instability of unknown origin should be followed up by diagnostic peritoneal aspiration (DPA). It the DPA is positive, patient should be taken to the operating room. Patients who are hemodynamically stable but inevaluable or with equivocal abdominal examination should be evaluated by CT scan (Flow chart 16.1).

CT scan provides crucial information for the need of laparotomy. It is more sensitive than ultrasound, equally sensitive as DPL and more specific than both.

CT has become an integral part of the decision making on the need for laparotomy. However, the value of clinical examination still remains undisputed. The indication for laparotomy should be made after full appreciation of the clinical condition. Even in the age of technological advancements, clinical examination

Flow chart 16.1: Decision making in blunt injury abdomen

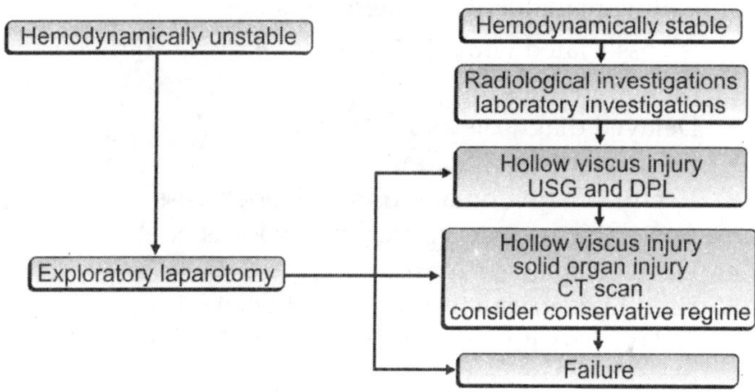

should be the primary tool determining the need of operation or observation.

Nonoperative management (NOM) of blunt abdominal injuries is well established and is based on hemodynamic stability and CT scan findings are now being widely used in the treatment of solid organ injuries including liver, spleen, kidney pancreas and pelvic injuries.[46] In blunt abdominal trauma (BAT) including severe solid organ injuries, selective NOM has been the standard of care.[47] If the decision has been made to observe the patient by NOM, the patient should be admitted to higher level of care for at least 48-72 hours with close monitoring on vital signs, hematocrit and repeated clinical examination. Serum lactic acid and base deficit can also help to determine if NOM is failing.

The general principles[47] of NOM are:

- Always keep mechanism of injury in mind
- Patient is alert awake and responding
- Hemodynamically stable and no coagulation disorders
- No other clear indication for laparotomy
- Maintain high index of clinical suspicion
- Caution in multiple injured patient
- Higher level of care with round-the-clock availability of laboratory, radiology and operation theater.

NOM to be abandoned[48] when there is:

- Deterioration of vital signs
- Development of new peritoneal signs

- Continued need for blood transfusions
- Falling hematocrit or progressing hematoma.

The risks[48] associated with NOM are:

- Missed injuries
- Delayed diagnosis and treatment
- Inadequate resuscitation
- Retained hematoma, sepsis and/or abscess
- Bowel/biliary/pancreatic/urinary leaks
- Delayed splenic rupture
- Pseudoaneurysm formation and delayed rupture
- Delayed treatment of vascular injuries and their complications
- Risks involved in blood transfusion.

Though hepatosplenic injuries still remain the most common solid organ injuries in BAT, liberal use of high resolution imaging techniques, such as CT scan revealed that the liver is the most common solid organ injured and not the spleen as popularly believed.[49] In the modern set up, the worldwide laparotomy rate for BAT is only about 20%.[50]

Nonoperative management in BAT is challenging owing to diversity of presentation and wide range of visceral injuries. However, it is quite satisfying to manage them by conservative approach which is highly successful in selective case. Although sophisticated imaging and availability of interventional radiologist has helped in decision making but even today, nothing surpasses the value of repeated clinical examination by an experienced surgeon in guiding the ultimate therapeutic decision "When in doubt it is better to open and see then to wait and watch" Grey-Turner.[50]

EVALUATION OF PENETRATING ABDOMINAL INJURIES (PAIs)

The incidence of penetrating injury will vary from hospital-to-hospital and region-to-region. It is vital that penetrating injury is treated differently as compared to blunt trauma. The mechanism and physical characteristics of injury are different as are the relevance and accuracy of investigations and the methods and timing of repair.

Penetrating abdominal injuries have been traditionally managed by routine laparotomy. New understanding of trajectories, potential for organ injury and correlation with advanced radiographic imaging has allowed a shift towards nonoperative management of appropriate cases. Although a selective approach has been established for stab wounds, the management of abdominal gunshot wounds remains a matter of controversy. The goal of any algorithm for penetrating abdominal trauma should be to identify injuries requiring surgical repair and avoid unnecessary laparotomy with its associated morbidity.

Stab wounds (SW) are encountered three times more often then gunshot wounds (GSW), but hove a lower mortality because of the lower energy transmitted. Prior to world war I, PAI was managed expectantly. During world war II, studies showed that early laparotomy improved survival. By the late 1950s, routine laparotomy was the standard treatment for PAI. Over the last 30 years the pendulum shifted towards selective management, initially involving only SW and later including GSW. The refinement of diagnostic procedures and imaging studies has contributed significantly in the new trends of PAI management.

Evaluation of hemodynamically stable patient will require use of one or more of the following diagnostic modalities after initial evaluation with chest X-ray and placement of nasogastric tube and urinary catheter (Table 16.3).

- Serial physical examination (PE)
- Local wound exploration (LWE)
- Diagnostic peritoneal lavage (DPL)
- Ultrasound (FAST)
- CT scan
- Laparoscopy
- Laparotomy

The decision on which method or combination of methods, to choose will depend, primarily on hospital factors such as trauma patient load access to in-patients beds, availability of in-house surgical teams, access to multislice CT scanners, etc. Sensitivity, specificity and negative predictive value (NPV) according to study is quoted as follows.[51]

Selective Nonoperative Management (SNOM) of SW

Stab wounds are classified in thirds. One-third do not penetrate the peritoneal cavity, one-third penetrate but do not damage and one-third penetrate causing significant injury.[52] Patients are

Table 16.3: Diagnostic modalities for penetrating injuries abdomen

	PE	*LWE*	*DPL*	*FAST*	*CT scan*	*Laparoscopy*	*Laparotomy*
Sensitivity (%) (for therapeutic intervention)	95-97	71	87-100	86-85	97	50-100	–
Specificity (%)	100	77	52-89	48-95	98	74-90	–
NPV(%)	92	79	78-100	60-98	98	100	–
Requires awake, cooperative Patient	+	–	–	–	–	–	–
Invasive	–	+	+	–	–	+	++
Requires admission	+	+/–	–	–	–	+	+
Evaluates retroperitoneum	+/–	–	-	–	+	–	–
High clinical workload	+	–	–	–	–	+/–	+/–
Complication rate	–	+	+/–	–	–	+	++

PE: Physical examination, LWE: Local wound exploration, DPL: Diagnostic peritoneal lavage

selected for nonoperative management based on the absence of hemodynamic instability and peritonitis. Both of these terms are selective and single value is inappropriate to define them. Therefore, the astute clinician needs to monitor the patient carefully, assess the situation as a whole picture and not as fragmented informational pieces, and determine the presence of hemodynamic instability or peritonitis based on knowledge, experience and the ability to practice the art of surgery.

Unlike trauma surgeons, a lower threshold for surgical exploration is not unreasonable for physicians who do not treat such patients frequently. Close monitoring and follow-up are mandatory in patients managed non-operatively. These patients should have repeat clinical exams-by preferably the same physician over the 12-24 hours ensuing arrival to the hospital.[53]

Anterior Abdomen

About 55% of stab wounds to the anterior abdomen can be managed non-operatively.[54] In a recent report Demetriades et al conducted a prospective study of 152 patients with penetrating injuries to abdominal solid viscera.[55] Forty-five patients (929.6%)

were stabbed. The liver was the most commonly injured solid organ (73%) followed by the kidney (30.3%) and the spleen (30.3%). Forty-one patients (27%) were successfully managed without a laparotomy and any abdominal complication.

Patients with isolated solid organ injuries treated non-operatively had significantly shorter hospital stay than patients treated operatively even though former group had more severe injuries.

Similarly another prospective randomized study by Lepparniem et al concluded the SNOM of abdominal SW, although resulting in delayed laparotomy in some patients is safe and the preferred strategy for minimizing the days in hospital as well as hospital costs.[56]

Posterior Abdomen (Back)

Penetrating injuries of the back may not be clinically detectable in the early stages but missed colonic or duodenal perforations, urinary tract and vascular wounds may have devastating outcomes. For these reasons many have raised concern about the safety of SNOM of penetrating injuries of the back (Figs 16.9 and 16.10).

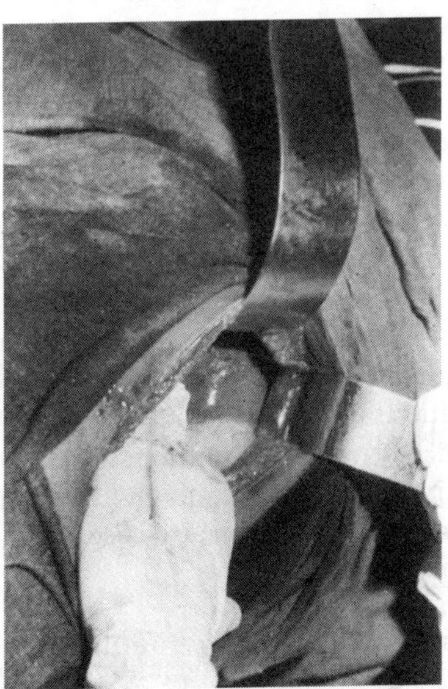

Fig. 16.9: Gunshot wound abdomen grazing the liver which could have been treated conservatively *(For color version, see Plate 5)*

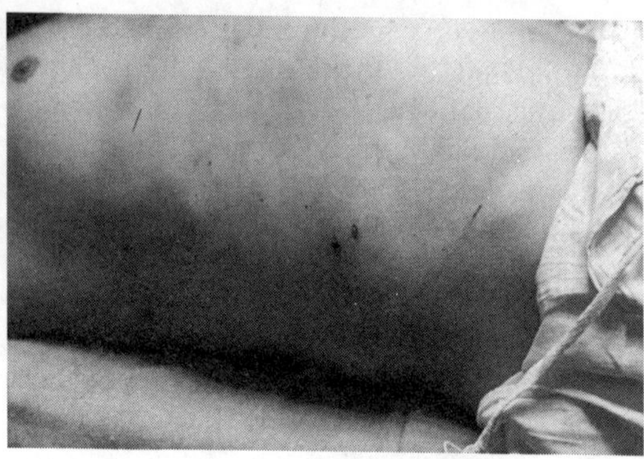

Fig. 16.10: Penetrating injury abdomen
(For color version, see Plate 5)

Demetriaides et al in a prospective study of 230 patients with penetrating injuries to the back showed that diagnostic accuracy of the initial abdominal examination was 95.2%.[57] Peritoneal lavage was mentioned only to be condemned. The authors concluded that penetrating injuries of the back should be assessed in the same way as those of the anterior abdomen. Peck and Berne in their series of 465 patients with penetrating, stab wound to the back showed that physical examination was extremely reliable in deciding when to do laparotomy.[58] Eighty percent of the patients were managed nonoperative. Colon, vascular and diaphragmatic injuries were more common. They concluded that SNOM for all patients with penetrating stab wound to the back was a reliable and prudent approach.

Therefore in the absence of obvious signs of significant organ or vascular injury, the best management plan for patients with stab wounds of the posterior abdomen is SNOM. Repeated physical examinations are the main stay of treatment, as indicated by many authors. Other studies such as diagnostic peritoneal lavage, angiography, intravenous pyelography and contrast CT scanninig are indicated on a case-by-case basis but as yet lack convincing justification for routine.[59]

Selective Nonoperative Management (SNOM) of GSW

Anterior Abdomen

Despite the initial disbelief, SNOM of anterior abdominal GSW has gained significant momentum and is widely used, particularly by experienced surgeons. SNOM of anterior abdominal gunshot wound was first introduced by Shafter in 1960, presenting the idea of "selective conservativism".[60] FAST can be useful initial diagnostic study after penetrating abdominal injury (PAI) but due to its low sensitivity it cannot be relied upon for distinguishing PAI patient who may or may not need surgical explorations.[56]

SNOM can be reliably evaluated with an abdominal CT scan.[60] Although careful and repeat clinical examination is the mainstay for non operative management of CT scan can be useful adjunct in identifying patients for operative management. New high quality helical CT scan with the ability to offer multiplanar reconstruction have assessed greatly in determine that trajectory of bullet is confirmatively outside the peritoneal cavity. Then such patient can be discharged immediately whereas others are observed closely and/or operated upon.

Back and Buttocks

The management of buttocks and back follows the same priniciples with anterior abdomen GSW. Velmahos et al in a prospective study evaluated 192 patients with GSW to the back and based on the initial negative clinical examination were successfully with SNPM of these patients.[61] The clinical examination had a sensitivity of 100% and specificity of 95%. A rigid sigmoidoscopy was introduced per routine in all cases.

Transpelvic GSW

Even in previous times, it would be almost impossible to believe that a transpelvic GSW could have been managed by SNOM, Velmahos et al have shown that principle of guiding surgical intervention on the basis of good clinical examination and appropriate imaging tests is valid even in this scenario.[62]

Management of Asymptomatic Left Thoracoabdominal Penetrating Injuries

Patients with penetrating injuries to the left thoracoabdominal area are at high risk of diaphragmatic injury. The natural history of unrepaired diaphragmatic lacerations is unknown. Although large lacerations may cause intrathoracic herniation and visceral strangulation, smaller lacerations must likely heal or are sealed by omentum. For patients without an indication for laparotomy, laparoscopy is considered a reasonable alternative to rule out diaphragmatic injuries if larger than 2 cm laceration is suspected. The excellent accuracy of CT (96%) to detect diaphragmatic injuries, as shown by the Maryland group, has not been duplicated by others. The groups conclude that with increasingly evolving technology, CT may become the standard of care for identifying such injuries.[63]

Primary Repair Vs Colostomy for Colon Injury

The management of colon injuries has undergone major change in the last three decades. From era of world war II wherein colon injuries were routinely managed by performing colostomy, transformation occurred by primary repair in selected cases in the late 1970's to the liberal primary repair in the most cases in 1990's. Stone and Fabian in 1979.[64]Concluded that patients that satisfied the specific criteria of: 1. preoperative shock being never profound, 2. blood loss less than 20% of estimated normal volume, 3. no more than two intra-abdominal organs injured, 4. minimal fecal contamination, 5. operation within 8 hours, and 6. wounds of colon and abdominal wall never so destructive as to require resection, should have primary closure as the preferred method of treatment.

Nelson et al in their meta-analysis study of randomized controlled trials of primary repair vs fecal diversion for penetrating colon injuries showed that there was no difference in mortality between the two groups. The two groups concluded that the currently published randomized controlled trials favor primary repair over fecal diversion for penetrating colon injuries.[65]

Prophylactic Antibiotics for Penetrating Abdominal Injuries

Presumptive antibiotic therapy is administered in PAI to reduce the incidence of postoperative infection. However, the appropriate timing duration and choice of antibiotics are still a matter of debate, although most clinicians lean towards broad spectrum antibiotics together with Metrogyl administered over a period of 5-7 days for most of the cases. However in a perspective randomized study, Cornwell et al treated 63 high risk patients with 24 hours vs 5 days of 2 gm cefoxitin. The authors concluded that even in the highest risk PAI patients extending prophylactic antibiotics to more than 24 hours is no benefit.[66]

Exploratory Laparotomy for Abdominal Trauma

Preferred incision is midline incision centered on the most likely area of injury. Advantages are easy extensibility, rapid to perform, minimal bleeding, and sound healing. Extension into the right side of the chest or median sternotomy will usually be required if extensive hepatic or retrohepatic venous injury is suspected and repair is to be performed, rather than packing. If on opening peritoneal cavity an explosive escape of blood occurs, the surgeon should expect to find a major vascular or solid visceral injury. Rapid removal of the blood by scooping with the gloved hand is done and at least two suckers are employed. As each quadrant of the abdomen is cleared of gross blood and clots, several laparotomy pads should be packed into the area to help absorb the remaining blood, and hopefully prevent new bleeding from refilling the abdomen. If bleeding is profuse, pressure should immediately be placed on the abdominal aorta as it traverses the diaphragm using an aortic compression device. If an experienced assistant is available, thumb and finger pressure works well and is faster. Venous bleeding can also be massive. Bleeding from the liver, spleen or a kidney is usually darker. Control can generally be attained by applying pressure to the fractured organ through several large lap sponges. Once temporarly control of hemorrhage is obtained considerations and questions to address include the following.[67] Should more blood be brought to operation theater? Are enough rapid infusion blood warmer set up? Should fresh frozen plasma and platelets be requested? Should additional help be called? Will a head lamp, special sutures, or more instruments such as vascular clamps or an argon beam coagulator be needed? Have all the needed sutures been opened and loaded on needle holders?

Exploration of the traumatized abdomen should include visualization of the entire gastrointestinal tract from the oesophagogastric junction to the peritoneal reflection over the rectum. Portions of this exploration must not be omitted in patients with penetrating injury based on the presumptions as to the course of a missile or knife. The liver spleen, and pancreas should be inspected. A Kocher's maneuver to mobilize the duodenum and exploration of the lesser peritoneal sac are essential steps. The later exploration involves division of the gastrocolic ligament. Bile staining of paraduodenal tissue can result from retroperitoneal duodenal injury or from bile duct injury. One may quickly temporary seal the perforations before exploration so that soiling does not continue while exploring.

Closure of the abdomen is done in single layer using prolene sutures. Skin may be kept open for delayed primary closure if there was heavy soling of the abdominal cavity. Opinion regarding drains vary from, to put drain as and when you think of it to drain only if you must. Continuous irrigation of the peritoneal cavity has fallen out of favor. However, a thorough irrigation, of the peritoneal cavity with copious saline till all particulate matter is removed and returning fluid is clear, must be done before closure. There are situations when the abdomen cannot be closed without tension or there is need to promptly and expeditiously terminate the operation. In either circumstances, closure of skin only or the placement of a prosthesis to temporarily fill the defect is indicated. In many instances, edema resolves and the abdomen can be closed primarily after 48-72 hours.

Intra-abdominal Hematomas

The intra-abdominal approach to any intra-abdominal hematoma depends on the mechanism of injury (blunt or penetrating) and the site and size of the hematoma. For practical purpose the retroperitoneal hematomas are classified into three zones:

Zone I—which includes the midline area between the aortic, hiatus of diaphragm and the sacral promontory, Zone II—which includes the left and right perirenal areas and Zone III—which includes all pelvic hematomas. As a general rule, routine exploration in blunt trauma should be considered only for pancreaticoduodenal hematomas. Stable retroperitoneal, pelvic or retrohepatic hematomas should be left undisturbed. Superior mesenteric artery hematomas in the root of mesentery should not be explored routinely unless hematoma is expanding or bowel appears ischemic.

In penetrating trauma as a general rule, all hematomas in all three zones should be explored. Often underneath a small hematoma there is an underlying vascular injury or hollow viscus perforation. The only exception to this rule is a stable retrohepatic hematoma because exploration in this area is technically difficult and dangerous with potentially lethal consequences. Stable perirenal hematomas are best left undisturbed although many authors advocate routine exploration.

Abdominal Drains

The role of abdominal drains following trauma is much debated. There is convincing evidence that the use of sump drains is associated with increased risk of sepsis. However, the used closed suction drains does not increase the risk of intra-abdominal complications and there is evidence that in major injuries of either the liver or pancreas, they reduce the risk of infection. It is believed that in trauma drain should be used liberally in areas with even minor oozing, especially in the presence of an associated hollow viscus perforation. Closed drains should also be placed in areas packed as part of damage control.

Abdominal Closure

The abdominal fascia is closed with continues nonabsorbable sutures provided there is no significant tension. Retention sutures have no role in at least during initial/first laparotomy. The management of the skin wound in the presence of extensive enteric contamination or colon perforation shows variable incidence of wound sepsis when primary closure is done rather than leaving the skin wound open. The role of primary skin closure over subcutaneous drain is not clear and needs further evaluation. In patients managed with damage-control laparotomy, primary closure of the abdomen should be avoided because of the high incidence of abdominal compartment syndrome.

Nontherapeutic Laparotomies

The incidence of nontherapeutic laparotomies for trauma varies depending on the experience and policies of individual trauma centers. However, this incidence for blunt abdominal trauma is similar to that in penetrating trauma and is about 20%.[68] Morbidity associated with unnecessary laparotomies is quoted varying between 3 to 25.9%.

Respiratory complications followed by prolonged paralytic ileus, surgical wound inection and small bowel obstruction are by far the most common complications.[69]

The costs associated with an unnecessary laparotomy are significant. Mean length of hospital stay also increases following unnecessary laparotomy.

Missed Abdominal Injuries

The benefits of successful nonoperative management of abdominal injuries should be weighed against the consequences of missed injuries and delayed treatment. The mainstay of selective nonoperative management is close continuous monitoring and immediate operation with the first signs of peritonitis. The delay beyond which the morbidity increases has not been defined. It is possible that in patients with excessive peritoneal contamination even a few hours delay may be associated with significant morbidity. On the other hand, in patients with small perforation and confined contamination, longer delays may be tolerated without morbidity.

REFERENCES

1. Enderson BL, Reath DB, Meadors J, et al. The tertiary trauma survey: a prospective study of missed injury. J Trauma June 1990;30(6):666-9, discussion 669-70[Medline].
2. Tso P, Rodriguez A, Cooper C, et al. Sonography in blunt abdominal trauma: a preliminary progress report. J Trauma July 1992;33(1):39-43; discussion 43-4[Medline].
3. McAnena OJ, Moore EE, Marx JA. Initial evaluation of the patient with blunt abdominal trauma. Surg Clin North Amer 1990;70:495-514.
4. Chattopadhayay U. Management of abdominal injuries in the forward areas (part II). MJAFI 1973;29:420-23.
5. Muhammad UB, Nikolaos Z, George CV. Penetrating abdominal injuries: management controversies. Sc and J Trauma Resusc Emerg Med.2009;17:19.
6. Tiling T, Boulin B, Schmid A, et al. Ultrasound in blunt abdominal thoracic trauma. In: Border JR, ed. Blunt multiple trauma: Comprehensive pathophysiology and care. Newyork: Mercel Dekker 1990;415-33.
7. Demetriaides D, Chan LS, Bhasri P, et al. Relative bradycardia in patients with traumatic hypotension. J Trauma 1998;45:534.
8. Shoemaker WC, Betzberg H, Wo CCJ, et al. Multicentric study of non-invasive monitoring systems as alternative to invasive monitoring of acutely ill emergency patients. Chest 1998;114:1643.
9. John Udeani, Sidney R Steinberg. Abdominal Trauma: Blunt. emedicine.medscape.com. Aug 22, 2008. [cited 15 July 2010] Available: http://emedicine.medscape.com/article/433:404-overview.

10. Kevin TC, Greg F. Abdominal Trauma: A review of prehospital assessment and management of blunt and penetrating abdominal trauma. EMS Magazine. March 2010. [cited 15 July 2010] Available: http://www.emsresponder.com/print/EMS-Magazine/CE-Article-Abdominal-Trauma/1$12262.
11. Root HD, Hauger CW, McKinley CR, et al. Diagnostic peritoneal lavage. Surgery 1965;57:633-7.
12. Biving BA, Sachatello CR, Daughtery ME, et al. Diagnostic peritoneal lavage is superior to clinical evaluation in blunt abdominal trauma. Am Surg 1978;44:637-41.
13. Alyono D, Perry JF. Value of quantitative cell count and amylase activity of peritoneal lavage fluid. J Trauma 1981;21:345.
14. McClellan BA, Hanna SS, Montoya DR, et al. Analysis of peritoneal lavage parameters in blunt abdominal. J Trauma 1989;29:494.
15. Henneman PL, Marx JA, Moore EE, et al. Diagnostic peritoneal lavage: accuracy in predicting necessary laparotomy following blunt and penetrating trauma. J Trauma 1990;30:1345-55.
16. Bilge A, Sahini M. Diagnostic peritoneal lavage in blunt abdominal trauma. Eur J Surg 1991;157:449-51.
17. Day AC, Rankin N, Charlesworth P. Diagnostic peritoneal lavage: integration with clinical information to improve diagnostic performance. J Trauma 1992;32:52-7.
18. Blow O, Bassan D, Butter K, et al. Speed and efficiency in the resuscitation of blunt trauma patients with multiple injuries: the advantage of diagnostic peritoneal lavage over abdominal computed tomography. J Trauma 1998;44:287-90.
19. Davis JW, Hoyt DB, Mackersie RC, et al. Complication in evaluating abdominal trauma: diagnostic peritoneal lavage versus computed axial tomography. J Trauma 1990;30:1506-9.
20. Mendez C, Gubler KD, Maier RV. Diagnostic accuracy of peritoneal lavage in patients with pelvic fractures. Arch Surg 1994;129:477-82.
21. Cochrane W, Sobat WS. Open versus closed diagnostic peritoneal lavage. A multiphasic prospective randomized comparison. Ann Surg 1984;200:24-8.
22. Meyer DM, Thal ER, Weigelt JA, et al. Evaluation of computed tomography and diagnostic peritoneal lavage in blunt abdominal trauma. J Trauma 1989;29:1168-70.
23. McAnena OJ, Murx JA, Moore EE. Contributions of peritoneal lavage enzymes determinations to the management of isolated hollow visceral abdominal injuries. Ann Emerg Med 1991;20:834-7.
24. Soyka JM, Martin M, Sloan EP, et al. Diagnostic peritoneal lavage: is an isolated WBC count greater than or equal to 500/mm^3 predictive of intra-abdominal injury requiring celiotomy in blunt trauma patients? J Trauma 1990;30:874-9.

25. Ceraldi CM, Waxman K. Computed tomography as an indicator of isolated mesenteric injury. A comparison with peritoneal lavage. Am Surg 1990;56:806-10.
26. Davis JR, MorrisonAL, Perkin SE, et al. Ultrasound impact on diagnostic peritoneal lavage, abdominal computed tomography and resident training. Am Surg 1999;65:555.
27. Rozycki GS, Gchsner MG, Jaffin JH, et al. Prospective evaluation of surgeons's use of ultrasound in the evaluation of trauma patients. J Trauma 1993;34:516-27.
28. Charleskrin, Karim Brohi, Kawaguchi. Penetrating Abdominal Trauma: Guidelines for evaluation. trauma.org, August 2004;9:8. [cited 15 July 2010] Available:http://www.trauma.org/index.php/main/article/414.
29. Tiling T, Boulin B, Schmid A, et al. Ultrasound in blunt abdominal thoracic trauma.In: Border JR, Ed. Blunt multiple trauma: Comprehensive pathophysiology and care. New York: Mercel Dekker; 1990;415-33.
30. Branney SW, Wolfe RE, Moore EE, et al. Quantitative sensitivity of ultrasound in detecting free intraperitoneal fluid. J Trauma 1995;39:375-80.
31. Shuman WP, Holtzman SR, Bree RL, Bettmann MA, Casciani T, Foley WD, Gay SB, Gomes AS, Rosen MP, Sacks D, Greene FL. Expert Panel on Gastrointestinal Imaging. Blunt abdominal trauma. [online publication]. Reston (VA): American College of Radiology (ACR); 2005.8p.[cited15July2010]Available:http://www.guideline.gov/summary/summary.aspx?doc_id=15726.
32. Boulanger BR, Brennemen FD, McLellan BA, et al. A prospective study of emergent abdominal sonography after blunt trauma. J Trauma 1995;39:325-30.
33. Healey MA, Simons RK, Winchell RJ, et al. A prospective evaluation of abdominal ultrasound in blunt trauma. Is it useful? J Trauma 1996;40:875-83.
34. Kern SJ, Smith RS, Fry WR, et al. Sonographic examination of abdominal trauma by senior surgery residents. Am Surg 1997;63:669-74.
35. Ochsner MG, Knudson MM, Pachter HL, et al. Significance of minimal or no intraperitoneal fluid visible on CT scan associated with blunt liver and splenic injuries. A multicenter analysis. J Trauma 2000;49:50F.
36. Selafai SJA. Imaging abdominal trauma in 1990's . in Campbell RE, Harie PS (Eds): Syllabus: Diagnostic categorical course in emergency department radiology. Chicago, RSNA publication. 1990;49-61.
37. Breten PN Jr, McAninch JW, Federle MP, et al. Computerized tomographic staging of renal trauma: 85 consequtive cases. J Urol 1986;136:561.

38. Frich EJ Jr, Pusquade MD, Cipolle MD, et al. Small bowel and mesenteric injuries in blunt trauma. J Trauma 1999;46:920.
39. Beirle EA, Chen MK, Whalen TV, et al. Free fluid on abdominal computed tomography scan after blunt trauma does not mandate exploratory laparotomy in children. J Ped Surg 2000;35:990.
40. Guizberg E, Carrillo EH, Kopelman T, et al. The role of computed tomography in selective management of gunshot wounds to the abdomen and flank. J Trauma 1998;45:1005.
41. McCunn M, Mirvis S, Reynolds M, et al. Physician utilization of a portable computed tomography scanner in the intensive care unit. Crit care Med 2000;28:3808.
42. Villavicencio RT, Aucar JA. Analysis of laparoscopy in trauma. J Am Coll Surg 1999;189:11.
43. Murray JA, Demetriades D, Cornwell EE, et al. Penetrating left thoracoabdominal truama, the incidence and clinical presentation of the diaphragm injuries. J Trauma 1997;43:624.
44. Murray JA, Demetriades D, Asensio J, et al. Occult injuries to the diaphragm: Prospective evaluation of laparoscopy in penetrating injuries to the left lower chest. J Am Coll Surg 1998;187:626.
45. Renz BM, Felicaino DV. Unnecessary laparotomies for trauma: A prospective study of morbidity. J Trauma 1995;38:350.
46. Stawicki SP. Trends in nonoperative management of traumatic injuries: A synopsis OPUS 12 scientist 2007;vol 1, No 1(s).
47. Schwab CW. Selection of nonoperative management candidates. World J Surg 2001;25:1382-95.
48. Mohpatra S, Pattanayak SP, et al. Option in the management of solid visceral injuries from blunt abdominal trauma. IJS 2003;65:263-8.
49. Knudson MM, Maull KI. Nonoperative management solid organ injuries - past, present and future. Surg Clin Noth Am 1999;79:1357-71.
50. Jurkovice GJ, Carrico CJ. Trauma: Management of the acutely injured patients. In: Sabiston DC J2, et al, editor, textbook of surgery. NOIDA: Jhonson Press (Indian)Ltd;1997:296-337.
51. Charleskrin, Karim Brohi. Penetrating abdominal trauma: Guidelines for evaluation. trauma.org, August 2004;9:8. [cited 15 July 2010] Available:http://www.trauma.org/index.php/main/article/414.
52. Doherty GM, Meko JB. Olson JA, Pepbsid GR, Worrral NK. Trauma Surgery in; McNevan MS, Bucheman. The Washington Manual of Surgery 2nd, 1999;404.
53. Muhammad UB, Nikolaos Z, George CV. Resuscitation and emergency medicine. Sc and, Journal of Trauma 2009;17:19.
54. Navsaria PH, Berli JU, Edu S, Nicol AJ. Nonoperative management of abdominal stab wounds–analysis of 186 patients. S Afr J Surg 2007;45:128-32. Pub Med Abstract.
55. Demetriades D, Hadjizacharia P, Constantinou C, Brown C, Inaba K, Rhee P, Salim A. Selective nonoperative management of penetrating

abdominal solid organ injuries. Ann Surg 2006;244:620-8. Pub Med Abstract.

56. Lepparniem AK, Haapiamen RK. Selective nonoperative management of abdominal stab wounds: prospective randomized study. World J Surg 1996;20:1101-5. Pub Med Extract.
57. Demetriaides D, Rabinorvitz B, Sofianos C, Da Silva J. The management of penetrating injuries to the back. A prospective study of 230 patients. Ann Surg 1988,207:72-4. Pub Med Abstract.
58. Peck JJ, Berne TV. Posterior abdominal stab wounds. J Trauma 1981;21:298-306. Pub Med Abstract.
59. Berne TV. Management of penetrating back trauma. Surg Clin North Am 1990;70:671-6. Pub Med Abstract.
60. Velmahos GC, Constantinor C, Tillor A, Brown CV, Salim A, Demetriaides D. Abdominal computed tomographic scan for patients with gunshot wounds to the abdomen selected for nonoperative management. J Trauma 2005;59:1155-61. Pub Med Abstract.
61. Velmahos GC, Demetriaides D, Foianini E, Tatedassian R, Cornnell EE 3rd, Asensio J, Beizberg H, Berne TV. A selective approach to the management of gunshot wounds to the back. Am J Surg 1997;174:342-46. Pub Med Abstract.
62. Velmahos GC, Demetriaides D, Corrnell EE III. Transpelvic gunshot wounds: Routine laparotomy or selective management? World J Surg 1998;22:1034-38. Pub Med Abstract.
63. Stein DM, York GB, Boswell S, Shanmuganathan K, Haan JM, Scalla TM. Accuracy of computed tomography (CT) scan in the detection of penetrating diaphragm injury. J Trauma 2007;63:538-43. Pub Med Abstract.
64. Stone HH, Fabian TC. Management of penetrating colon trauma: randomization between primary closure and exteriorization. Ann Surg 1979;190:430-36. Pub Med Abstract.
65. Nelson R, Singer M. Primary repair for penetrating colon injuries. Cochrane Database Syst Rev 2002;(3):CD002247 Pub Med Abstract/ Published full text.
66. Cornwell EE 3rd, Dougherty WR, Berne TV, Velmahos G, Murray JA, Cahwan S, et al. Duration of antibiotic prophylaxis in high risk patients with penetrating abdominal trauma: A prospective randomized trail. J Gastr Intest Surg 1999;3:648-53. Pub Med Abstract/ Published full text.
67. Moore EE, Moore JB, Van Duzer-Moore S, et al. Mandatory laparotomy for gunshot wounds penetrating the abdomen. Am J Surg 1980;140:847.
68. Sober JL, Baker M, Peute I, et al. Negative laparotomy in abdominal gunshot wounds: Potential impact of laparoscopy. J Trauma 1995;38:194.
69. Reinz BM, Feliciano DV. Unnecessary laparotomies in Trauma: A prospective study of morbidity. J Trauma 1995;38:350.

Chapter

17

Management of Hepatic Trauma

SK Kochar

INCIDENCE AND MECHANISM OF INJURY

The liver is injured in 5-10% of patients with abdominal trauma. However, the incidence of hepatic injuries detected in patients undergoing laparotomy for blunt/penetrating trauma varies from 15 to 45% at different centers.[1] Blunt hepatic injuries can result from direct blow, compression from the injury in right lower chest or shearing at fixed points secondary to deceleration. The large size of the liver and its location in both upper quadrant of the abdomen make it vulnerable to injury in patients with penetrating wounds.

ANATOMY

Details of the liver anatomy as described by Chouinard (Fig. 17.1) is of particular importance in trauma to the liver. Division of the liver into right and left lobe is in a plane that passes from the gallbladder across the dome of the liver to the vena cava. The traditional left lobe of the liver, that portion to the left of the falciform ligament (Chouinard II and III) is the lateral segment of the left hepatic lobe and the medial segment of the left lobe (Chouinard IV) is the traditionally described quadrate lobe. The right hepatic vein drains the right lobe of the liver. The middle hepatic vein which lies in the interlobar plane, drains the medial segment of the left lobe (Chouinard IV) and a portion of segment V. The left hepatic vein drains the lateral segments of the left lobe (Chouinard II and III) and usually enters the vena cava in conjunction with the middle hepatic vein. The left branch of the portal vein passes to the left near the under surface of the liver

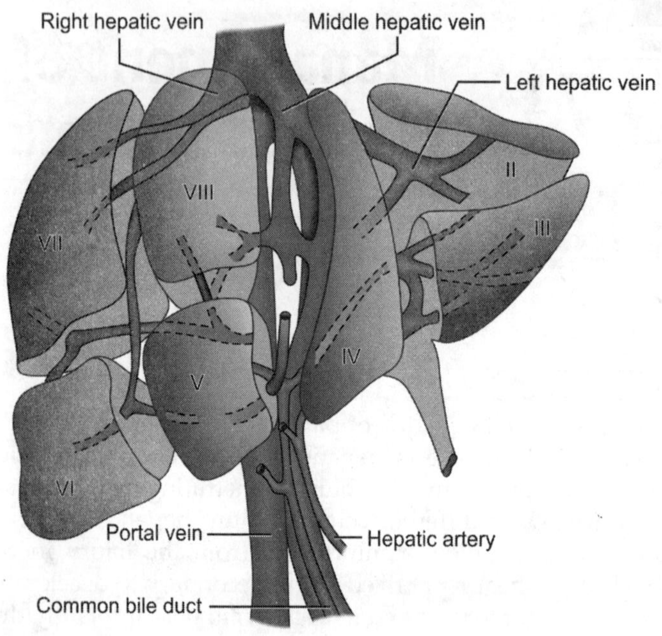

Fig. 17.1: Segmental anatomy of liver

to the plane of the falciform ligament, where it curves forward in an umbilical fashion. Branches from the convex aspect supply segments II and III, whereas segment IV is supplied by its terminal branches. The caudate lobe (Chouinard I) is independent of either right or left lobe in its blood supply. The liver receives an average blood flow of 25% of the cardiac output in man. The hepatic artery with an oxygen saturation of 95% provides 25% of this flow, while the portal vein provides the remaining 75% with an oxygen saturation of approximately 80%. It has been shown that hepatic arteries are not end arteries and that as many as 20 collateral channels exists in man. Occasionally, right hepatic artery may arise from superior mesentery and left from the left gastric artery.

Classification of Hepatic Trauma

Several classification of liver injuries have been proposed but organ injury scaling is being adopted universally. Liver injury scale is as follows in Table 17.1.[2]

Table 17.1: Liver injury scale

Grade		*Injury description*
I	Hematoma	Subcapsular < 10% surface area.
	Laceration	Capsular tear < 1 cm parenchymal depth.
II	Hematoma	Subcapsular 10-50% of surface area. Intraparenchymal < 10 cm diameter
	Laceration	Capsular tear 1-3 cm parenchymal depth and <10 cm in length.
III	Hematoma	Subcapsular > 50% surface area or expanding ruptured subcapsular or parenchymal hematoma; intraparenchymal hematoma > 10 cm or expanding.
	Laceration	> 3 cm parenchymal
IV	Laceration	Parenchymal disruption involving 25-75% of hepatic lobe or I-III Chouinard segments within a single lobe.
V	Laceration	Parenchyma disruption involving > 75% of hepatic lobe or > 3 Chouinard segments within a single lobe.
	Vascular	Juxtahepatic venous injuries, retrohepatic vena cava/central major hepatic veins.
	Vascular	Hepatic avulsion.

Advance one grade for multiple injuries up to grade III.

Diagnosis

Although a history and physical examination will always be gold standard during the primary assessment period, these parameters may be of limited value for those patients who have alcoholic intoxication, drug ingestion, intracranial injury or injury to the spinal cord. The most frequent sign of injury on physical examination are profound hypotension and peritonitis. Other findings are varying grades of abdominal tenderness, guarding, distention and hypoactive or absent bowel sounds. The presence of penetrating wounds, upper abdominal bruising or ecchymosis or lower chest injury may be an indication of hepatic trauma. Many of the patients with minor or moderate hepatic injuries are hemodynamically stable when first evaluated in the emergency room and may have minimal physical findings. Investigations are required not only to arrive at the diagnosis but also to evaluate the injury.

In hemodynamically unstable patient with blunt trauma, the sole diagnostic studies performed in the center should be X-ray of the chest and pelvis to rule out other obvious injuries that might account for the patient's hypotension and an intravenous pyelogram in the patients with hematuria. In the profoundly hypotension with penetrating trauma thought to be involving liver, a rapid sequence intravenous pyelogram is used to verify the presence of two functional kidneys. In hemodynamically stable patient with blunt trauma, hematocrit and WBC count, diagnostic peritoneal lavage, USG of the abdomen and CT scan are the investigations of choice. The reliability of peritoneal lavage as a diagnostic tool is, in general excellent but it is invasive and it may make USG evaluation of the injury and hemoperitoneum quantification difficult. Computed tomography scanning allows for precise definition of the presence and magnitude of hepatic injury (Fig. 17.2). CT scan grading of hepatic trauma is useful for evaluation for nonoperative management protocol and follow-up of patients. Injury grading as per CT scan[3] findings is as follows in Table 17.2.

CT scan is most helpful in evaluating stable patients whose history strongly suggests major trauma to the abdomen and who are difficult to assess due to: (i) head/spinal injury, (ii) drug abuse/alcohol intoxication, and (iii) associated retroperitoneal hematoma/pelvic fracture. It is also helpful in evaluating stable patients who come to the emergency department at a delayed interval after trauma and those patients who are going to be managed by nonoperative protocol.

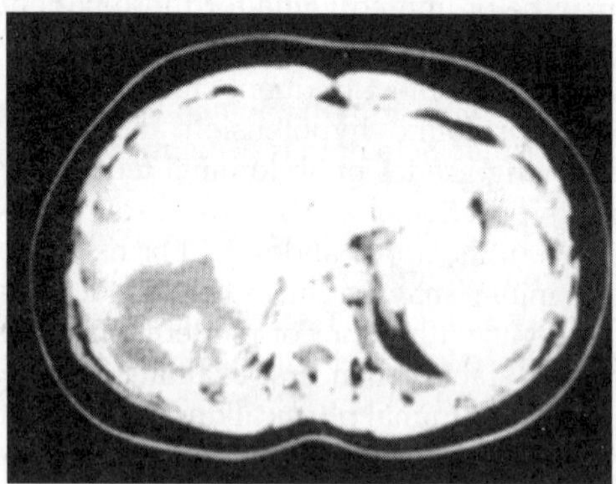

Fig. 17.2: CT scan showing grade III hepatic injury

Table 17.2: Injury grading as per CT scan

Grade I	Capsular avulsion; superficial laceration < I cm deep. Subcapsular hematoma < 1 cm maximum. Periportal blood tracking only.
Grade II	Laceration 1-3 cm deep. Central/subcapsular hematoma 1-3 cm diameter.
Grade III	Laceration >3 cm deep. Central/subcapsular hematoma > 3 cm diameter.
Grade IV	Massive central/subcapsular hematoma > 10 cm. Lobar tissue destruction or devascularization.
Grade V	Bilobar tissue destruction (maceration) or devascularization.

In penetrating trauma to the right lower portion of the chest/ back and right upper quadrant there is always some question whether the hemodynamically stable asymptomatic patient has or does not have hepatic injury. Most commonly used technique for its diagnosis are repeated physical examination, local wound exploration, DPL and USG. Center with extensive experience with DPL have used a standard red blood count greater than 100,000 RBC/mm^3 or white blood count greater than 500/mm^3 as a criteria of abdominal positive lavage as an indication for emergency laparotomy. False positive lavage secondary to intraperitoneal collection of blood from the stab wound site in the abdominal wall occurs in approximately 4-5% of all patients. Another 5-19% of all patients will be found to have injuries that are no longer bleeding by the time operation is performed.

CT scan findings include the following:

- Subcapsular hematoma
  - This is usually seen in a lenticular configuration; most subcapsular hematomas are anterolateral to the right lobe of the liver.
  - Subcapsular hematomas cause direct compression and deformity of the shape of the underlying liver.
  - On nonenhanced CT scans, the liver appears hyperattenuating compared with a subcapsular hematoma.[17]
  - On enhanced CT scans, a subcapsular hematoma appears as a low-attenuating, lenticular collection between the liver capsule and the enhancing liver parenchyma.
  - Unless bleeding recurs, attenuation of the subcapsular hematoma decreases with time. Subcapsular hematomas resolve within 6-8 weeks.

- Intraparenchymal hematomas
  - On contrast-enhanced CT scans, acute hematomas appear as irregular, high-attenuation areas, which represent clotted blood, surrounded by low-attenuating un-clotted blood or bile.
  - Over time, the attenuation of the hematoma is reduced, and the hematoma eventually forms a well-defined serous fluid collection that may expand slightly.
  - A focal, intrahepatic, hyperattenuating area with attenuation of 80-350 HU may represent an active hemorrhage or pseudoaneurysm.
  - Focal or diffuse periportal low attenuation is believed to be secondary to tracking of blood around the portal vessels, although other possibilities include bile leaks, edema, and dilated periportal lymphatics resulting from increased central venous pressure or injury to the lymphatics.
  - A low-attenuating periportal collar is seen in children with nonhepatic blunt abdominal trauma and also in the absence of intra-abdominal injury. Thus, without other ancillary findings within the liver, the presence of a low-attenuating periportal collar is not indicative of hepatic injury. However, the presence of this sign in documented abdominal trauma correlates with the severity of trauma, physiologic instability, and a higher mortality rate.
  - CT scan findings in approximately 25% of children with blunt abdominal trauma show periportal low attenuation. That only 40% of these children have evidence of liver injury has been shown.
- Laceration
  - Laceration of the liver appears as a nonenhancing linear or branching structure, usually at the liver periphery.
  - Acute lacerations have a sharp or jagged margin, but with time, lacerations may enlarge, and the margins may develop rolled edges.
  - Multiple parallel lacerations occur as result of compressive forces (bear claw lacerations).
  - Lacerations may communicate with hepatic vessels and/or biliary radicles.

- Vascular injuries
  - Injuries to the major hepatic veins and the retrohepatic inferior vena cava are uncommon after blunt abdominal trauma.
  - Retrohepatic vena caval injuries are suggested on CT scans when lacerations extend into the major hepatic veins and the inferior vena cava or when profuse retrohepatic hemorrhage extends into the lesser sac or near the diaphragm.
  - Perihilar liver tissue may become partially devascularized by a deep laceration or complete avulsion of the dual hepatic blood supply. These devascularized areas of the liver appear as wedge-shaped regions extending toward the liver periphery, and they fail to enhance after the administration of contrast material.
  - Pseudoaneurysms are better depicted by using spiral or multisection CT scanning because of the ability to image during peak contrast enhancement.
- Acute hemorrhage
  - Acute, intrahepatic hemorrhage is seen as irregular areas of contrast agent extravasation.
  - Measurement of attenuation values is useful in differentiating extravasated contrast from hematoma. Extravasated contrast material has an attenuation value of 85-350 HU (mean, 132 HU), whereas hemorrhage has an attenuation value of 40-70 HU (mean, 51 HU).
  - CT scans can be useful in depicting recurrent bleeding after surgery or radiologic intervention.
- Gallbladder injury
  - Gallbladder injury is uncommon, occurring in 2-8% patients with blunt liver trauma. Prior to the availability of CT scanning and ultrasonography, gallbladder injuries were rarely diagnosed before surgery.[18]
  - CT findings in gallbladder injuries include ill-defined or irregular wall contour, pericholecystic or subserosal fluid, collapsed gallbladder, wall thickening, intraluminal blood, free intraluminal mucosal flap, contrast enhancement of the gallbladder wall or mucosa, free intraperitoneal fluid isoattenuating with bile, mass effect on the duodenum, and displacement of the gallbladder toward the midline.

- Biloma and bile peritonitis.
- Biloma
  - As a result of the slow rate of leaking, a biloma may take weeks or months to develop after trauma; hence, it usually is diagnosed by using follow-up scans.
  - CT scan findings of a post-traumatic biloma demonstrate a cystic structure of low attenuation in or around the liver.
  - Bilomas may contain debris or septa.
  - Bile peritonitis is an uncommon complication of blunt liver trauma. CT scan findings of bile peritonitis include persistence or increasing amounts of low-attenuating, free peritoneal fluid and thickening of a peritoneum that shows evidence of enhancement.
- Ultrasonograms can demonstrate a number of traumatic lesions, such as hematomas, contusions, bilomas, and hemoperitoneum.[22]
- Hepatic hematomas are grouped into three categories, as follows:
  - Rupture into the liver and its capsule
  - Separation of the capsule by a subcapsular hematoma
  - Central hepatic ruptures.
- A subcapsular hematoma usually appears as a curvilinear fluid collection; its echogenicity varies with age.
  - Initially, hematomas are anechoic, becoming progressively more echogenic over the course of 24 hours.
  - With the passage of time, echogenicity of the hematoma once again begins to decrease, and within 4-5 days, the hematoma becomes hypoechoic or anechoic.
  - Septa and internal echoes often develop within the hemorrhagic collection by 1-4 weeks.
- Appearances of hepatic laceration change with time. Lacerations appear slightly echogenic, becoming hypoechoic or cystic when scanned days after the injury.
- Similar to hematomas, contusions usually are hypoechoic initially, becoming transiently hyperechoic and then hypoechoic.
- The most common ultrasonographic pattern observed with liver parenchymal injuries is a discrete hyperechoic area; however, a diffuse hyperechoic and occasionally a discrete hypoechoic pattern may be observed (Fig. 17.3).[17,22]

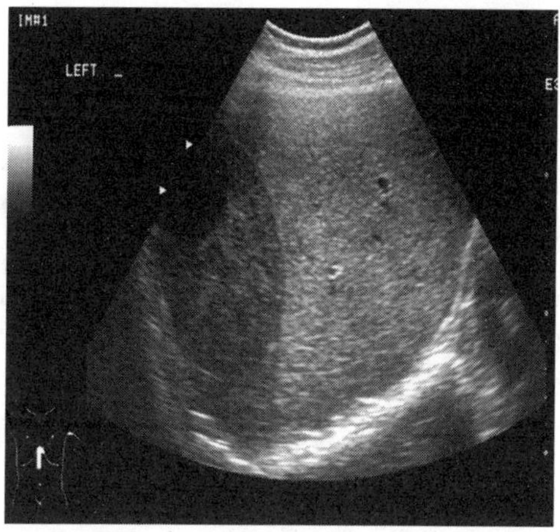

Fig. 17.3: Abdominal sonogram in blunt abdominal injury shows a crescent-shaped hyperechoic collection along the right lateral aspect of the liver consistent with subcapsular hematoma

- An echogenic clot often is seen surrounding the liver, and hypoechoic fluid may be observed in other parts of the abdomen.
- Bilomas appear as rounded or ellipsoid, anechoic, loculated structures that are fairly well defined in close proximity to the liver and bile duct.
- Diaphragmatic ruptures appear as a discontinuous line of echoes.
- A number of studies have suggested that ultrasonography can replace the invasive procedure of peritoneal lavage in the evaluation of blunt abdominal trauma.

Management

Resuscitation

Approximately 80% of all patients who die of hepatic injuries do so in the perioperative period from hemorrhage and hypovolemic shock. Profound hypothermia is frequently present in patients with severe hepatic trauma, particularly after repeated transfusion of nonwarmed blood. Maneuvers to prevent or decrease hypothermia in patients with major hepatic injuries are:

i. Resuscitation with warm (37°C) crystalloid solution.
ii. Resuscitation with high flow blood warmers.

iii. Covering of patients head, placement of patients on heating blankets or covering of lower extremity with plastic bags or space blankets.
iv. Irrigation of nasogastric tube with warm saline.
v. Irrigation of open body cavity with warm saline.
vi. Using of heating cascade on anesthetic machine.

The most important resuscitative technique in the patient with a major hepatic injury includes insertion of large bore intravenous lines in the upper extremities, rapid transfusion with warm crystalloid solution and type specific blood and early operation for controlling of ongoing hemorrhage.

Determination of Operation Need

Indication of exploratory laparotomies are:

i. All patients of hepatic trauma whatever may be grade of injury if they are hemodynamically unstable or become unstable after being stable initially.
ii. Patients who are hemodynamically stable and detected to have hepatic injury on USG or CT scan but the facilities for nonoperative protocol does not exists.
iii. Patients of hepatic trauma who have been put on nonoperative protocol (vide infra) and develops: (a) deterioration in vital signs or continuing need of transfusion, (b) increased abdominal tenderness or the development of new peritoneal signs, (c) progressive expansion of the hematoma or laceration as documented by repeat CT scan, and (d) an intrahepatic or subcapsular hematoma thought to represent septic focus.

Exposure

The most versatile incision for abdominal trauma is a full vertical incision. The falciform, coronary and triangular ligaments should be divided to the extent necessary to mobilize the liver and expose the site of injury. If injury to the hepatic veins is suspected, exploration of the region of the hepatic veins should not be attempted through the abdominal incision. The exposure necessary to explore the region of the hepatic veins and to repair major venous injury will almost always require a thoracotomy, made by extending the incision into the right chest, or by a median sternotomy. If the peritoneal cavity is contaminated with fecal contents, extending the abdominal incision into the chest is justifiable only under life-threatening conditions.

Management of Actively Bleeding Liver

First and foremost aim at exploration is to stop active bleeding from the liver. Various techniques are: (i) manual compression, (ii) portal triad occlusion, (iii) placement of perihepatic packs, (iv) direct clamping of liver parenchyma, (v) direct suture of the liver, and (vi) application of liver tourniquet.

Manual compression: Once the abdomen is entered and serious bleeding is encountered, manual compression is the first life saving maneuver the surgeon should attempt. It is applied from right and left margins of the liver towards the center. At the same time, a posterior directional force may help tamponade bleeding in the retrohepatic surface and posterior perihepatic space. While the senior surgeon maintains compression, the first assistant continues the management by aspirating blood from the peritoneal cavity, dissecting the ligamentous attachments of the liver, extending the incision, controlling the portal triad or applying clamps or tourniquet's directly to the liver.

Portal triad occlusion: The Pringle maneuver is usually the first step in attempting to stop hepatic bleeding by means of artery occlusion/interruption. Digital compression of the portal triad may control the bleeding from the common bile duct, portal vein and hepatic artery. A Rumel tourniquet can occlude the structures just as easily, leaving the surgeon hand free for other maneuvers. The results are observable in 10 minutes. The Rumel tourniquet can be placed rapidly by finger dissection through the foramen of Winslow. One should avoid clamping the portal triad as it may cause inadvertent damage. The upper limit of normothermic occlusion of the liver is presently unknown, although it has been successfully extended up to one hour in elective cancer surgery. The two methods of extending hepatic ischemia time are topical hypothermia and large doses of steroids (30-40 mg/kg of solumedrol),[4] however, it has not been verified by randomized prospective trials.[5]

Perihepatic packing: Recently there has been a resurgence of interest in using gauze packs as a temporary expedient in treatment of hepatic injuries. Packs are used when a surgeon is not prepared to handle the injury and wishes to defer treatment until a more experienced surgeon arrives or to transfer the patient elsewhere. When the patients is becoming hypothermic, acidotic, or coagulopathic or is likely to require massive transfusion and when the surgeon is unable to control hemorrhage surgically. The technique consists of placing dry folded laparotomy pads between the diaphragm and the liver, below the liver and laterally until sufficient pressure is generated to achieve hemostasis. Importantly, excessive packing should be avoided because it may compromise cardiac inflow from the inferior vena cava. When packing is on a raw surface, a small steri-drape is placed between the packs and the liver. This prevents disruption of hemostasis when the pack pads are removed during re-exploration. Closed suction drains are placed and the patient is transferred to the intensive care unit where vigorous rewarming is instituted and attempts are made to treat the coagulopathy. It consists of the following: (a) maintenance of tissue perfusion by ensuring adequate blood and extracellular fluid volumes guided by appropriate monitoring, (b) rapid rewarming of the patient using thermal blankets, warm intravenous fluids and warm, humidified gases in the ventilator, and (c) the empirical use of fresh frozen plasma and platelets transfusions. When hemodynamic instability, acidosis, hypothermia and coagulopathy have been corrected the patient may be returned to the operation theater for pack removal. These events usually don't occur until 24 to 72 hours after the original surgery. Reoperation serves not only to remove the packs, but also to debride nonviable hepatic tissue, suture ligate specific bleeding point and lacerated bile ducts, irrigate the abdomen of clots and establish new drainage.

Surgical clamps: The various surgical clamps for liver falls into two categories: (i) occluding, noncrushing clamps, and (ii) crushing clamps. These clamps are large enough to encompass fully the thickest part of the liver, both posteriorly and anteriorly. Successful placement of these clamps, which often requires previous dissection of the ligamentous attachments of the liver, stops the bleeding dramatically. This rapid cessation of bleeding permits further patient resuscitation and definitive ongoing treatment of the anatomic injury in a dry surgical field.

Surgical hemostasis: With either blunt or a penetrating injury to the liver and a wound upto 3 cm in depth (Grades I or II injury), a gentle distraction of the wound with pressure on the edges of the liver usually exposes the depth of the wound. A vessel may be seen and homeostasis can be secured with a clip, a tie or by a suture ligature. With a deeper injury (Grade II or greater) or multiple injuries to the liver, a greater degree of hemostasis is desirable before attempting to identify and occlude severed blood vessel by methods enumerated above. Direct suturing is almost ingrained instinct to the surgeon, but direct suture for the liver should be an adjunctive procedure, not a first step. In the liver suture placement, one must avoid creating a dead space, which may lead to abscess formation or to hemobilia. Ideally liver sutures should be placed parallel to any laceration to control the bleeding by compression of the hepatic substance rather than apposition of cut edges. Parallel sutures control the hemorrhage and leave the wound open, permitting proper drainage of the wound without dead space. With a deeper fracture in the liver and, in particular, with an injury that passes across the dome of the liver and down towards its posterior aspect, exposure and exploration of the depth of the wound is likely to produce daunting hemorrhage, despite using the Pringle maneuver. Under such circumstances liver suture may be life saving. This is a heavy absorbable suture on a large, curved, blunt tipped needle. The suture enters hepatic substance several centimetres from the site of the injury, passes deeply through the hepatic substance outside of the wound, and exits on the opposite side. Bolsters of surgicel may be used with the sutures. The sutures may be passed twice through hepatic substance in an over and over fashion (Fig. 17.4). The suture is tied snugly but not so tight as to cause strangulation of hepatic substance. Coaptation of hepatic substance by a series of liver sutures usually controls bleeding unless there is a major venous injury.

Debridement

Small fragments of amputated and devitalized hepatic substance should be removed. The resulting defect does not require closure. Occasionally, hepatic injury is of such severity as to require a major resection of devitalized tissue, a resectional debridement. This usually is an avulsion injury (Grade IV) and will often

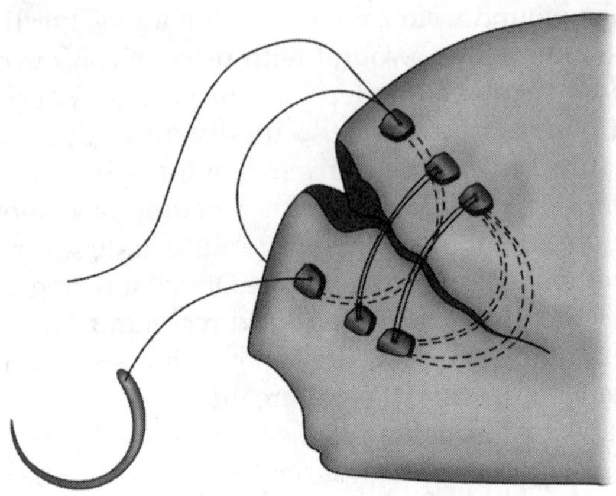

Fig. 17.4: Liver sutures being placed over the bolster

involves the right lobe of the liver and results from blunt trauma. Major injuries of the lateral segment of the left lobe of the liver (Segments II and III) are usually treated by resection debridement. If a major resectional debridement is required planes of the injury in the liver are followed. When it is necessary to resect major portions of hepatic substance, there are two planes to be avoided within the liver: (i) the interlobar plane, and (ii) the plane of the falciform ligament. Resection through the interlobar plane invites injury to the middle hepatic vein. If the right lobe is resected, this jeopardizes the venous drainage of the medial segment of the left lobe (Segment IV). If the resection is of the left lobe, ligation of the middle hepatic vein will jeopardize the drainage of segment V. A resection of the lateral segment of the left lobe through the plane of the falciform ligament invites injury to the umbilical portion of the portal vein, and the portal venous supply to the medial segment of the left that is being preserved is jeopardized.

Viable Omental Pack

The finger fracture technique of splitting the liver to achieve hemostasis under direct vision and subsequent debridement of nonviable parenchyma will usually result in a fair sized dead space within the hepatic parenchyma. Few surgeons prefer to fill the dead space within the liver with a pedicle of omentum, nourished by either the right or left gastroepiploic vessels. The liver edges are coapted loosely around the omentum with chromic sutures. There are several advantage of using a viable omentum pedicle: (i) the omentum's ability to tamponade major bleeding and minor oozing is well recognized, (ii) by filling large defects within the liver, dead space is decreased and the chances of developing an abscess is decreased, and (iii) the omentum is a rich source of macrophages and when introduced in the traumatized liver, may be beneficial in combating sepsis.[6]

Hepatic Resection

Major hepatic resections for trauma carry an excessive mortality. Indication for major hepatic resection for trauma do however exist. Major resection should be reserved for the following instances: (i) patients with total destruction of the normal hepatic parenchyma, (ii) when the extent of the injury precludes, "perihepatic packing, (iii) instances where the injury has virtually performed the resection and completion can be achieved with several additional clamps, and (iv) when hepatic resection is the sole method of controlling exsanguinating hemorrhage.

Juxtahepatic Venous Injuries

If there is injury to major hepatic veins or the juxtahepatic vena cava (Grades V and VI injuries) the surgeon must decide whether to proceed with definitive therapy or to attempt temporary control of hemorrhage with a pack. Definitive repair usually requires vascular isolation of the liver. Venous injuries that can be repaired without vascular isolation are most often in the juxtahepatic vena cava and result from penetrating trauma. In this situation it may be possible to apply a vascular clamp to the vena cava or to control bleeding with direct pressure while injury is repaired. Vascular isolation is necessary for definitive repair of most grade vascular injuries and in essentially all grade VI injuries. There are three techniques for vascular isolation of the liver: (i) placement of atrial-caval shunt through the right atrium (Fig. 17.5), (ii) placement of an intracaval shunt from below the liver (Fig. 17.6), and (iii) use of multiple occlusive clamps (Fig. 17.7). The intra-atrial[7] shunt is established with a no 8F endotracheal tube. A purse string suture is placed in the right atrial appendage. An opening is made in the atrium and the tube is passed downward through the vena cava behind the liver to an infrahepatic location. The balloon on the

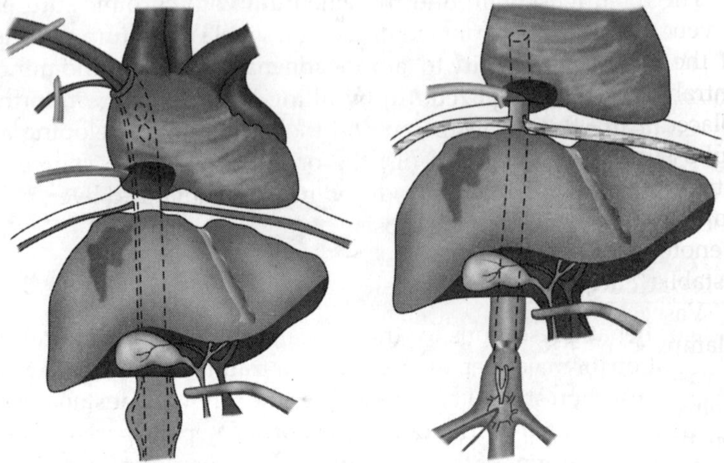

Fig. 17.5: Diagrammatic representation of atrial caval shunt

Fig. 17.6: Placement of intracaval shunt

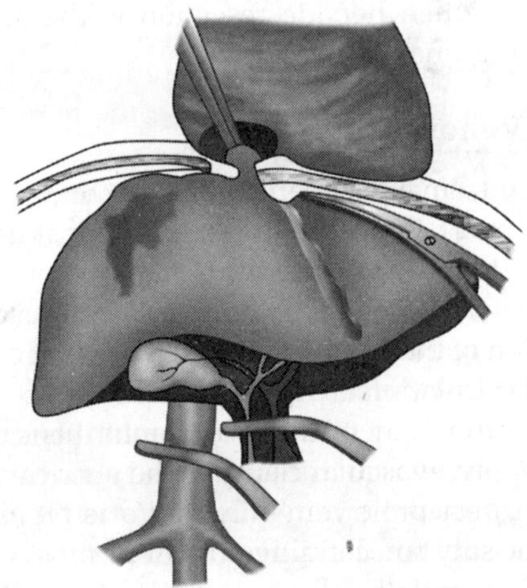

Fig. 17.7: Use of multiple clamps for vascular isolation of the liver

end of the tube is inflated. Extra hole are cut in the portion of the tube that will lie within the atrium. The pericardium is opened just above the diaphragm, and a Rumel tourniquet is placed about the vena cava just above the liver. A shunt is thus established from the infrahepatic vena cava to the atrium. A Pringle maneuver is also performed.

The intracaval shunt[8] is established by inserting a tube through a venotomy in the infrahepatic cava or sphenofemoral junction. If the vena cava is used, a purse string suture is placed in the intrahepatic but suprarenal vena cava. Rumel tourniquet are placed about the vena cava above and below the liver. A no 28 F tube is inserted into the vena cava and passed upward to the atrium through an infrahepatic venotomy. A tape is attached to the inferior aspect of the tube and brought out through the venotomy that is temporarily closed. An intracaval shunt is thus established. A Pringle maneuver is also performed.

Vascular isolation of the liver by using multiple occlusive clamps[9] consists of: (i) a Pringle maneuver, (ii) the placement of a vascular occlusive clamp across the vena cava above the renal veins but below the liver, (iii) placement of an occlusive clamp on the suprahepatic vena cava through the open pericardium, and (iv) occlusion of the aorta at or just above the level of the diaphragm, either with a vascular clamp or an aortic compression device. A clamp is preferable. This method is recommended for those surgeons who are not familiar with cardiac surgery. When the liver has been isolated, the rate of bleeding usually decreases to a point where it is possible to expose the hepatic venous or retrocaval injury and to proceed with its treatment. If one or more hepatic veins have been avulsed from the vena cava or are divided, occlusion of the hepatic vein is indicated. A vascular clamp should be applied to the torn vein or vena cava and the vessel over sewn with a 5/0 or 6/0, vascular suture rather than to attempt a ligature that will tend to tear the vein. If there is a caval defect, a Satinsky clamp can be applied. If it is necessary to mobilize the right lobe of the liver, small venous tributaries from the liver to the vena cava are identified and divided between ligatures. If a major hepatic vein is ligated often it is necessary to resect the hepatic substance drained by them.[10]

Drains

If hemostasis has been adequate and no bile leak exists after repairing grade I and grade II injury, a drainage may not be instituted. Hepatic lacerations of grade III or greater should be drained. Deep stab wounds that are not bleeding at the time of operation may result in a bile leak and should be drained. Closed suction drainage allows for the elimination of blood, perihepatic fluid, and bile collections. Concomitant injuries to the gastrointestinal tract, the presence of shock and the amount of blood transfusion required, play a significant role in the perioperative sepsis rate and are factors independent of the presence or absence of drains.[11]

Selective Hepatic Artery Ligation

The safety of selective hepatic artery ligation has been well documented. The high oxygen saturation in the portal veins of human, along with the absence of bacteria and coupled with an extensive collateral arterial flow, has allowed hepatic artery ligation to be done without significant impairment of liver function or subsequent hepatic necrosis.[12] Ligation of hepatic artery is indicated in less than 2% of cases. Hepatic artery ligation is ineffective in controlling hemorrhage from either lobar branch of portal vein, or from the major hepatic vein or their intrahepatic tributaries. The addition of hepatic artery ligation in a hypotensive patient with a resultant decrease in perfusion to the liver may tender the liver sufficiently ischemic to result in subsequent necrosis and sepsis. A 54% mortality exists in patients in whom hepatic artery ligation has failed to control hemorrhage.[13] Although hepatic artery ligation can safely be performed electively, its role in hepatic trauma appears to be at best, limited. Some authors prefer to ligate the right or the left hepatic artery rather than the proper hepatic artery.

Perihepatic Mesh Encasement

The goal of prosthetic encapsulation of the liver is to obtain sufficient compression of the liver parenchyma, and thus to achieve hemostasis. The injured lobe is freed of its peritoneal attachments by dividing the falciform ligament along the diaphragm until the suprahepatic portion of the inferior vena cava is reached. In addition, the triangular ligament and the two leaves of the coronary ligament are divided until the borders of the retrohepatic inferior vena cava are reached. During the entire dissection, the first assistant compress the liver to minimize the bleeding. The mesh is placed around the injured hepatic lobe so that the larger of the two free edges come into contact with the falciform ligament on the upper aspect. A running Vicryl suture is placed through the falciform ligament to secure the mesh to the liver. The parenchyma is then compressed progressively. The first purse string is inserted medial to lateral along the anterior edge of the liver, securing the mesh to the previously divided round ligament. The purchase must be sufficiently distant from the edge to ensure that adequate compression is achieved. As the running suture is inserted, the reinserted purse strings are tightened until plication on the liver surface is created. By virtue of their different directions and their deep location, the main portal and hepatic pedicles are not compressed by the purse strings. When the border of the liver is reached, the end of the running suture is attached to the last purse string.[14] Two silicone drains are placed one above the other below the liver. The use of mesh seems best adopted to grade III and grade IV and lobar tears.

Hemostatic Products

The massively traumatized liver after surgery is seldom completely dry and replacement of clotting factors is a key factor in managing the patient. Microfibrillar collagen is one of the most useful synthetic agent available to control some of the persistent oozing that often continues inspite of normalization of the coagulation profile. It may be applied with large caliber syringe or along with surgical as a sandwich. Another invaluable adjunctive hemostatic agent is fibrin glue. Fibrin glue can either be sprayed onto the injury or directly injected into the hepatic parenchyma when deep and inaccessible injuries are present. Reported complications are postoperative intra-abdominal sepsis, rebleed and fatal reaction.[15]

Complications

Recurrent bleeding: The incidence of postoperative bleeding varies from 3 to 7%. If coagulopathy can be confidently ruled out recurrent bleeding in the early postoperative period is as a result of inadequate hemostasis. The patient's condition permitting, reoperation and definitive control of specific bleeding site is the operation of choice. If the patient is unstable to tolerate a laparotomy at this time, consideration should be given to angiography and selective embolization of the bleeding vessel.

Hemobilia: Mild form of hemobilia is fairly common following endoscopic papillotomy and surgery on the biliary tract but hemobilia following blunt hepatic trauma is extremely uncommon. Approximately one-third of patients present with the classic triad of hematemesis/melena, pain right hypochondrium and jaundice. Signs and symptoms may occur as early as the fourth post injury day or may manifest itself weeks to a month later. Upper GI endoscopy is diagnostic most of the times. The diagnosis is confirmed by angiography and the treatment is best accomplished by embolization of the offending vessel. The therapeutic efficacy of embolization in instances of hemobilia has clearly been established.[24] Failure of embolization or nondemonstration of the offending vessel, or when associated with large intrahepatic cavity are the indications for surgery.

Intra-abdominal abscess: The frequency of intra-abdominal abscess varies from 1.9 to 09%.[25,26] Factors which influence are: the extent of hepatic injury; associated gut injury, the number of transfusion required and the type of drains used. Percutaneous USG/CT guided drainage has been reported to have a success rate of 95%. Failure of percutaneous drainage is an indication for reoperation. Extraperitoneal approach/formal laparotomy will depend on site of abscess and the condition of the patient. Extraperitoneal approach is preferred initially.

Biliary fistulae: The persistence of greater than 50 ml of biliary drainage for 2 weeks constitute a biliary fistula. The reported incidence of biliary fistula is 10%. If adequate drainage had been accomplished at the initial surgery and the flow of bile into the duodenum is unimbedded, these fistulae usually close spontaneously. Persistence of bile drainage in excess of 300 ml per day should lead to the performance of a fistulogram to determine the anatomy of the fistula. If it is found that a major intrahepatic duct has been lacerated, spontaneous closure is unlikely. ERCP is performed and placement of stent endoscopically obviates the need of major surgery. The advantage of initial nonoperative methods are: (i) it allows the better preparation of the patient if the surgery becomes necessary, (ii) it can at times be therapeutic, and (iii) ERCP serves as an invaluable road map if hepaticojejunostomy is required.

Subcapsular and intrahepatic hematoma: The management of intrahepatic hematoma and subcapsular hematoma have been controversial. If the diagnosis is made preoperatively generally nonoperative approach is favored. Criteria for operative interventions during observation are: evidence of ongoing hemorrhage, progressive expansion of hematoma, sign of sepsis and deterioration of liver function. When subcapsular and intrahepatic hematoma are encountered at operation the management should be individualized. Factors to be considered are site and size of hematoma, general condition of the patient and the expertise available.

Nonoperative Management

Use of ultrasonography and abdominal CT scan in the initial evaluation of blunt trauma patients allows the detection of liver injuries that previously might have remained occult and therefore have historically been unintentionally treated nonoperatively. Thirty to seventy percent of liver injuries are not bleeding at the time of laparotomy and don't require any surgical treatment. The recognition of these subset of patients with liver injuries who are hemodynamically stable or become stable following resuscitation has led a few surgeons to recommend selective nonoperative management for these patients.[16,17] It has been demonstrated by multiple investigators that nonoperative management of most children with blunt hepatic injury yields satisfactory results.[18,19] The nonoperative management scheme has been retrospectively and recently prospectively been reviewed for adult population and the results are quite favorable with a few liver related failures.[20-22]

Selection Criteria for Nonoperative Protocol

- Hemodynamically stable patient
- Blunt abdominal trauma
- Awake, alert and responding patient
- Grades I to III injury (CT evaluation)
- No clinical/CT evidence of continued bleeding or expanding hematoma
- No other indication for surgery
- Ready access to CT scan and operation theater
- Availability of surgeon / radiologist with extensive experience in interpreting the CT scan
- Blood requirement less than 40 ml/kg in children and 20 ml/kg in adults.

Once a decision is reached to use a nonoperative approach the patient is placed on strict bed rest and repeated physical examination by the same surgeon is performed. Blood count and hematocrit is done 12 hourly. USG is done daily. After 5-7 days of observation a repeat CT scan is performed. If the second scan reveals no change in the injury or some worsening, the surgeon must decide whether further inhospital observation is warranted or immediate laparotomy. If nonoperative care is chosen, the patient continues bed rest for a period of 5-7 days and then discharged to home for further bed rest for 4 weeks. After 4 weeks CT scan is repeated and by this time 95% of lesion have healed (Figs 17.8 to 17.11.). Individual is then permitted to return to his previous profession. Contact sports should be forbidden for 3 months.

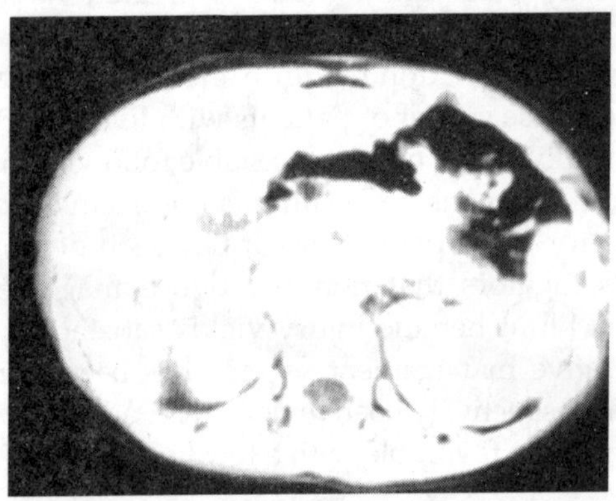

Fig. 17.8: CT scan of a child showing hepatic trauma grade II treated conservatively

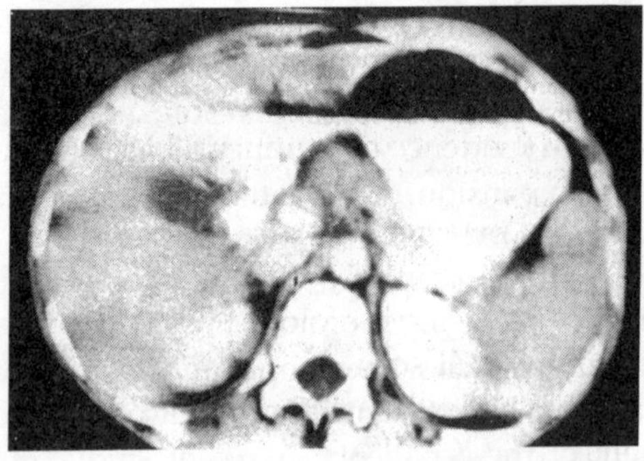

Fig. 17.9: Follow-up CT scan showing resolution in progress of Figure 17.8

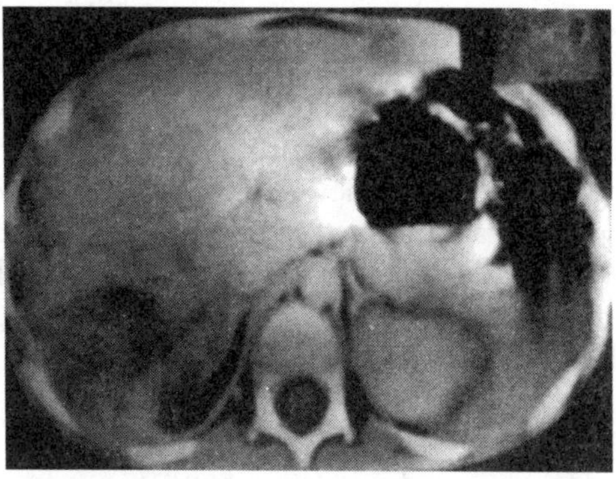

Fig. 17.10: CT scan in a young boy treated conservatively

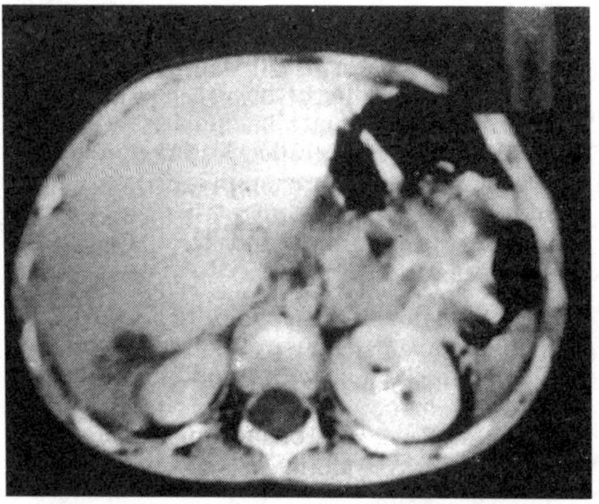

Fig. 17.11: Follow-up CT scan showing complete healing of Figure 17.10

Nonoperative management is abandoned when there is:

- Deterioration of vital signs
- Continued requirement of blood transfusion
- Increasing abdominal tenderness or the development of new peritoneal signs
- Progressive expansion of hematoma or laceration as documented by repeated USG/CT scan
- An intrahepatic/subcapsular hematoma thought to be present as septic focus.

The current success rate with nonoperative management of stable hepatic injuries stem from trauma centers with extensive experience in management of these patients. A recent study concluded that nonoperative management is safe for hemodynamically stable patients with blunt hepatic injury regardless of injury severity. There are fewer abdominal complications and less transfusions when compared with a matched cohort of operated patients.[23]

Nonoperative management should neither lead to excessive blood transfusion nor to inordinate delay in operative interventions. The weakness of nonoperative management of blunt hepatic injuries is the possibility of missing an associated intra-abdominal injury. The rate of missed injuries in published literature is about 3-5% mainly being small bowel injury and diaphragmatic tear.[23a]

Penetrating Injuries

Selected patients with isolated grades I and II gunshot wounds to the liver can be managed nonoperatively.[23b] Patients with penetrating injuries to the liver are divided grossly into two categories: (1) those who are hemodynamically stable, and (2) those who are in shock. 28% of patients with penetrating injuries to the abdomen can be managed nonoperatively. Most of these involve injuries to the liver. Most are low-velocity gunshot wounds and stab wounds. The caveat is that the patient cannot have a hollow viscus injury, including the gallbladder.[23c] The NOM of appropriately selected patients with liver gunshot injuries is feasible, safe, and effective, regardless of the liver injury severity.[23d]

INTERVENTION RADIOLOGY

Angiographic findings in patients with liver trauma include the following:

- Liver contusion
  - Stretching and elongation of arterial branches around an avascular mass may be observed.
  - Delay in hepatic blood flow to the involved segments may occur.
  - A transient attenuation difference in uninvolved segments may be depicted.
  - Mottled accumulation of contrast material in the parenchymal phase may be noted.
  - The portal venous phase may confirm a parenchymal defect.

   - Peripheral portal venous filling may be unusually well demonstrated in the presence of contusions.
- Liver lacerations (Fig. 17.12)
   - Arterial collaterals may bypass arterial occlusions.
   - Contrast material extravasation may occur.
   - Discrete lacerations may appear as linear or complex lucent defects.
   - Intrahepatic hematomas may appear as poorly defined lucent defects.
   - Arterioportal fistulas may be obvious.
   - Contrast material may pass into the biliary tree, identifying the site of hemobilia.
- Subcapsular hematoma
   - Subcapsular hematomas compress normal parenchyma and may appear as sharply defined, lucent defects against the increased contrast accumulation in the compressed parenchyma.
   - Arterial displacement may be seen.
   - Contrast material extravasation may occur.

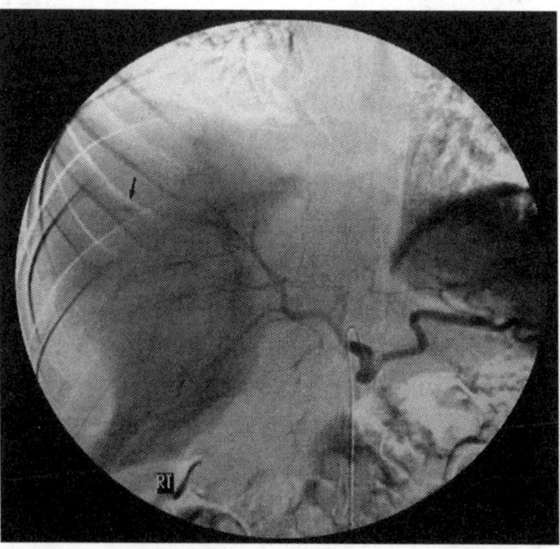

Fig. 17.12: The image shows a focal area of hemorrhage in the right lobe of the liver (arrow) due to the stabbing injury. The well-demarcated filling defect seen in the lateral aspect of the right lobe of the liver is due to compression of normal liver parenchyma by the subcapsular hematoma

- High-velocity bullet injuries
  - High-velocity bullets tend to cause burst injuries with distant contusions and parenchymal disruption.
  - Occasionally, these injuries are associated with aortic and renal injuries.
  - All of the angiographic findings of blunt liver trauma can be seen in this group of patients.
- Low-velocity penetrating injury (stab wounds, liver biopsy, and biliary drainage TIPS procedure)
  - Arterial aneurysms and arterial pseudoaneurysms
  - Arteriovenous fistulas
  - Hematomas.

Blunt hepatic trauma more often causes venous injury and hemorrhage. Most arterial injuries are increasingly being caused by radiologic interventional procedures, such as liver biopsy, TIPS, PTC, and biliary drainage. The typical injury is a small pseudoaneurysm, which may require meticulous, superselective angiography. A combined surgical and radiologic approach may be required in the treatment of patients with high-grade liver lacerations with injury to the retrohepatic inferior vena cava.[25] Initially, the surgeon attempts to control the hemorrhage with temporary perihepatic packing.

Recurrent liver parenchymal bleeding can be successfully treated by using transcatheter embolization, and bleeding from a major hepatic vein can be controlled by placing an intravenous stent.[26] Embolization can be performed in persistent arterial hemorrhage, as may occur with stab wounds of the liver, and in the occlusion of pseudoaneurysms. Transcatheter arterial embolization may reduce transfusion requirements and allow healing of hepatic injuries without surgery.

Because hepatic arteries are not end arteries, occlusive devices should be deployed distal to the lesion to prevent collateral backdoor filling. The entire hepatic artery may be occluded, if required, as long as the portal vein is patent. If the portal vein is occluded, only selective embolization can be performed; this should prevent liver infarction due the presence of intrahepatic collaterals. The uncommon complication of bile peritonitis can be confirmed by means of diagnostic aspiration under ultrasonographic or CT scan guidance.

REFERENCES

1. Feliciano DV, Pachter HL. Hepatic trauma revisited. Curr Probl Surg 1989;26: 453-524.
2. Moore EE, Cogbill TH, Malangoni MA, Jurkovich GJ, Shackford SR, Champion HR, McAninch JW. Organ injury scaling. Surg Clin North Am 1995;75:293-305.
3. Mirvis SE, Whitley NO, Vainwright JR, Gens DR. Blunt hepatic trauma in adults: CT based classification and correlation with prognosis and treatment. Radiol 1989;171:27-32.
4. Depin EA, Figueroa I, Lopez R, Vazquez J. Protective effects of steroids on liver ischaemia: 142 cases. Am Surg 1975;41:683.
5. Pachter HL, Spencer FC, Hofstetter SR. The management of juxtahepatic venous injuries without an atrial caval shunt: Preliminary clinical observations. Surg 1986;99:569.
6. Jurkiewicz MJ, Nahai F. The omentum: Its use as a free vascularised graft for reconstruction of the head and neck. Ann Surg 1982;195:756.
7. Schrock T, Blaisdell FW, Mathewson C. Management of blunt trauma liver injuries and hepatic veins. Arch Surg 1968; 96:698-704.
8. Buckberg GD, et al. Hypotension following revascularisation of the anoxic liver: Factors influencing its occurrence and prevention. Surg 1968;63: 446-58.
9. Heaney JP, et al. An improved technique for vascular isolation of the liver: Experimental study and case reports. Ann Surg 1966;163:237-41.
10. Donovan AJ, Berne TV. Liver in Donovan AJ (ed). Trauma Surgery, ed 1. St Louis, Mosby, 1994;111-35.
11. Pachter HL, Liang HG, Hofstetter SR. Liver and biliary tract trauma. In Moore EE, Mattox KL, Feliciano DV (Eds). Trauma, second edition. East Norwalk, CT, Appleton & Lange, 1991;441-63.
12. Waltz AJ. The mythology of hepatic trauma, or babel revisited. Am J Surg 1978;135:12.
13. Flint Lm Jr, Polk HC. Selective hepatic artery ligation: Limitaion and failure. J Trauma 1979;19:319.
14. Brunet C, Sielezneff I, Thomas P, Thirion X, Sastre B, Farisse J. Treatment of hepatic trauma with perihepatic mesh: 35 cases. J Trauma 1994;37:200-4.
15. Kram HB, Nathan RC, Klein SR, et al. Clinical use of nonautologous fibrin glue. Am Surg 1988;54:570.
16. Vock P, Kehrer B, Tscheppeler H. Blunt liver trauma in children: The role of computed tomography in diagnosis and treatment. J Pediatr Surg 1986;21:413.
17. Brick SH, Taylor GA, Potter BM, et al. Hepatic and splenic injury in children: Role of CT in the decision for laparotomy. Radiol 1987;163:643.

18. Oldham KT, Guice KS, Ryckman F, et al. Blunt injury in childhood: Evaluation of therapy and current perspective. Surg 1986;100:542-9.
19. Amroch D, Schiavon G, Carmignola G, et al. Isolated blunt liver trauma: Is nonoperative treatment justified? J Pediatr Surg 1992;27:466-8.
20. Knudson MM, Lim RD Jr, Oakes DD, et al. Nonoperative management of blunt liver injuries in adults: The need of continued surveillance. J Trauma 1990;30:1494-1500.
21. Durham RM, Buckley J, Keegan M, et al. Management of blunt hepatic injuries. Am J Surg 1992;164:477-81.
22. Meredith JW, Young JS, Bowling J, et al. Nonoperative, management of blunt hepatic trauma: The exception or the rule? J Trauma 1994;36: 529-35.
23. Croce MA, Fabian TC, Menke PG, et al. Nonoperative management of blunt hepatic trauma is the treatment of choice for haemodynamically stable patients. Ann Surg 1995;221:744-55.
23a. Atef El-Gamal, Hamid Labib, Hussein M, Hussein, Liljana Petkovska, Ziad Daouk, Neema Al-Awadi. Liver injury after blunt abdominal trauma: Role of nonoperative management. PAN Arab Medical Journal 51 SURGERY2005.
23b. Demetriaides D, Gomez H, Chahwan S, Charalambides K, Velmahos G, Murray J, Asensio J, Berne TV. Gunshot injuries to the liver: the role of selective nonoperative management. J Am Coll Surg 1999;188(4):343-8.
23c. Donald D Trunkey. Penetrating liver injuries. Medscape General Surgery. 2002;4(2) © 2002 Medscape
23d. Demetriaides D, Hadjizacharia P, Constantinou C, Brown C, Inaba K, Rhee P, Salim A. Selective nonoperative management of penetrating abdominal solid organ injuries. Ann Surg 2006;244(4):620-8.
24. Cyret P, Baumar R, Roche A. Hepatic haemobilia of traumatic or iatrogenic origin. Recent advances of diagnosis and therapy. Review of the literature from 1976-1981. World J Surg 1984;8:2.
25. Feliciano DV, Mattox KL, Jordan Gl, Jr, et al. Management of 1000 consecutive cases of hepatic trauma (1979-1984). Ann Surg 1986; 204:438.
26. Cogbill TH, Moore EE, Jurkovich GJ, et al. Severe hepatic trauma: A multicenter experience with 1,335 liver injuries. J Trauma 1988; 28:1433.

Chapter

18

Injuries of Spleen

SK Kochar

INTRODUCTION

The spleen is the most common abdominal organ injured by blunt abdominal trauma. It is frequently involved in penetrating injuries of the lower chest, abdomen and flank. Iatrogenic trauma may cause injuries to the spleen in a variety of situations. Traction on the stomach or colon during laparotomy, inadvertent placement of chest tube below the left diaphragm and percutaneous catheter drainage of the intra-abdominal abscess have resulted in splenic injuries in the literature.

Classification

Organ injury scale proposed by Moore et al 1994[1] is widely being used for classification of injuries of the spleen. It is based on CT scan and operative observations (Table 18.1).

ANATOMY

The spleen arises as a localized cellular collection in the left layer of the dorsal mesogastrium. The later is divided by the spleen into an anterior gastrosplenic portion and a posterior splenoaortic portion within which courses the splenic artery. As the growth takes place, the spleen and stomach migrate to the left and the medial segment of the splenoaortic mesogastrium apposes and fuse into the parietal peritoneum overlying the posterior abdominal wall and the left kidney. The most lateral unfused segment of the dorsal mesogastrium becomes the splenorenal ligament. The gastrosplenic omentum or ligament derives from the anterior portion of the dorsal mesogastrium and contains the left gastroepiploic artery and

Table 18.1: Injury severity score

Grade	Type	Description
Grade I		
	Hematoma:	Subcapsular 10% surface area
	Laceration:	Capsular tear <1 cm parenchymal depth
Grade II		
	Hematoma:	Subcapsular 10-50% surface area, intraparenchymal (5 cm diamter)
	Laceration:	Capsular tear, 1-3 cm parenchymal depth which does not involve a trabecular vessel
Grade III		
	Hematoma:	Subcapsular 50% surface area or expanding, ruptured subcapsular or parenchymal hematoma, intraparenchymal hematoma > 5 cm or expanding
	Laceration:	3 cm parenchymal depth or involving trabecular vessels
Grade IV		
	Laceration:	Laceration involving segmental or hilar vessels producing major devascularization (25% of spleen)
Grade V		
	Laceration:	Completely shattered spleen
	Vascular:	Hilar vascular injury which devascularizes spleen

(*Note:* Advance one grade for multiple injuries up to grade III)

the short gastric vessels. The spleen is attached to the diaphragm through the phrenicolienal ligament and the splenic flexure of the colon through lienocolic ligament, the later occasionally containing vessels which may require ligation during splenectomy. The splenic artery commonly divides into a major superior pole branch and an inferior pole branch, each of which gives rise to a variable number of terminal vessels that provide discrete segmental splenic perfusion. This arrangement constitutes the anatomical bases for partial resection of the spleen. Pancreatic tail is intimately related to the splenic vessels and the hilum of the spleen and may get injured while doing splenectomy. There is more functional smooth muscle and elastase in the spleen of the children than the adults.

Physiology

The spleen plays an exceedingly active role in the reticulo-endothelial system. In the spleen microcirculation is the primary site of clearance of blood born bacteria and particulate antigen.

The spleen is also a major synthetic site for the opsonic proteins, tuftsin and properdin, which are essential for the processing of antigens. It has a role in the modification of reticulocytes and destruction of senescent red blood cells.[2] Following splenectomy, IgM levels falls and remains low for a year or more. There is also a reduction in phagocytic capacity with resultant inability to clear encapsulated bacteria from the blood stream. These factors may result in overwhelming postsplenectomy infection. Meningitis, pneumonia or septicemia may occur days to years following splenectomy. The majority of serious infections occur within 2 years and almost half within 2 months. Postsplenectomy sepsis resulting in death occurs in approximately 1 in 2000 children and 1 in 4000 adults undergoing splenectomy for injury.[3] Postsplenic sepsis is usually quite sudden with nausea, vomiting, headache and confusion progressing to coma. Fever as high as 104°F has been noted. Most commonly the organism is *Streptococcus pneumoniae* (50%), other organism are *Neisseria meningitidis, Haemophilus influenzae, E. coli*. The overall mortality is 50-80%.[4]

Diagnosis

History of blunt or penetrating trauma to left hypochondrium or left lower chest, signs of peritonism in the form of pain, tenderness in the left hypochondrium, features of oligemic shock in the form of low blood pressure, tachycardia, giddiness, fainting attack may be presenting features.

Kehr's sign: Kehr's sign is elicited by bimanual compression of the upper quadrant, after the patient has been in Trendelenburg's position for several minutes proceeding the maneuver. It is inconstant and may vary in incidence from 15 to 75%.

Ballance sign: On occasions patients with splenic injury will have a palpable mass in the left upper quadrant, resulting from an extracapsular hematoma with omentum adherent to the injured spleen.

Diagnostic peritoneal lavage: Peritoneal lavage has an accuracy of 95 to 98% in the diagnosis of intra-abdominal injuries due to blunt trauma and similar sensitivity has been reported for stab wounds. It is not organ specific and it only indicates intra-abdominal hemorrhage.

Radiological Evaluation

Conventional radiography: Chest radiograph may show fracture of tenth and eleventh rib. Left pleural effusion, elevated hemidiaphragm and pulmonary contusion are additional evidence of significant injury to the left hypochondrium. Abdomen X-ray done in supine position may provide clues to the diagnosis of splenic trauma though none of these are specific. At least 800 ml of intraperitoneal blood is required to be evident on plain X-ray of the abdomen. The following finding may be observed:

i. The flank strip sign is a fluid dense zone separating the ascending or descending colon from a distinctly outlined lateral peritoneal wall, the colon is displaced medially.
ii. The dog ear sign results from accumulations of blood that gravitates between viscera and side walls on each side of the bladder.
iii. The injured spleen may cause displacement of the gastric bubble medially or indentation of the splenic flexure of the colon.
   - Ultrasound is generally used in the diagnosis of blunt abdominal injury as the focused abdominal sonography for trauma (FAST) examination. This exam uses four views (subxiphoid, suprapubic, left and right upper quadrants) with a 3.5 mHz probe to detect hemoperitoneum and/or hemopericardium. Evaluation of the left upper quadrant can detect hemoperitoneum associated with possible splenic injury. In the sagittal view, an anechoic (dark black area without echoes) may be seen in the splenorenal recess, indicating hemoperitoneum. Parenchymal abnormalities commonly are subtle:
     - Lacerations appear as hypoechoic regions, which can be irregular or linear in configuration.
     - Splenic infarct has a similar appearance, but it is usually better defined. Infarcts are wedge shaped, with the apex toward the hilum, compared to traumatic injury in which a more complex distribution is seen.
     - Subtlety of parenchymal injury probably relates to associated local hemorrhage. Any trapped blood soon coagulates, becoming isoechoic with the surrounding tissue.

With multiple views, the FAST exam has been shown to have 80–85%[5] sensitivity for detecting hemoperitoneum. The false negative rate may be higher in patients with hematuria, spine fractures, or pelvic fracture.

CT Scan (Figs 18.1 and 18.2)

- Blunt splenic trauma can result in subcapsular hematoma, intraparenchymal hematoma, laceration, or fragmentation with autosplenectomy.

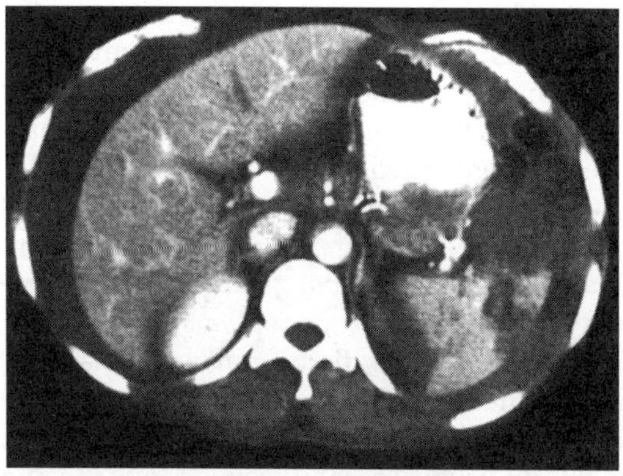

Fig. 18.1: CT scan showing complex laceration extending to the hilum grade IV injury

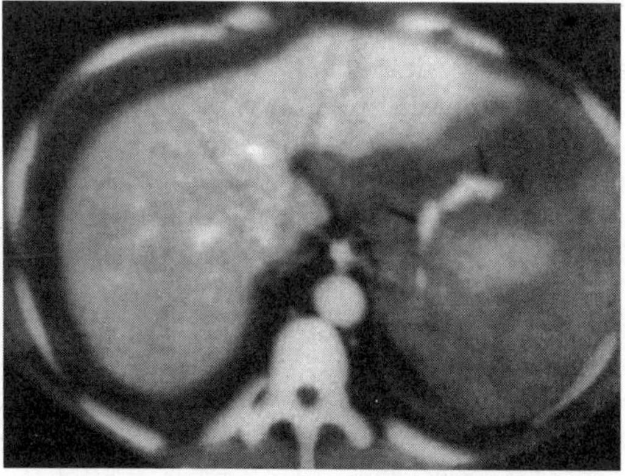

Fig. 18.2: Contrast enhanced CT scan showing localized area of dense contrast in the splenic hilum with massive amount of surrounding fluid blood indicating autosplenectomy, grade V injury

- Laceration appears as an irregular hypodense area of nonenhancement, with somewhat indistinct borders compared to the margin in an unlacerated spleen.
- Subcapsular hematomas are regularly shaped, crescentic, hypoattenuating collections closely applied to the perceived splenic margin. The margins are usually sharp in distinction to a perisplenic clot. Underlying deformity or indentation of the parenchyma is appreciated.
- Intraparenchymal hematoma is a broader, more irregular, hypoattenuating area with mass effect and enlargement of the spleen. A parenchymal hematoma, which is contained within the spleen, should have a discernible rim of surrounding splenic tissue on contrast-enhanced images. On nonenhanced images, the hematoma can appear hypoattenuating, isoattenuating, or hyperattenuating compared with the parenchyma.

- Hemoperitoneum almost always accompanies splenic injury. Uncommonly, a perisplenic clot is present without evidence for capsular disruption, which has been reported in approximately 9% of patients and is termed the sentinel clot. The sentinel clot is a sensitive sign of visceral injury and should prompt careful inspection of the images for an etiology; however, a small laceration can be compressed by perisplenic clot, rendering it invisible.
- The CT appearance of intraperitoneal blood depends on the age and physical state of the clot.
  - Immediately after hemorrhage, intraperitoneal blood has the same attenuation as circulating blood of 20-30 HU. However, attenuation values less than 20 HU are a frequent finding in the acute setting. The proposed reason for this is that blood, being a strong peritoneal irritant, causes a local inflammatory response with transudation of fluid across the peritoneum.
  - Transudate fluid mixes with and dilutes the blood before coagulation begins, decreasing the attenuation. Within hours, a clot forms.
  - Attenuation increases as hemoglobin concentrates, and values in the range of 50-75 HU are seen.
  - Densely clotted blood may have attenuation values upwards of 100 HU.

- Clot lysis begins within 48-72 hours, and attenuation decreases to fluid values. Lysis proceeds more rapidly for intraperitoneal hematomas than visceral hematomas secondary to abdominal and respiratory motion and bowel peristalsis.
- After a few weeks, most hematomas have attenuation values approaching those of water, namely, 0-20 HU.
- Hemoperitoneum does not indicate whether active hemorrhage is present. Repeat imaging, as clinically warranted, can aid in detecting ongoing hemorrhage. Increasing hematoma size or changes in character contrary to the expected sequence are indications of continued hemorrhage.

• On contrast-enhanced CT, extrasplenic extravasation of contrast material rarely is seen. When extravasation occurs, patients most likely have hemodynamic instability and proceed to laparotomy. However, an intraparenchymal vascular blush may appear as single or multiple well-defined areas of contrast material collection when a bolus injection is performed.
  - Hyperattenuating areas represent localized areas of contrast material extravasation from pseudoaneurysms or arteriovenous fistulas.
  - Pseudoaneurysm formation is reportedly a delayed finding in 10% of patients with splenic injury. The presence of a pseudoaneurysm is a strong predictor of nonoperative failure.

• Many authors have attempted to develop grading systems and delineate specific findings to predict the need for laparotomy and assess the success of conservative treatment. Resciniti et al proposed a CT scoring system to address the need.[6]

CT scoring system is as follows:

• Splenic parenchyma
  - Intact - 0
  - Laceration (thin, linear defect) - 1
  - Fracture (thick, irregular defect) - 2
  - Shattered - 3

• Splenic capsule
  - Intact - 0
  - Perisplenic fluid present - 1

- Abdominal fluid
  - No fluid - 0
  - Any fluid except perisplenic - 1
- Pelvic fluid
  - No fluid - 0
  - Any pelvic fluid - 1

In adult patients with a total CT score of less than 2.5, nonsurgical treatment was successful in all patients.[7]

Radioactive scintiscan: Spleen scanning with technetium 99m sulfur colloid has become a reliable noninvasive technique to delineate splenic parenchymal injury where facility of this modality exists. Scintiphotographs are obtained in anterior, posterior, lateral and oblique positions. Evidence of splenic injury includes focal area devoid of radioactivity as well as overt splenic fragmentation. The overall sensitivity of technetium spleen scanning for acute injury is 98%. It is less specific in grading splenic injuries and obviously cannot quantitate intraperitoneal hemorrhage. Radioisotopes scan are useful during healing and are indirect measures of residual splenic function.

ANGIOGRAPHY

Splenic trauma can produce a wide variety of angiographic findings, either directly or indirectly (Figs 18.3 and 18.4).

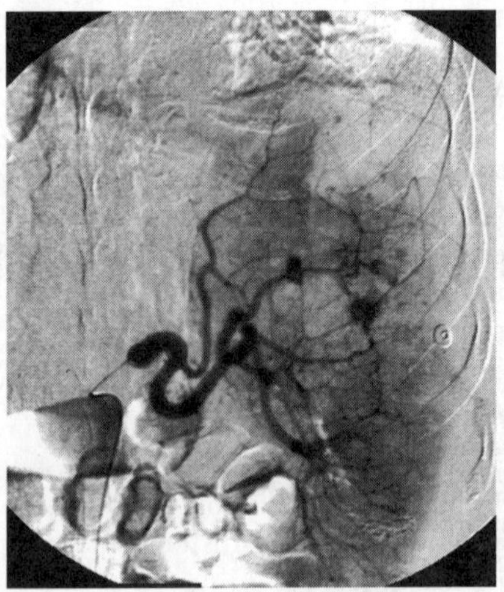

Fig. 18.3: Splenic artery angiography showing multiple areas of parenchymal contrast extravasation

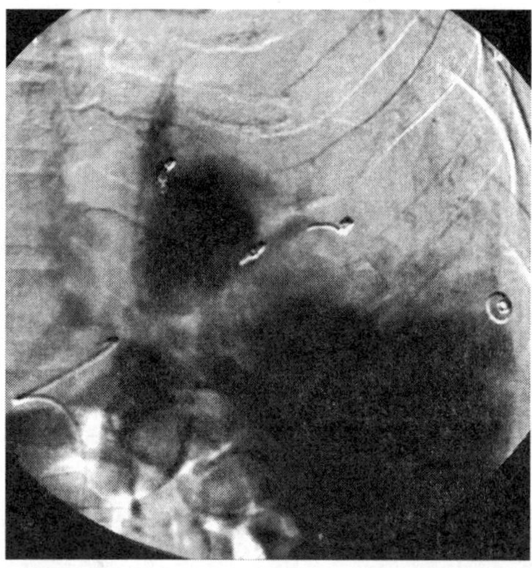

Fig. 18.4: Spleen, trauma. Final arteriographic image from a main splenic artery catheter injection after selective/superselective coil embolization. Approximately 50% of the spleen has been devascularized. No residual arterial vascular injury or extravasation is present. The patient recovered uneventfully

- Indirect signs include displacement of the spleen from the abdominal wall and avascular parenchymal areas from hematoma.
- Peripheral parenchymal defects may represent subcapsular hematomas, but care must be taken not to confuse traumatic change with developmental notching or lobulation.
- Mass effect can be identified with traumatic injury.
- Compression of the vascular pattern along the defect margin is characteristic of subcapsular hematoma.
- Defects from chronic change, such as infarct, should have clear margins that are more regular in contour without mass effect.
- Parenchymal hematoma usually demonstrates hazy borders with splaying of the surrounding vessels. Hematoma age affects the degree to which these characteristics are visualized.
- Parenchymal irregularity or mottling may result from localized edema of a contusion without apparent vessel abnormalities.

- The most reliable angiographic sign of splenic trauma is contrast-material extravasation, either parenchymal or extrasplenic. At times, extravasation may be observed only after the administration of vasopressin or epinephrine. These medications enhance detection of vascular injury by increasing precapillary arteriolar resistance.
- Abrupt cutoff of vessels, vessel wall irregularity, pseudo aneurysms, and early filling of splenic veins are findings of traumatic injury.

Clinical Examination

High index of suspicion aided by USG can clinch the diagnosis in 90% of the patients of blunt abdominal trauma. Any penetrating injury in the area of midclavicular line anteriorly to the tip of scapula posteriorly in the lower chest and upper abdomen left side should be thoroughly evaluated to rule out injury to the spleen. Often patient is a victim of polytrauma and associated injury may either dominate or alter the presentation.

Management

Appreciation of the postsplenectomy overwhelming infection, advances in technique used for monitoring physiological status, development of ultrasonography and CT scan which can delineate the injury of the spleen and quantify the hemoperitoneum have led to recent changes in the management protocols for splenic trauma. From mandatory splenectomy the pendulum has swung to organ preservation. The specific management of the patient with splenic trauma is governed by:

- Hemodynamic status
- Mechanism of injury
- Patient's age
- Interval from time of injury
- Associated injuries
- Grade of injury (CT grading)
- Pre-existing disease.

Patients who is hemodynamically stable or become stable after resuscitation is subjected to further investigation to assess the grade of injury and to decide whether to follow the nonoperative protocol or choose mandatory laparotomy. Patients who are hemodynamically unstable or become unstable are subjected to

Flow chart 18.1: Management of splenic trauma

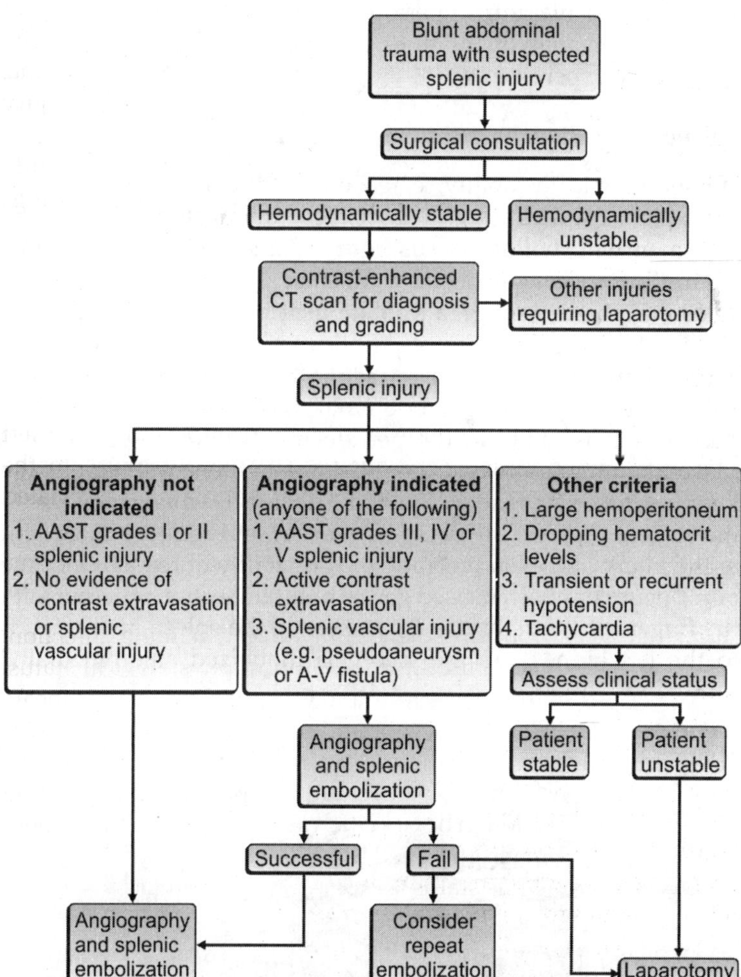

exploratory laparotomy after baseline investigations. Patients who sustain gunshot wounds are subjected to exploratory laparotomy while those who sustain stab wounds are selectively managed (Flow chart. 18.1). Pediatric age group favors a selective laparotomy while associated trauma and pre-existing disease tilts the balance to mandatory laparotomy. At exploration the type of procedure to be performed will depend on:

- Extent of injury
- The availability of perioperative care
- The availability of glues, absorbable mesh
- The expertise.

Splenectomy

Hemodynamic instability, extensive devascularization or fragmentation of the spleen, associated injuries, soiling of the abdomen with hollow viscus injury along with splenic trauma are indications for splenectomy. In emergency circumstances, the spleen, exposed through a midline incision is rapidly mobilized by dividing the left leaf of the lienorenal ligament, which is exposed and made taut by retracting the spleen medially while an assistant retract the abdominal wall laterally (Fig. 18.5). An incision is made in the peritoneum lateral to spleen, with Metzenbaum scissors and the incision lengthened to parallel the longitudinal axis of the spleen. If this incision is made too close to the spleen, capsular stripping may occur and increase the extent of the injury and even preclude the possibility of repair. Once the peritoneum has been incised gentle blunt dissection is begun with the fingers of the right hand posterior to the spleen and anterior to the left kidney. As the spleen is mobilized anteromedially,

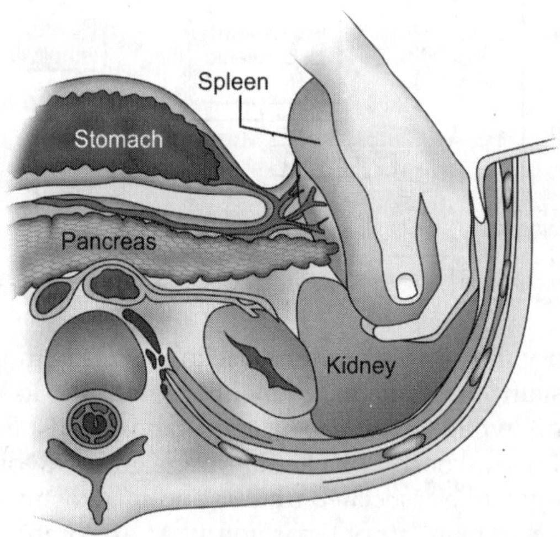

Fig. 18.5: Mobilization of spleen

attachment to the diaphragm (phrenicolienal ligament) and the splenic flexure of the colon (lienocolic ligament) are encountered and divided. The attachment of the colon may contain vessels that require ligation. With complete mobilization of the spleen to the midline, the splenic vessels are visualized, divided and ligated. Care should be taken to avoid injury to the tail of the pancreas, which frequently extends to the hilum of the spleen. Division of the splenic vessels exposes the adjacent short gastric arteries that courses within the gastrosplenic omentum. The later structure, with its contained vessels, is the remaining attachment of the spleen and must be divided carefully to avoid injury to the greater curvature of the stomach by clamp or ligature. If there is persistent oozing or if there is concern over injury to the tail of the pancreas, closed suction drainage of the left upper quadrant is performed. Drain should be removed as soon as drainage ceases or by the 5th postoperative day to avoid subphrenic abscess.

Splenorrhaphy

When the condition of the patient and initial examination of the spleen at laparotomy does not mandate immediate splenectomy, consideration is given to the splenic repair and organ preservation. Proper assessment of the splenic injury requires complete mobilization of the spleen (division of the lienorenal, phrenicorenal and lienorenal ligament) and removal of all thrombus from the site of injury. The order of dissection is influenced by the condition of the spleen. When there is minimal bleeding it may be worthwhile to first divide the gastrosplenic omentum and the short gastric vessels. This maneuver exposes the pancreas along the superior border of which courses the proximal portion of the splenic artery, which can be temporarily occluded. With complete mobilization and clearance of thrombus the splenic injury can be assessed and graded. Grade I injuries may be managed with compression, cautery or suture ligation with 0 or 2-0 absorbable sutures, but often no intervention is required. Bleeding from grade II injuries is frequently responsive to the application of topical hemostatic agents such as oxidized regenerated cellulose, microfibrillar collagen, or absorbable gelatin sponge alone or saturated with topical thrombin. Reapproximation of parenchymal edges with interrupted horizontal mattress sutures of absorbable material, usually 0 or 00 may be required. Compression packing with a vascularized omental pedicle is useful in deeper parenchymal laceration after visible vessels are ligated. Deeper parenchymal tears producing devitalized tissue may be treated by selective ligation of the segmental arterial branches and then partial splenectomy performed at the line of ischemic demarcation (Figs 18.6 and 18.7). Division of the injured splenic segment can be done with scalpel or cautery or by finger fracture technique. The oozing from cut surface of the spleen is managed with mattress sutures buttressed with pledgets of teflon or absorbable mesh. An atraumatic technique to fix the omentum after partial splenectomy consists of passing horizontal catgut mattress sutures, keeping the loop end free and long. A vascularized portion of the omentum is advanced over the edge of the spleen. The ends of the sutures are passed through the loose loops and compression is warranted in two dimensions: vertically and perpendicular, when one end of each suture is tied with the end of the adjoining stitch.[8]

Splenic capping has been described as a technique for controlling persistent bleeding after ligation of visible bleeding intraparenchymal vessels. Here absorbable polyglycoline mesh is wrapped around part or all of the spleen to tamponade the injury

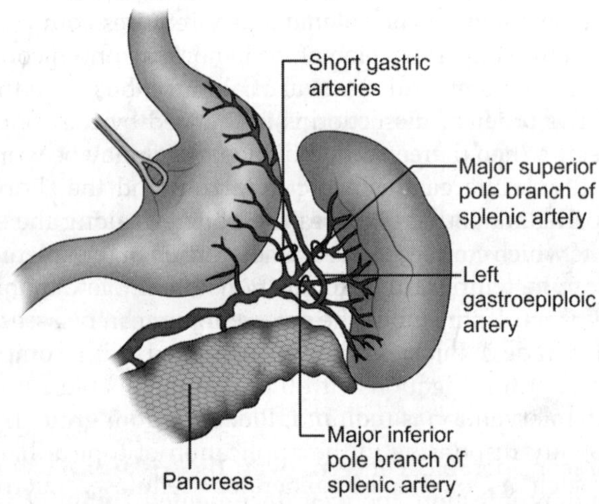

Fig. 18.6: Segmental ligation of splenic vessel in preparation of partial splenectomy

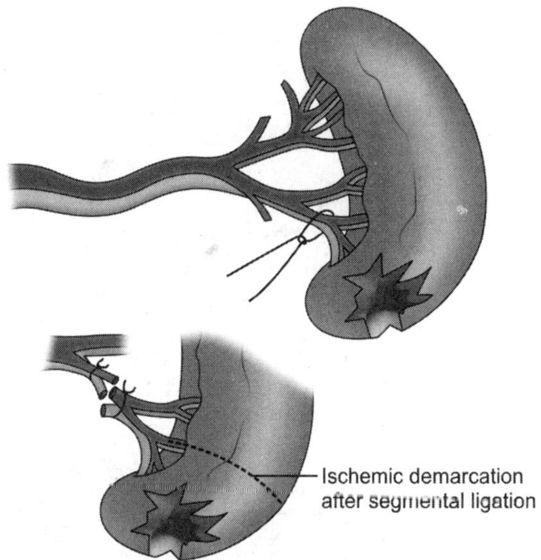

Fig. 18.7: Partial splenectomy on the line of demarcation

and restore normal architecture (Fig. 18.8).[9] Although some authors have reported ligation of the main splenic artery just proximal to terminal bifurcation, this technique is not recommended as it may result in impairment of the normal phagocytic function of the spleen. Splenic infarction manifested by pain and fever has been reported. These patients subsequently required operation for removal of an infarcted spleen. It is estimated that approximately 6% of patients will have inadequate collateral, and patients who had extensive mobilization of the spleen are not candidates for this procedure. Contraindications for splenorrhaphy are: (i) polytrauma patient who is hemodynamically unstable, (ii) extensive devascularization, and (iii) fragmentation of the spleen.

Splenic Autotransplantation in Human

Despite considerable concern over the risk of postoperative splenectomy infection, the well documented ability of spleen to regenerate, and the simplicity of carrying out the procedure remarkably few reports of splenic autotransplantation appear in the literature.[10,11] The majority of authors placed implants into omental pouch but there is no uniform number or size of implants.

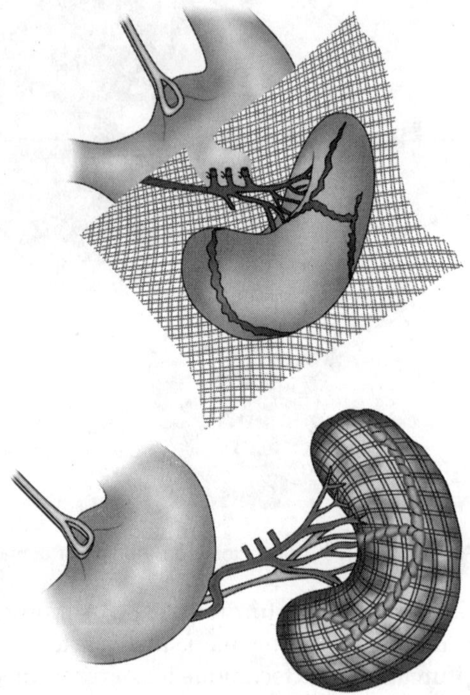

Fig. 18.8: Capping of injured spleen with woven polyglycolic acid mesh

Methods range from the use of homogenized spleen through the use of small cubes, thin and thick rectangular slices of different dimensions[11,12] to thin slices (approximately 3 mm) of the whole of middle of the spleen. Proof of successful regeneration is usually confirmed by either scintiscan, normal platelet numbers or a restoration of peripheral blood film to normal. Reported complication includes intestinal obstruction, chronic abscess and torsion.

Functional Ability of Regenerated Splenic Tissue

There is now a considerable amount of evidence that regenerated splenic tissue can restore the filtering function of the spleen. Platelets numbers have also been shown to be within normal range after transplantation in both humans and experimental animals. Normal levels of immunoglobin M were widely reported in those with regenerated spleen.[10,12,13] Many additional factors which are reported to be abnormal following splenectomy are also claimed to be restored by splenic autotransplantation. These includes circulating antibodies, levels of phagocytosis stimulating α_2 glycoproteins, fibrinolecithins, leucokinins levels and opsonin activity.

Does Reimplanted Spleen Protect Against Infection

There is little evidence by which to state categorically that the regenerated splenic fragments are capable of protection of the host against pneumococcal infection.[13,14] Splenic salvage with preservation of intact vascular supply to even a small amount of spleen is a more effective method of preserving splenic function than autotransplantation.

Nonoperative Management

Nonoperative management is not a conservative management of splenic injuries but a selective management in a well defined setting. The prerequisites are:[3]

- Hemodynamically stable patient
- Awake alert individual
- Minimal or no abdominal findings
- Minimal laboratory evidence of blood loss
- Low energy trauma
- Isolated splenic injury on CT scan
- No associated injury on CT scan
- No hilar involvement/massive destruction on CT scan.

In those centers treating both adults and children approximately 18% of patients with splenic injury were eligible for nonoperative management and approximately 80-94.2% were successfully treated without operation.[15] The advocated protocol is: The diagnosis and degree of injury is obtained by CT scan.[6] Only grade I and grade II injuries are entered into nonoperative method. The patient is admitted to the intensive care unit and vitals are closely monitored. The patient is kept ready for the operative room, should there be evidence of hemodynamic instability or persistent bleed from spleen. Stay in the ICU is for 48-72 hours and CT scan is repeated. Adults receive a maximum of 2 units of blood and children to a maximum of 40 ml/kg body weight. Patient is discharged after 7 days and called upon for follow-up at 4 weeks and 12 weeks. Restricted activity is followed for 12 months. Only 12-15% of adults will be eligible for nonoperative management with success rate of 70%.[16,17] Nonoperative management is abandoned when there is:

- Deterioration of vital signs
- Continued requirement of blood transfusion
- Increasing abdominal tenderness or the development of new peritoneal signs
- USG/CT scan/angiographic evidence of continuing hemorrhage.

Angiography and Embolization

Angiography and embolization has been reported as useful adjunct to nonoperative management of the injured spleen. Its use in selected patients has been reported to increase the overall splenic salvage rate to 87–92%[18] of attempted NOM. As reported in the EAST multicenter study, the vast majority (> 90%) of grade V splenic injuries in adults requires immediate operation.[19]

Lower rates of splenic salvage are seen in high grade injuries. However, there are no uniformly accepted indications for either angiography or embolization and its use is applied differently across centers. In some centers, angiography with subsequent embolization is liberally applied as a means to cease active hemorrhage in order to avoid laparotomy. Most often, angiography is used in stable patients when CT reveals a contrast blush or high grade splenic injuries as an adjunct to nonoperative treatment. In addition, SAE is generally used for documented vascular abnormality at the time of angiography.[18]

Additional controversy exists over the preferred method of embolization, main splenic artery coiling versus distal (superselective) embolization. Proponents of main artery coiling cite a decrease in splenic perfusion pressure, while maintaining splenic blood flow through short gastric vessels and collaterals to prevent infarcts. Superselective embolization addresses the vascular injury encountered, but was associated with a higher rate of splenic infarction on follow-up CT. A combination of both techniques may be employed for higher grade injuries. Use of SAE is not risk free. As reported in the multicenter series of SAE, 20% of patients developed major complications: delayed bleeding, missed abdominal injury, and splenic abscess. Two-thirds of this group (19 of 27 patients) required laparotomy.[18] There exists a significant concern in employing SAE, especially in higher grade injuries where active bleeding may be occurring. There may be a significant delay in the availability of the angiographic resources necessary to do these complex procedures. Radiology can be a dangerous location for a multiply-injured trauma patient for a prolonged procedure to obtain angiographic control of hemorrhage.

SAE should probably not be offered as an option if the procedure is likely to result in excessive splenic tissue loss, because splenectomy is associated with lower relative risk. A patient who has significant or total splenic volume infarction after SAE requires close observation for the development of complications. When the data are considered, continuing with splenectomy when the patient is stabilized may be prudent if complete splenic infarction occurs after SAE.[19]

REFERENCES

1. Moore EE, Cogbill TM, Malangoni MA, Jurkovich GJ, Shackford SR, Champion HR, Mc Aninch. Organ Injury Scaling. Surg Clin North Amer 1995;75:293-303.
2. Eicher HR. Splenic function. Normal, too much and too little. Am J Med 1979;66:311-20.
3. Wisner DH, Blaisdell FW. When to save the ruptured spleen. Surgery 1992;111:121-2.
4. Sherman R. Management of trauma to the spleen. Adv Surg 1984;17:37-71.
5. Ballard RB, Rozycki GS, Newman PG, et al. An algorithm to reduce the incidence of false-negative FAST examinations in patients at high risk for occult injury. Focused assessment for the sonographic examination of the trauma patient. J Am Coll Surg 1999;189.
6. Resciniti A, Fink MP, Raptopoulos V, et al. Nonoperative treatment of adult splenic trauma: development of a computed tomographic scoring system that detects appropriate candidates for expectant management. J Trauma. Jun 1988;28(6):828-31.
7. Steven R Klepac, Evan J Samett. Spleen, Trauma Jan 16, 2009. www.medscape.com
8. Sarmiento JM, Yugueros P. An atraumatic technique to fix the omentum after partial splenectomy. J Trauma. 1996;41:160.
9. Delany HM, Rudaviky AZ, Lan S. Preliminary clinical experience with the use of absorbable mesh splenorrhaphy. J Trauma 1985;25:909-13.
10. Patel J, Willians JS, Shmigel B, Hinshaw JR. Preservation of splenic function by autotransplantation of traumatized spleen in Ann. Surgery 1981;90:683-8.

11. Milliken JS, Moore EE, Moore GE, Stevens RE. Alternatives to splenectomy in adults after trauma repair, partial resection and reimplantation of splenic tissue. Am J Surg 1982;144:711-6.
12. Velcik FT, Jongco B, Shaftan GW, et al. Post-traumatic splenic reimplantation in children. J Pediatr Surg 1982;17:879-83.
13. Nielson JL, Sakso P, Soresen FH, Hausen HH. Demonstration of splenic function following splenectomy and autologous splenic implantation. Acta Chir Scand 1984;150:469-73.
14. Moore GE, Stenns RE, Moore EE, Aragan GF. Failure of splenic implants to protect against fatal post splenectomy infection. Am J Surg 1983;146:413-4.
15. Coburn MC, Pfeifer J, DeLuca FG. Nonoperative management of splenic and hepatic trauma in the multiply injured pediatric and adolescent patient. Arch Surg 1995;130:332-8.
16. Shackford SR, Molin M. Management of splenic injuries. Surg Clin North Amer 1991;595-620.
17. Cogbill TH, Moore EE, Jurkovich GJ, et al. Nonoperative management of blunt splenic trauma. A multicenter experience. J Trauma 1989;29:1312-17.
18. Haan JM, Biffl W, Knudson M, et al. Western Trauma Association Multi-Institutional Trials Committee: Splenic embolization revisited:a multicenter review. J Trauma 2004;56:542-7.
19. Peitzman AB, Heil B, Rivera L, et al. Blunt splenic injury in adults: multi-institutional study of the Eastern Association for the Surgery of Trauma. J Trauma 2000;49:177-89.

Chapter

Injuries of Pancreas

SK Kochar

INCIDENCE AND MECHANISM OF INJURY

Injuries to the pancreas are uncommon. A recent study from Sweden[1] reported an incidence of only 4 per 100,000 population. Incidence of pancreatic damage in abdominal trauma may range from under 1 to 12%.[2] Damage to the pancreas is caused by either blunt or penetrating injuries. Blunt injury is following road traffic accidents while penetrating could be due to gun-shot wounds or stab injuries. Relative incidence of this varies from place to place. In rural areas penetrating injuries are more common while in cities blunt injuries have higher incidence. In blunt trauma there are three general pattern of injury to the pancreas,[3] depending on the vector of frontal force applied to the gland in relation to spine. When applied to the right to the spine, injury to the head of the pancreas and duodenum can be expected. Midline force will result in disruption of the body, while those to the left of midline will cause damage to the tail of the pancreas. Isolated injuries to the pancreas are uncommon. There is a high incidence of associated injuries, with figures of 50-98% widely reported.[4] These associated injuries lead to most of the morbidity and mortality linked with pancreatic trauma. The liver, spleen, stomach, duodenum, colon are the organs most commonly injured. These injuries may be more obvious at laparotomy and injured pancreas may be missed.

Classification of Injuries[5]

A classification of pancreatic injuries are given in Table 9.1.

Table 19.1: Organ injury scale for pancreas

Grade I	
Hematoma/laceration:	Minor contusions or lacerations without duct injury
Grade II	
Hematoma/laceration:	Major contusion or laceration without duct injury or tissue loss
Grade III	
Laceration:	Distal transection or parenchymal injury with duct injury
Grade IV	
Laceration:	Proximal transection or parenchymal injury involving ampulla
Grade V	
	Massive destruction of pancreatic head

DIAGNOSIS

Blunt Abdominal Trauma

The diagnosis requires a high index of suspicion since symptoms of abdominal pain are often minimal or absent during initial phase of management in blunt abdominal trauma. If there is no significant surrounding retroperitoneal injury to activate pancreatic enzymes, days may pass before the build up of pancreatic secretions result in symptoms suggestive of pancreatitis or pseudocyst formation. The minimal abdominal pain and tenderness present immediately after injury often decreases over the next 1-2 hours only to worse again within 6 hours. This feature will result in a missed diagnosis unless repeated subsequent examination is carried out. Serum amylase is often normal in the immediate post-trauma period, serial determination will be elevated in at least 70% of patients with later proven blunt pancreatic injury.

The finding of an elevated amylase in the lavage fluid is once again suggestive of significant pancreatic injury, although a normal level does not rule out the injury. A plain radiograph should be taken to identify retroperitoneal air, which may be present in duodenum rupture. In a study of 152 cases it has been found to be positive in 18% of cases.[6] USG may show diffuse swelling of the pancreas or fluid collection around pancreas in some cases. CT scan is of more value in assessing the stable patient, but again its usefulness is limited. A CT scan may appear normal in 40% of significant pancreatic injuries. Unexplained thickening of the anterior renal fascia should alert the examiner to possible pancreatic trauma.[7] CT scan in the acute stage may be more useful for diagnosis of associated injuries. ERCP although advocated by some authors[8] for stable patients, probably has no place in acute stage because of its invasive nature.

Computed tomography (CT) is commonly employed as the initial imaging modality in blunt trauma patients and affords a timely diagnosis of pancreatic trauma. The CT findings of pancreatic trauma can be broadly categorized as direct signs, such as a pancreatic laceration, which tend to be specific but lack sensitivity and indirect signs, such as peripancreatic fluid, which tend to be sensitive but lack specificity.

CT findings may be subtle, and sometimes the pancreas may appear normal. The integrity of the pancreatic duct is the most important factor in the decision whether or not to operate. CT is limited in detection of pancreatic injuries when only little peripancreatic fat tissue is present and in detection of subtle pancreatic duct injuries. Specific signs of pancreatic injuries on CT scans are fractures or lacerations of the pancreas, edema or hematoma of the pancreatic parenchyma, active hemorrhage from the pancreas, and blood collections between the parenchyma and the splenic vein (Figs 19.1 and 19.6).

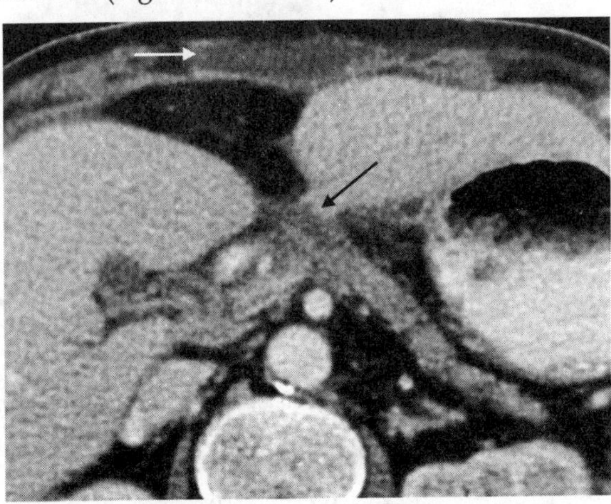

Fig. 19.1: Grade I pancreatic injury. Axial CT image shows a minor contusion of the pancreatic body (black arrow). There is no pancreatic duct injury and no active bleeding. Note the hematoma of the anterior abdominal wall at the site of the injury (white arrow)

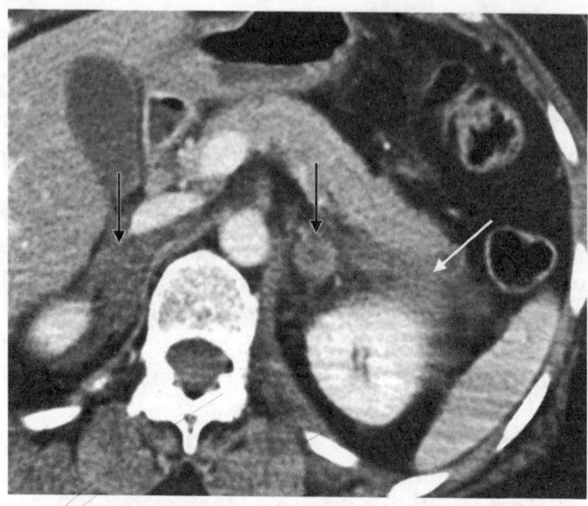

Fig. 19.2: Grade II pancreatic injury. Axial CT image shows a major contusion of the pancreatic tail (white arrow). The pancreatic tail is slightly displaced anteriorly because of a peripancreatic hematoma. Both adrenal glands are thickened (black arrows), a finding suggestive of contusions

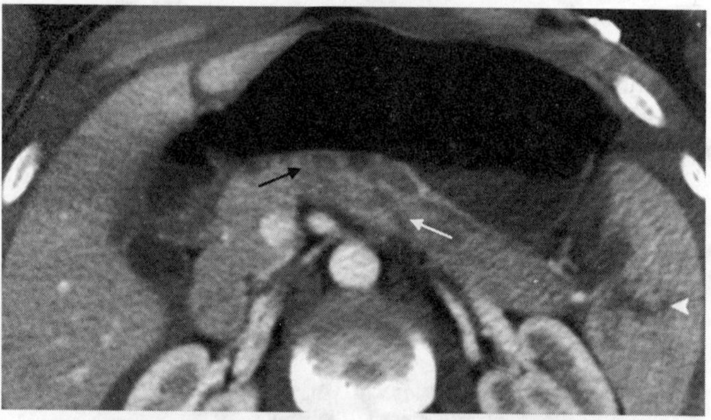

Fig. 19.3: Grade III pancreatic injury. Axial CT image shows diffuse edema of the pancreatic parenchyma with some defined areas of contusion (black arrow). There is a transection across the pancreatic body (white arrow). A grade II splenic laceration is also present (arrowhead)

In patients with equivocal CT findings or ongoing clinical suspicion of pancreatic trauma, magnetic resonance cholangiopancreatography (MRCP) may be employed for further evaluation. The integrity of the main pancreatic duct is of crucial importance,

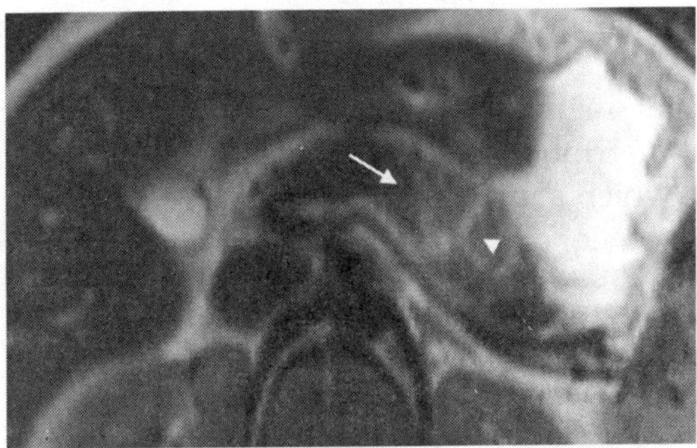

Fig. 19.4: Grade III pancreatic injury. Axial T2-weighted MR image shows the contusions to the pancreatic body (arrow) and the distal transection (arrowhead)

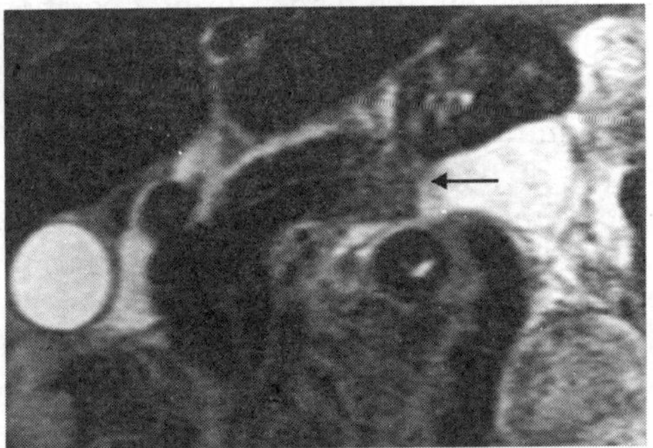

Fig. 19.5: Grade III pancreatic injury. Coronal T2-weighted MR image shows an injury to the pancreatic duct (arrow)

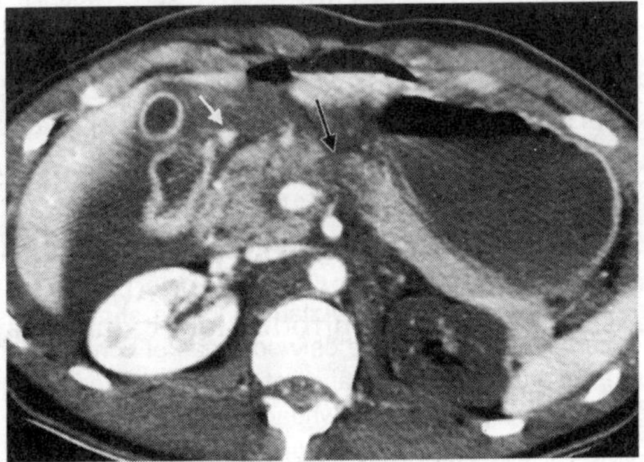

Fig. 19.6: Grade IV pancreatic injury. Axial CT image shows a proximal pancreatic transection (black arrow) with a large peripancreatic hematoma. There is also active bleeding (white arrow). The left kidney demonstrates no enhancement because of an occlusion of the renal artery (grade IV)

and though injury of the duct may be strongly suggested upon initial CT, MRCP provides clear delineation of the duct and any potential injuries.[9a] The major advantage of the prompt retrograde discription of the pancreatobiliary system after an accident in which pancreas involvement is suspected is the more precise assessment of the extent of the injuries. If a stent is placed in the same session, it is possible to carry out definitive and interventional treatment.[9b]

Penetrating Injuries

In all gunshot wounds and some stab wounds to the abdomen a laparotomy is mandatory. In these cases the diagnosis of pancreatic trauma should be made during operation. However, even at laparotomy, injuries to the pancreas may be missed, with potentially disastrous consequences. If pancreatic trauma is a possibility, intraoperative examination require an adequate exposure of entire pancreas. It entails a Kochar's maneuver, complete mobilization of the spleen, exploration of the lesser sac by division of gastrocolic omentum, incision of the retroperitoneal attachment inferior to the pancreas to allow mobilization of the body for purpose of inspection and bimanual palpation of that part of the gland not previously exposed (Fig. 19.7). If a hematoma around the pancreas is encountered it must be explored. Failure to do so can result in missed injuries to the pancreatic duct. Although contusions and lacerations to the pancreas are readily diagnosed, ductal damage can easily be missed even with thorough exploration. Because of this some surgeons[9] advocate intraoperative pancreatography to outline the main pancreatic duct. It is performed in two ways: (1) Tail of the pancreas is amputated and a cannula is inserted into the main duct, (2) The more popular method is to cannulate the ampulla of Vater through a duodenostomy using a 5F gauge pediatric catheter. In one of the series the rate of major complications dropped from 55 to 15% and death from 11 to 0% after the introduction of ductography.[9]

MANAGEMENT

Major injuries of the pancreas are uncommon, but may result in considerable morbidity and mortality because of the magnitude of associated vascular and duodenal injuries or underestimation of the extent of the pancreatic injury. Prognosis is influenced by

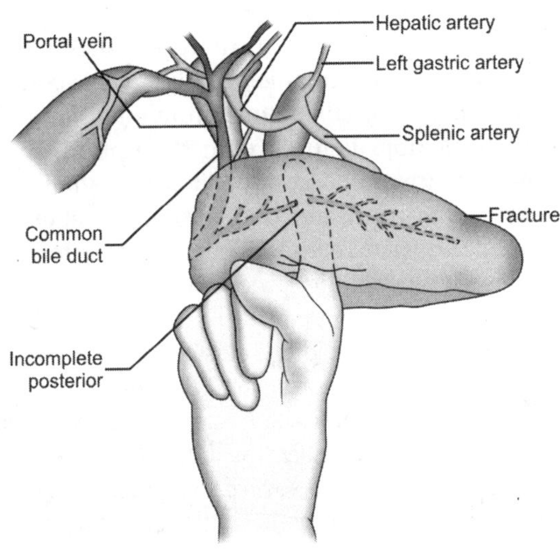

Fig. 19.7: Palpating the posterior aspect of the gland for injury to the posterior wall and duct

the cause and complexity of the pancreatic injury, the amount of blood lost, duration of shock, speed of resuscitation and quality and nature of surgical intervention. Early mortality usually results from uncontrolled or massive bleeding due to associated vascular and adjacent organ injuries. Late mortality is a consequence of infection or multiple organ failure. Neglect of major pancreatic duct injury may lead to life-threatening complications including pseudocysts, fistulas, pancreatitis, sepsis and secondary hemorrhage. Careful operative assessment to determine the extent of gland damage and the likelihood of duct injury is usually sufficient to allow planning of further management. This strategy provides a simple approach to the management of pancreatic injuries regardless of the cause.

Four situations are defined by the extent and site of injury:

i. Minor lacerations, stabs or gunshot wounds of the superior or inferior border of the body or tail of the pancreas (i.e. remote from the main pancreatic duct), without visible duct involvement, are best managed by external drainage;
ii. Major lacerations or gunshot or stab wounds in the body or tail with visible duct involvement or transection of more than half the width of the pancreas are treated by distal pancreatectomy;

iii. Stab wounds, gunshot wounds and contusions of the head of the pancreas without devitalization of pancreatic tissue are managed by external drainage, provided that any associated duodenal injury is amenable to simple repair; and

iv. Non-reconstructable injuries with disruption of the ampullary-biliary-pancreatic union or major devitalizing injuries of the pancreatic head and duodenum in stable patients are best treated by pancreatoduodenectomy. Internal drainage or complex defunctioning procedures are not useful in the emergency management of pancreatic injuries, and can be avoided without increasing morbidity. Unstable patients may require initial damage control before later definitive surgery. Successful treatment of complex injuries of the head of the pancreas depends largely on initial correct assessment and appropriate treatment. The management of these severe proximal pancreatic injuries remains one of the most difficult challenges in abdominal trauma surgery, and optimal results are most likely to be obtained by an experienced multidisciplinary team.[10a]

Grade I Injuries

The most common type of injuries and the easiest to treat are these injuries. Hemorrhage from superficial pancreatic vessel is usually the major feature, and control is achieved with direct, shallow simple or mattress 4/0 silk sutures. Attempts to clamp bleeding vessels prior to ligation should be restrained because of the inevitable crushing of surrounding pancreatic parenchyma. Wide based, deeply placed sutures may injure major ductal or vascular structures, further complicating matters. Disrupted capsule overlaying the pancreatic injuries should not be reapproximated and the area is drained. Although suction drains have been used by many authors successfully but currently sump drains are favored. In one of study the morbidity fell from 64 to 36% with use of sump drains.[4] The risk of erosion with sump drain may be diminished by the use of softer material in drains or interposition of a leaf of omentum between the drain and surrounding tissues. Between 2 and 15% of the patients with grade I injuries will develop a pancreatic fistula, but most are low output (< 500 ml/day) minimally affected by oral intake, and mostly close spontaneously within 2 weeks.

Grades II and III Injuries

Drainage alone is adequate for grade II injuries if the main duct is intact. Suturing the parenchyma and capsule although suggested by some is unnecessary and may be dangerous. A variety of opinions exist to deal with pancreatic duct damage when it occurs in the body or tail, to the left of the mesenteric vessels. The best method for dealing with the problem is distal pancreatectomy and drainage (Fig. 19.8). Some suggest splenic preservation but this involves a tedious dissection and added operation time, which could be considered inappropriate in an acute situation. There is also the possible risk of late complication of splenic vein thrombosis. Distal pancreatic resection are classified as extended, major or limited. Extended resection are those to the right of the superior mesenteric vessels for a grade IV injury (vide infra), major are those with transaction between the superior mesenteric vessels and the inferior mesenteric vein and limited resection are those with transaction to the left of the inferior mesenteric vein. The last two are performed for grade III injuries.

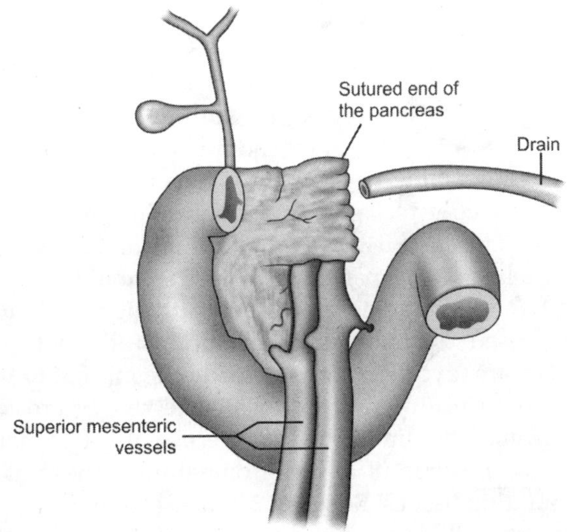

Fig. 19.8: Distal pancreatectomy for injury to the tail of the pancreas

Grades IV and V Injuries

These injuries have following spectrum:

- There may be major injuries to the pancreatic head with or without ductal damage.
- There may be injury to the pancreatic duct or the common bile duct in the juxtaduodenal location or both.
- There may be pancreatic injury with major duct disruption combined with a very severe duodenal injury.

Severe damage to the head of the pancreas, even in the absence of duodenum injury is particularly serious. Hemorrhage from the portal vein, vena cava, aorta or mesenteric vessel will often result in exsanguation during or shortly after surgical attempts at control of the injuries. Presuming that such injuries either are not present or are adequately controlled, there are several options to deal with grades IV and V injuries.

Onlays Roux-en-Y: Major injuries to the pancreatic head without ductal damage are best treated conservatively by sump drainage. If the duct is damaged, an onlay Roux-en-Y loop is probably the best procedure (Fig. 19.9).

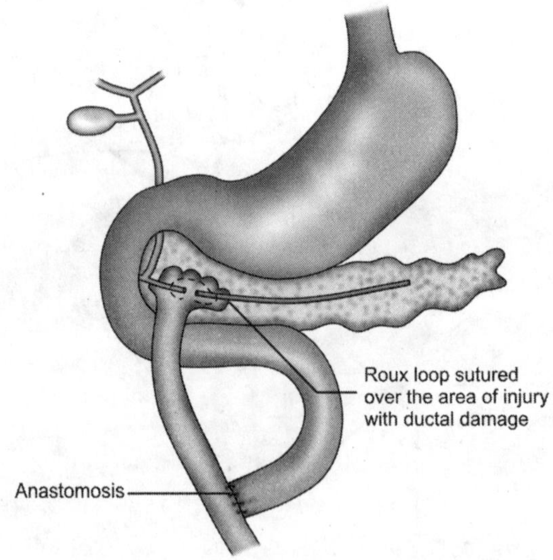

Fig. 19.9: Management of ductal injury in the head of the pancreas by Roux-en-Y loop suture over the ductal damage site

Duodenal diversion: These are more suited when the duodenal injuries are complex with pancreatic head injury. There are two ways of achieving this:

a. *Pyloric exclusion:* After repair of duodenal tear, a 4 cm gastrotomy is made along the distal greater curve. Through this the pylorus is approached and a polyglactin or chromic catgut suture is inserted to close the pylorus. A gastrojejunostomy is then constructed using the same gastrotomy.
b. *Duodenal diverticulization:* This is a more extensive procedure requiring duodenal repair, vagotomy, antrectomy, gastrojejunostomy, pancreatic resection, T tube drainage of CBD and tube duodenostomy (Fig. 19.10)

Pancreaticoduodenectomy: This carries an unacceptably high mortality rate in the acute situation. The overall mortality rate is 30-40%. A Whipple's procedure should therefore be performed only in the most severe injuries where the missile has effectively performed the resection and the operation is essentially debridement of devitalized tissue. The incidence of such procedure is no more than 2%.[4]

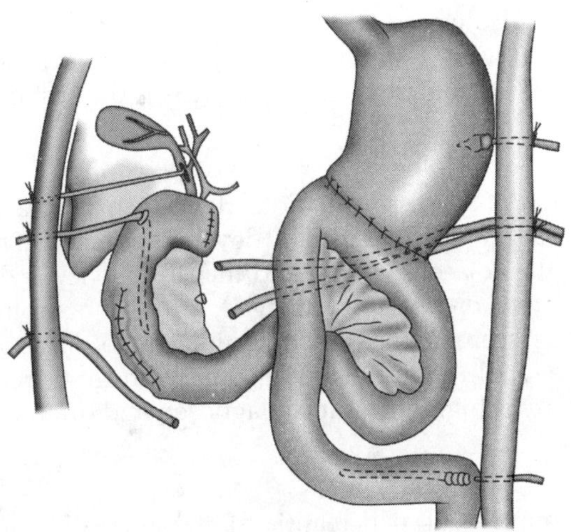

Fig. 19.10: Duodenal diverticulization for complex injuries of pancreas and duodenum

Complications

Morbidity rates are high and vary according to the nature of associated injuries. Complication rates range from 30-64%.[4,10]

Fistula

This is the most common complication arising from pancreatic trauma. The incidence may be from 7-20% rising to 26% after combined pancreaticoduodenal injury. Generally fistula are more common after injuries to the pancreatic head and mostly develop within the first 3 weeks. Abscess or fistula was seen in 9% of grade I injuries, 17% in grade II injuries and 36% in grades III, and IV and 50% in grade V injuries.[10] Fistula may drain up to 1000 ml/day depending on size. Most fistula can be managed conservatively. This involves good drainage, protection of the skin, and nutritional support. Each liter of fluid lost must be replaced with a liter of normal saline. Supplemental replacement of potassium bicarbonate and in prolonged cases zinc and magnesium may be necessary. Recently a somatostatin analogue, octreotide has been used. This may be administered as an intravenous infusion with TPN or as a twice daily subcutaneous injections.[11] In many series all fistulae closed spontaneously. and the maximum rate of reoperation was 7%. If the operation is necessary, a Roux-en-Y loop to the offending areas of the pancreas is the best treatment.

Abscess

The incidence of abscess formation after pancreatic trauma range from 10 to 25%.[10,12] Abscess usually develops as result of associated injuries to the adjacent viscera and their frequency is dependent on which other organs are damaged. Ultrasonography and CT scan are very useful in the early detection and localization of these abscess. They all require percutaneous drainage or reoperation. The mortality is high unless it is diagnosed and drained early.

Pancreatitis

The development of pancreatitis after pancreatic trauma is a common and serious complication and may carry a high risk of death. The mortality rate varies depending on the severity of the pancreatitis. The treatment is the same as for any patient with pancreatitis.

Pseudocyst

With early diagnosis and treatment of pancreatic trauma, the incidence of pseudocyst is below 5%. The rate depends on the adequacy of control of pancreatic secretions achieved by internal or external drainage or resection. The treatment of pseudocyst is internal drainage by surgery as percutaneous drainage is often unsatisfactory.

Postoperative Hemorrhage

This occurs in 5-10% of cases. After trauma, leakage of pancreatic juice or abscess development may result in erosion of an adjacent vessel resulting in major hemorrhage. Emergency operative intervention was required in 75-100% of cases of bleeding.[4]

Wound Sepsis

The incidence of this is between 10-30%. The rate varies according to the nature of any associated injuries and is particularly common with colonic involvement.

Exocrine and Endocrine Insufficiency

This is rare. In a series of 30 patients reported by Balasegaram no pancreatic insufficiency occurred after up to 90% resection.[6]

Death

Mortality rate varies from 3 to 22%. The type of injury, presence and type of associated injury and the cause of injury blunt or penetrating, GSW or stab injury influence the outcome.

REFERENCES

1. Nilsson E, Nooby S, Skullman S, Sjodahl R. Pancreatic trauma in a defined population. Acta Chir Scand 1986;152:647-51.
2. Wilson RH, Moorehead RJ. Current management of trauma to the pancreas. Br J Surg.1991;78:1196-1202.
3. Stone HH, Fabian TC, Satian B, Turklesion ML. Experience in the management of pancreatic trauma. J Trauma 1981;21:257-62.
4. Cogbill TH, Moore EE, Kashuti JL. Changing trends in the management of pancreatic trauma. Arch Surg 1982;117:722-28.
5. Moore EE, Cogbill TM, Malangoni MA, et al. Organ injury scaling. Surg Clin North Am 1995;75:293-303.

6. Balasegram M. Surgical management of pancreatic trauma. Curr Probl Surg 1979;16:11-59.
7. Jeffrey RB Jr, Federle MP, Crass RA. Computed tomography of pancreatic trauma. Radiol 1983;147:491-4.
8. Barkin JS, Ferstenberg RM, Panullo W, et al. Endoscopic retrograde cholangiopancreatography in pancreatic trauma. Gastrointest Endosc 1988;34:102-5.
9. Barni GA, Bardyk DF, Oreskovich MR, Carrico CJ. Role of intraoperative pancreatography in patients with injury to the pancreas. Am J Surg 1982;143:602-5.

9a. Rekhi S, Anderson SW, Rhea JT, Soto JA. Imaging of blunt pancreatic trauma. Emerg Radiol. 2010;17(1):13-9. Epub 2009 Apr 25.

9b. Wolf A, Bernhardt J, Patrzyk M, Heidecke CD. The value of endoscopic diagnosis and the treatment of pancreas injuries following blunt abdominal trauma. Surg Endosc. 2005;19(5):665-9. Epub 2005 Mar 11.

10. Smego DR, Richardson JD, Flint LM. Determinates of outcome in pancreatic trauma. J Trauma 1985;25:771-6.

10a. Krige JE, Beningfield SJ, Nicol AJ, Navsaria P. The management of complex pancreatic injuries. S Afr J Surg. 2005;43(3):92-102.

11. Prinz RA, Pickkleman J, Hoffman JP. Treatment of pancreatic cutaneous fistula with a somatostatin analog. Am J Surg 1988;155:36-42.
12. Feliciano DV Martin TD, Cruse PA, et al. Management of combined pancreaticoduodenal injuries. Ann Surg 1987;205:673-80.

Injuries of Stomach

SK Kochar

Incidence of injury to stomach following blunt trauma is 0.09 to 1.8% while penetrating injuries in any large series do account for 7%.[1] The first operative repair of gastric injury was reported by Nolleson in the 18th century, and the first case of gastric injury, as well as resultant fistula, is credited to Schenk in the 16th century.[1] Blunt gastric injury is uncommon and is associated with other injuries of greater magnitude, which generally influence mortality.[1a]

PATHOPHYSIOLOGY

The stomach in adults is protected by the overlying rib cage and well developed abdominal musculature. Inherent strength of the gastric wall is reinforced by a strong submucosa and its muscular coats. In addition, the stomach is naturally fixed in position solely by the pylorus and esophagus, thereby allowing considerable mobility. Esophageal and pylorus outlet serves as safety valve. These factors account for the low incidence of injury to stomach following blunt trauma.[1b] Younger children and full stomach is more prone to injury. The injury to the stomach may be partial or full thickness. Experimental studies using canine stomachs exposed to blunt trauma have shown that the tears generally initiate in the seromuscular layer and are followed by mucosal injury.[2] Gastric perforation secondary to blunt abdominal trauma in adults is most commonly located on the greater curvature. Presumably, this is because, a sudden increase in either intraluminal or wall tension will cause rupture at the point of greatest radius, in accordance with the law of Laplace.[3] The mechanism of blunt injuries is felt to be one of sudden gastric compression between the anterior parities and vertebral column due to sharp epigastric blow.

The injury to stomach may be partial thickness or full thickness. These may be classified according to extent of mural damage, as following (Table 20.1):

- Mucosal/submucosal lacerations
- Devascularization injury
- Perforations.

In penetrating injuries a single small perforation will be visualized on the anterior surface of the stomach when caused by stab wounds or low velocity firearm. High velocity usually cause paired perforations and are associated with areas of tissue damage and frank necrosis. Missile causes injury not only by direct contact but also by dissipation of energy lateral to the path of missile (blast effect).

DIAGNOSIS

Trauma to upper abdomen or lower thorax should alert the surgeon to the possibility of gastric trauma. Presence of hematemesis, altered blood on nasogastric aspiration, contusion upper abdomen, tenderness, rigidity, guarding in upper abdomen are the indicators that stomach may be the site of injury. More often than not the source of blood in the stomach is from swallowed blood from injury to face or oral cavity. A diagnostic gastric lavage is then performed using 250 ml of normal saline. Return of clear fluid rules out significant gastric injury. If the patient is hemodynamically stable upper GI endoscopy is the procedure of

Table 20.1: Stomach injury scale

Grade*	Description of injury
I	Contusion/hematoma
II	Partial thickness laceration
III	Laceration <2 cm in GE junction or pylorus
	<5 cm in proximal 1/3 stomach
	<10 cm in distal 2/3 stomach
IV	Laceration >2 cm in GE junction or pylorus
	>5 cm in proximal 1/3 stomach
	>10 cm in distal 2/3 stomach
V	Tissue loss or devascularization <2/3 stomach
	Tissue loss or devascularization >2/3 stomach

**Advance one grade for multiple lesions up to grade III. GE—Gastroesophageal.*

choice. A careful, thorough inspection of a maximally insufflated stomach is required. Lacerations may be small or hidden between the rugae; multiple tears are frequent. While most are found along the magenstrasse, Mallory-Weiss-type tears have been documented. Rarely, segmental pallor may be indicative of devascularization. When guarding, rigidity, hypotension, tachycardia in various combination is present it is indicative of perforation/partial transection and the necessity of emergency exploratory laparotomy. Diagnosis in penetrating injury is obvious but assessment for emergency laparotomy is occasionally difficult.

MANAGEMENT

Blunt Gastric Injury

Mucosal/Submucosal Lacerations

Not all lacerations require emergency surgical intervention.[4] Nonoperative management consists of gastric lavage with ice cold saline followed by check aspirate 4 hourly, H_2 receptor antagonists, ranitidine 12.5 mg 2 hourly or 50 mg 8 hourly has been recommended. If the gastric aspirate remains free of blood the nasogastric tube is removed and feeding started. The endoscopy may be repeated after four weeks. The indications for surgical intervention for mucosal/submucosal lacerations are:

- Massive gastric hemorrhage with hemodynamic instability.
- Endoscopic visualization of an actively bleeding laceration.
- Endoscopic evidence of active blood pooling in the stomach despite the inability to visualize a specific bleeding point.
- Recurrent hemorrhage despite medical management.

A generous longitudinal mid body gastrotomy is given. All clots are evacuated and large moist sponges are placed into the proximal and distal stomach. Distal sponges are removed initially, because most tears are found in this area. All lacerations are sutured over and over, using a running 2-0 or 3-0 chromic catgut placed at a depth necessary to incorporate both mucosal and submucosal layers. The distal stomach is then irrigated with normal saline to ensure that no sources of hemorrhage have been missed. The identical protocol is then repeated as the more proximal portion of the stomach is inspected.[5] Once hemostasis has been achieved, the gastrotomy is closed in layers. Drains are not indicated.

Devascularization Injury

The diagnosis of acute segmental gastric ischemia is typically unsuspected until emergency exploratory laparotomy is performed for blunt trauma. With upper GI endoscopy being freely available and forming a part of the protocol for upper GI bleed more and more cases are being diagnosed when the gastric wall is merely ischemic. At laparotomy careful examination of stomach wall will reveal segmental pallor. This most often occurs along the greater curvature; a hallmark of injury at this site is avulsion of the gastroepiploic vessels. Sleeve resection of the nonviable and doubtful area is done. When diagnosed late or not recognized at laparotomy, the ischemia progresses to full thickness gastric necrosis. Massive gastric hemorrhage/signs of intra-abdominal sepsis, few days following blunt trauma to the abdomen heralds the onset of full thickness gastric necrosis, culminating in exploratory laparotomy. At operation the involved gastric segment will demonstrate obvious necrosis with associated perforation, abscess formation, and dense visceral adhesions. Debridement and excision of the involved segment is done and the defect repaired in two layers. Closed system drains are instituted and nasogastric aspiration with broad spectrum antibiotic continued in postoperative period. Inspite of aggressive treatment mortality remains very high.

Perforation

Perforation following blunt trauma is different than the ones after penetrating injuries. Two types are: (i) Partial transection, and (ii) Complete gastric transection. Incidence is less than 1% in those who undergo surgical intervention for suspected intra-abdominal injury secondary to blunt trauma.[6] The more common injury is partial transection.

Partial transection: It classically occurs in fully distended stomach and as a result of impact which compresses the stomach enough to give rise to blow out. The majority of these patient have severe diffuse abdominal pain in close temporal association with receiving an epigastric blow. On examination there is diffuse tenderness, guarding, and rigidity. With the onset of peritonitis, hypotension and tachycardia may be a marked feature. X-ray chest may show air under the dome of diaphragm, gastrograffin swallow in doubtful cases may be helpful. At times the diagnosis is arrived at exploratory laparotomy. Ruptures are typically solitary, linear defects less than 10 cm in length. Two layers closure after debridement of the edges should be performed. Drains are optional.

Complete transection: This classically occurs in empty stomach when it get crushed against the vertebral column resulting in compete transection. Shock, hypotension, tachycardia with abdominal features suggestive of peritonitis are invariably present. At operation, the transected margins are debrided and reapproximated in two layers. The outer being silk/linen. If injury is extensive proximal and distal ends are closed/stapled and gastrojejunostomy performed, mortality remains high.

Penetrating Injuries

Penetrating injuries may be stab wounds or gunshot wounds. It is more common than blunt injuries. The diagnosis is obvious but assessment of the injury may be difficult. Nasogastric aspiration will have altered blood. Signs and symptoms of chemical peritonitis may be present. Evidence of breach of peritoneum is enough to proceed for laparotomy in stab wounds while some authors[7] go for selective conservative management and opting for laparotomy only when sign of peritonitis develops. In gunshot wounds emergency laparotomy is accepted norm.

The successful incorporation of diagnostic laparoscopy into the management of patients with penetrating abdominal trauma depends on the selection of hemodynamically stable patients, the availability and ease of use of quality laparoscopic equipment, and the experience of the surgeon in using the technique for diagnostic purposes in traumatic injuries.[8a]

Shotgun injuries pose unique problems and situations in diagnosis and treatment. Shotgun injuries from close range are associated with massive destruction of the abdomen wall and severe intra-abdominal injury.[8] Long range shotgun blast injuries are characterized by a large scatter pattern and shallow pellet penetration.[9] In absence of sign of peritonitis/peritonism some authors believe that penetration by more than four pellets are indicative of intra-abdominal injury, and therefore, mandates exploratory laparotomy[9] while others explore all cases where even one pellet has violated the peritoneum.[10] At laparotomy a careful inspection of all aspects of stomach must be done including gastrohepatic and gastroduodenal ligaments, anterior and posterior surfaces (Fig. 20.1), lesser and greater curvature. If required stomach may be mobilized from spleen by division of vasa brevia, one must be careful not to injury middle colic and spleen during mobilization for inspection. Gunshot wounds on the anterior wall of the stomach usually exit on the posterior surface. If an exit wound cannot be found on the posterior surface, gastrotomy must be performed and the internal inspection of the entire stomach is performed before assuming that there is no exit wound. All gastric injuries are debrided and closed in two layers.

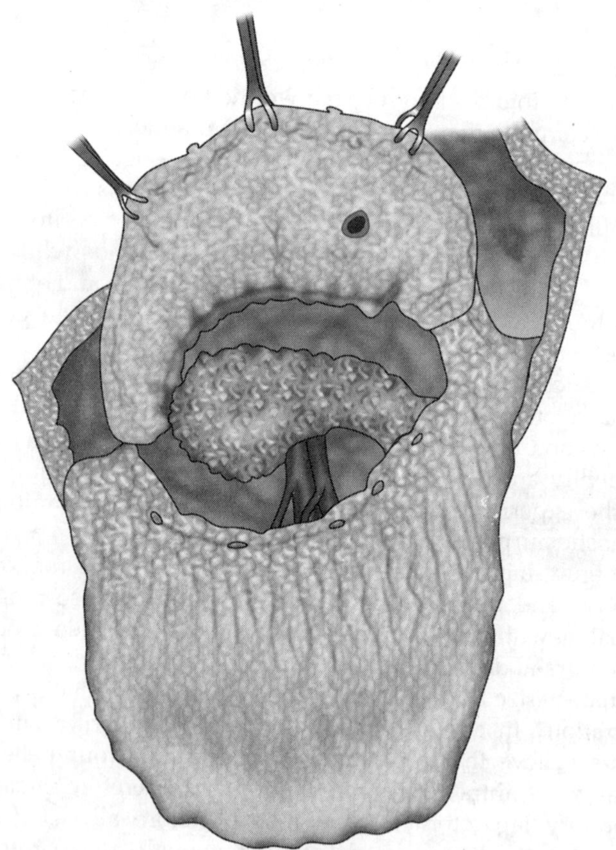

Fig. 20.1: Mobilization and visualization of posterior surface of the stomach for perforation

Surgical site infection commonly follow penetrating stomach and small bowel trauma. Risk factors for SSI include associated duodenal or colon injury. Delay to operating room, blood loss, and type and length of antibiotic prophylaxis were not associated with an increased risk of SSI.[11]

REFERENCES

1. Blaisdell FW, Trunkey DD (Eds). Trauma Management Vol I: Abdominal Trauma. New York, Thieme-Stratton, 1982.

1a. Drumondb DAF, JR Ribas Jrd. Blunt gastric injury. A multicentre experience. Injury Volume 32, Issue 10, Pages 761-764 (December 2001).

1b. Oncel D, Malinoski D, Brown C, Demetriaides D, Salim A. Blunt gastric injuries. Am Surg. 2007;73(9):880-3.

2. Silbergleit A, Berkas E. Neonatal gastric rupture. Min Med 1966; 49:65-7.

3. Yajko RD, Seydel F, Trimble C. Rupture of the stomach from blunt abdominal trauma. J Trauma 1975;15:177-92.

4. Tan DTD, Kim HS, Richmond D. Gastric mucosal lacerations from blunt trauma to the abdomen. Am J Gastroenterol 1975;63:246-8.

5. Ferrara JJ, Curreri PW. Gastrointestinal trauma. In. Trauma Surgery (ed) Moylan JA. Lippincott &Co. Philadelphia 1988;239.

6. Courcy PA, Soderstrom C, Brotman S. Gastric rupture from blunt trauma: A plea for minimal diagnostics and early surgery. Am Surg 1984;50:424-7.

7. Demetriaides D, Rabinowitz B. Indications for operation in abdominal stab wounds. A prospective study of 651 patients. Ann Surg. 1987; 205:129-32.

8. Demuth WE, Nicholas GG, Munger BL. Buckshot wounds. J Trauma 1076;18:53.

8a Katie Jo Stanton-Maxey, H Scott Bjerke. Abdominal Trauma, Penetrating Updated: Feb 19, 2010 (http://www.medscape.com/public/copyrig).

9. Flint LM, Cryer HM, Howard DA, et al. Approaches to the management of shot gun injuries. J Trauma 1984;24:415.

10. Schwab CW, Shaikh KA, Talucci RC. Injury to the stomach and small bowel. In Moore EE, Feliciano DV, Mattox KL (Eds). Trauma. Norwalk, CT, Appleton & Lange, 1991;485-98.

11. Salim A, Teixeira PG, Inaba K, Brown C, Browder T, Demetriaides D. Analysis of 178 penetrating stomach and small bowel injuries. World J Surg. 2008;32(3):471-5.

Injuries of Duodenum

SK Kochar

Though duodenum is a retroperitoneal structure well protected as compared to other intra-abdominal organs, blunt injuries are relatively fairly common. Two important factors are: (i) It lies in front of upper lumbar vertebrae and is predisposed to a crushing type of blunt force, and (ii) Its mobility is restricted being a retroperitoneal structure and further fixation imparted to it by pylorus, ligament of Treitz and mesenteric vessels. Morbidity and mortality is fairly high in duodenum trauma as diagnosis is often delayed due to scant clinical features owing to its retroperitoneal location. In penetrating trauma associated injuries to closely lying vital structures, viz. aorta, vena cava, portal vein, superior mesenteric vessels often leads to exsanguinating hemorrhage.

Duodenum trauma occurs following blunt injuries or penetrating injuries. Blunt injuries are common in road traffic accidents; impact with a steering wheel, faulty seat belt and bludgeoning assault during fights or rural bull injuries. Penetrating injuries are mostly due to gunshot wounds or stab injuries.

CLASSIFICATION

Duodenum injury has been classified[1] in Table 21.1.

Diagnosis

History of severe frontal force applied to upper abdomen; impact against steering wheel, seat belt or a swift kick is available in case of blunt injuries. In penetrating injuries often there is a gunshot wound/stab wound in the epigastrium or right hypochondrium but any wound in the upper abdomen may be the offending agent entry point. Though retroperitoneal containment may initially cause

Table 21.1: Classification of duodenum injuries

Grade		*Injury descriptions*
I	Hematoma	Involving single portion
	Laceration	Partial thickness; no perforation
II	Hematoma	Involving more than one portion
	Laceration	Disruption < 50% of circumference
III	Laceration	Disruption 50 to 75% of circumference of second portion
		Disruption 50 to 100% of circumference of first, third or fourth portion
IV	Laceration	Disruption of >75% of circumference of second portion
		Involving ampulla or distal common bile duct
V	Laceration	Massive disruption of duodenopancreatic complex
	Vascular	Devascularization of the duodenum

Advance one grade for multiple injuries up to grade III

a delay in the onset of symptoms, the majority of patients will complain of acute abdominal and back pain, which on occasions radiates to the right iliac fossa. Initial signs are diffuse tenderness and decrease bowel sounds. In matters of few hours depending on size and site of perforation, guarding and rigidity will be present. In altered sensorium, deep pressure in the epigastrium may illicit restlessness or agitation. Contained intramural hematoma, an injury peculiar to duodenum has got two distinct clinical scenarios.[2] An acute onset of severe epigastric discomfort and abdominal tenderness, in close temporal relationship to a traumatic insult, occurs most frequently in the adult population. In children, the development of symptoms is more insidious and is characterized by the gradual onset of abdominal pain followed by protracted vomiting. Physical examination typically reveals mild abdominal tenderness, gastric succussion splash, and an abdominal mass (present in up to 40% of cases).[3]

Investigations

Laboratory analysis is generally nonspecific although the presence of an elevated amylase should alert one to the possibility of pancreatoduodenum injury. Plane X-rays of the abdomen may demonstrate free intraperitoneal air (gas under the dome of the diaphragm in upright view) retroperitoneal gas outlining the kidney or right psoas shadow. In stable patients with minimal symptoms who are suspected to have duodenum injuries, water soluble contrast upper gastroduodenum studies may demonstrate leak or show the classic picture of "coiled spring" in a case of intramural hematoma. Where available computed tomography (CT) of the abdomen is becoming the initial investigation of choice due to its capacity to demonstrate retroperitoneal structures. Diagnostic peritoneal lavage is often negative. When clinical suspicion is very strong and all these noninvasive investigation are inconclusive exploratory laparotomy remains a valid diagnostic procedure.

CT Findings in Duodenum Injuries[3a]

In duodenum injuries, differentiation between a contusion of the duodenum wall or mural hematoma and a duodenum perforation is vital. Duodenum perforation is suspected if there is a retroperitoneal collection of contrast medium, extraluminal gas, or a lack of continuity of the duodenum wall. Duodenum contusion is suspected with edema or hematoma of the duodenum wall, intramural gas accumulations, and focal duodenum wall thickening (>4 mm) as findings of small bowel injury. Fluid or a hematoma in the retroperitoneum, stranding of retroperitoneal fatty tissue, or pancreatic transection can be present in both conditions. Mixed attenuation is a sign of duodenum wall hematoma. However, fluid collections in the anterior pararenal space only and thickening of the duodenum wall have been seen in both perforations and duodenum wall contusions (Figs 21.1 to 21.7).

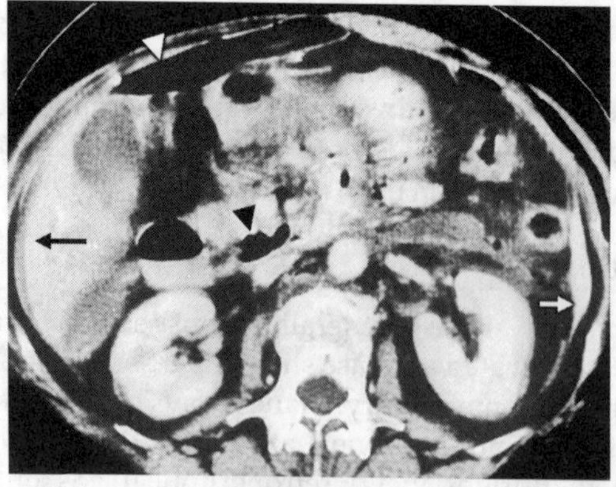

Fig. 21.1: Abdominal CT scan reveals free fluid (black arrow), free intraperitoneal air (white arrowhead), retroperitoneal air (black arrowhead), and intraperitoneal contrast material (white arrow). Case of duodenum and jejunal perforation

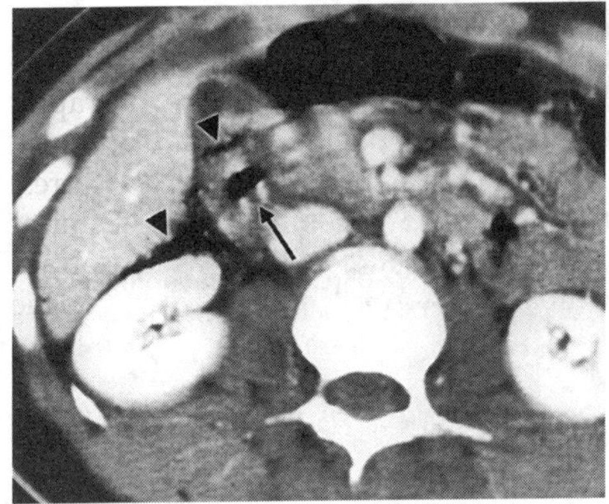

Fig. 21.2: Perforation of the duodenal "C" loop. Abdominal CT scan shows a thick-walled duodenum (black arrow), outlined by extraluminal retroperitoneal air (arrowheads)

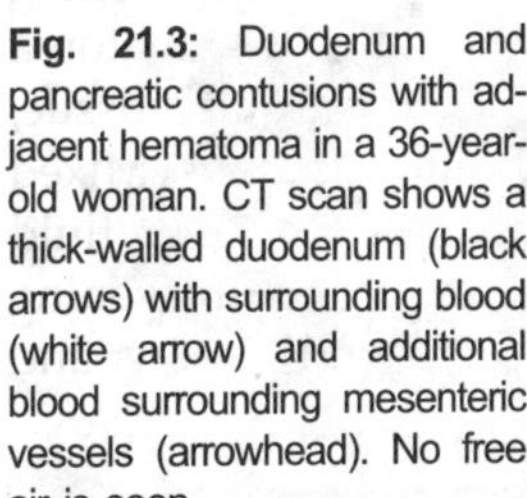

Fig. 21.3: Duodenum and pancreatic contusions with adjacent hematoma in a 36-year-old woman. CT scan shows a thick-walled duodenum (black arrows) with surrounding blood (white arrow) and additional blood surrounding mesenteric vessels (arrowhead). No free air is seen

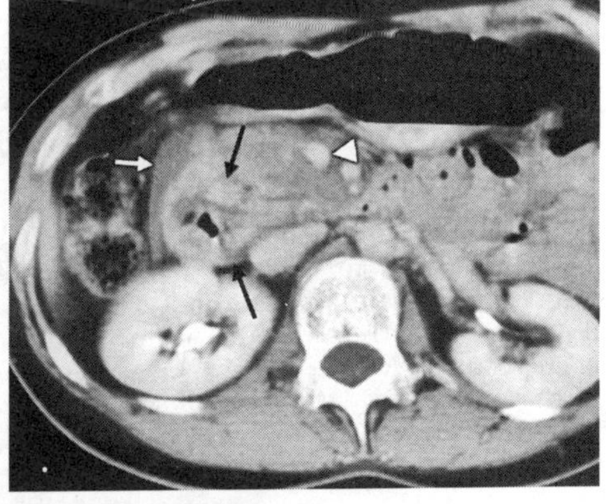

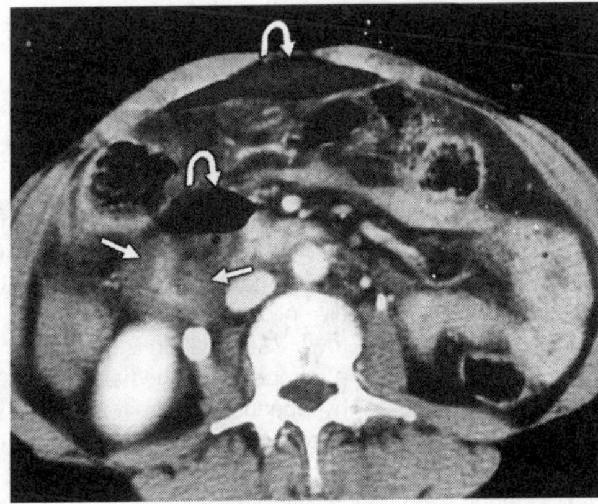

Fig. 21.4: Transection of the second portion of the duodenum and full-thickness perforation of the right colon. Abdominal CT scan reveals a thick-walled and ill-defined duodenum (straight arrows) and free and retroperitoneal air (curved arrows), findings that suggest duodenum injury

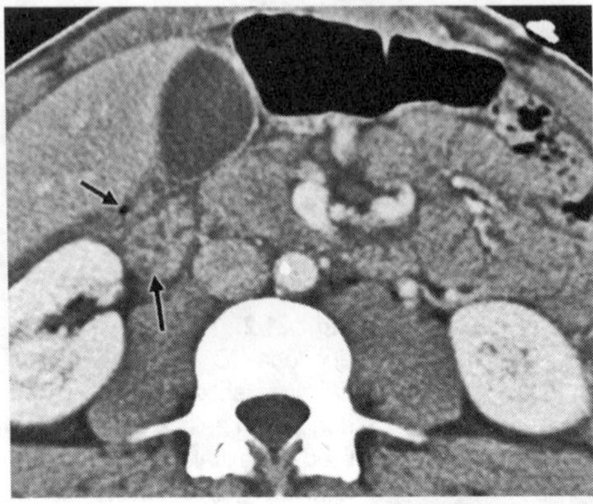

Fig. 21.5: Grade I duodenum injury. Axial CT image shows thickening of the duodenum wall (arrows) in the descending part without evidence of free air. There is stranding of the peripancreatic fat

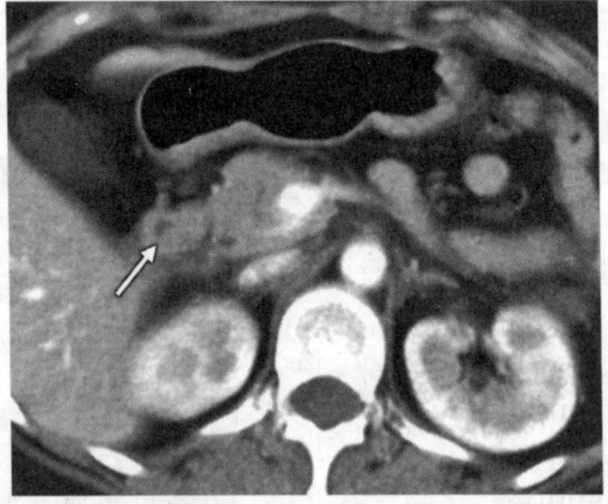

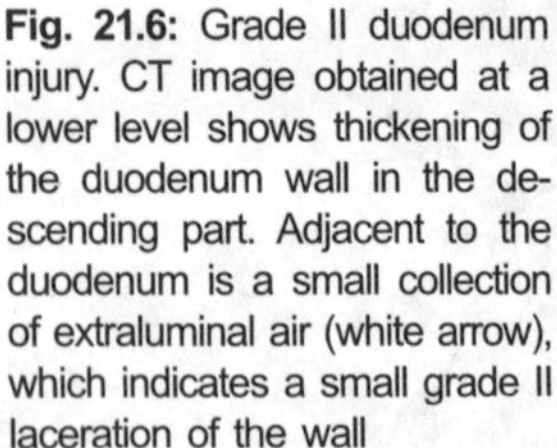

Fig. 21.6: Grade II duodenum injury. CT image obtained at a lower level shows thickening of the duodenum wall in the descending part. Adjacent to the duodenum is a small collection of extraluminal air (white arrow), which indicates a small grade II laceration of the wall

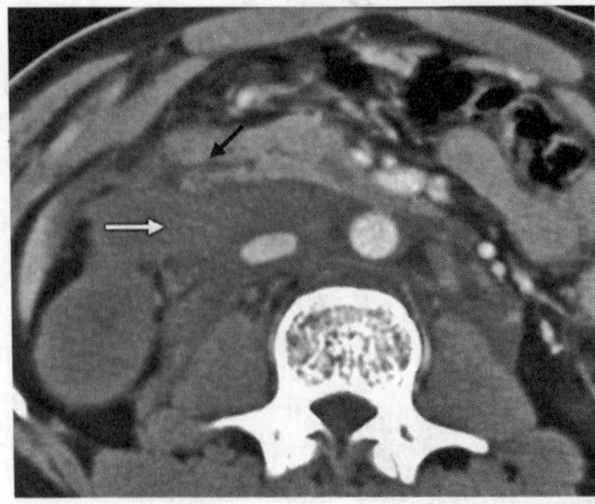

Fig. 21.7A: Grade III duodenum injury. Axial CT image shows thickening of the duodenum wall in the descending part (black arrow). At the transition zone to the horizontal part, there is disruption of the wall (white arrow). Additional findings include a retroperitoneal hematoma and hypoperfusion of the right kidney due to right renal artery occlusion

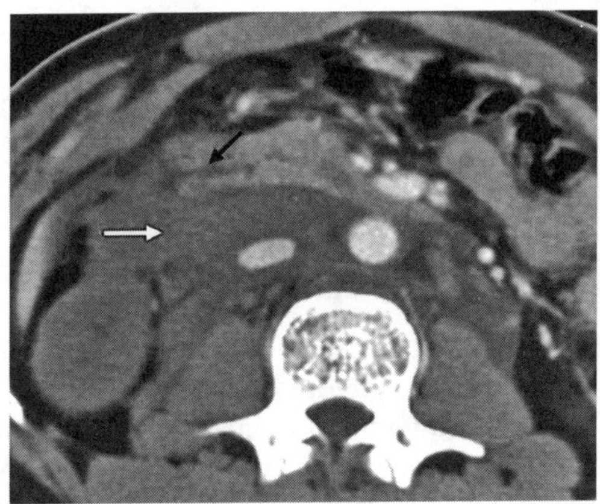

Fig. 21.7B: Grade III duodenum injury. CT image shows the disruption (black arrow) with a large surrounding extraluminal hematoma (white arrow)

Management

Intramural Hematoma (Grades I and II)

History and clinical features as described above and upper gastrointestinal contrast studies help to arrive at the diagnosis. Initial treatment is nonoperative, and operative intervention is reserved for persistent obstruction. Two to three weeks period of conservative treatment is acceptable by most of the authors before laparotomy is indicated. When an operation is necessary, the entire duodenum is mobilized by a Kochar's maneuver to allow careful inspection and palpation. An antimesenteric incision is made through the serosa and muscularis into the hematoma and the clot evacuated. The incised duodenum wall may or may not be sutured. If the abdomen is explored soon after the injury and a large bulging intramural hematoma is encountered, the hematoma should be evacuated. Patients who remain obstructed following an initial attempt at simple evacuation of the hematoma, gastrojejunostomy with vagotomy is the treatment of choice.

Lacerations–Grades I, II and Selected III

Blunt injuries without major loss of duodenum wall or viability, perforations from stab wounds, circumscribed injuries from low velocity gunshot wounds that do not involve pancreas are dealt with primary closure and closed suction drainage. The duodenum is closed in two layers. The inner being an absorbable suture and the outer is of interrupted 3-O silk sutures. A wide Kocher maneuver is always necessary to adequately examine the duodenum and to ensure tension free closure. In case viability is in doubt or the closure cannot be done without tension one should adopt the procedures mentioned below.

Lacerations—Grades III, IV and V

These injuries frequently involve varying degree of loss of duodenum substance. Attempts at repair often results in narrowing of the duodenum lumen. Involvement of ampulla of Vater, pancreas or distal bile ducts adds to the problem and directly influences the mortality and morbidity. Grade V injuries are often associated with major hemorrhage. Traditional method of resection and end-to-end anastomosis cannot be employed due to attachment of duodenum to pancreas. Increased morbidity/ mortality when combined with pancreas has prompted for a separate classification for combined injuries as shown in Table 21.2.[4]

Management of these injuries entails procedures to protect the repair from dehiscence as this complication at or distal to ampulla of Vater carried mortality in excess of 50%.[5] Options are:

- End to end gastroduodenostomy
- End to end duodenojejunostomy
- Jejunal patch/serosal jejunal onlay
- Side to side duodenojejunostomy Roux-en-Y
- Duodenum diverticulization
- Pyloric exclusion
- Distal pancreatectomy with one of the above
- Pancreatoduodenectomy

Table 21.2: Classification of duodenopancreatic injuries

Grades	*Injury descriptions*
I	Partial thickness duodenum injury without pancreatic duct involvement
II	Full thickness duodenum injury without pancreatic duct involvement
III	Full thickness duodenum injury with distal pancreatic duct injury
IV	Duodenum wounds > 20% of circumference with proximal pancreatic duct injury
V	Devitalizing injury to both the duodenum and pancreas

Factors which influences the choice of procedure are:

1. Primary closure under tension
2. Primary closure difficult or not possible to close due to tissue loss
3. Injury to duodenum at or below the ampulla of Vater
4. Injury to bile duct, ampulla, pancreas
5. Associated hemorrhage.

Grade III injuries to the first portion of the duodenum may be repaired by end-to-end gastroduodenostomy and injury to the fourth portion of the duodenum by end-to-end duodenojejunostomy. When grades III/IV injury is confined to the area proximal to ampulla of Vater a distal gastrectomy, gastrojejunostomy, primary closure of the injury with tube duodenostomy is preferred by many surgeons. If the wound is large and closure somewhat tenuous, a loop of jejunum may be placed over a duodenum closure and sutured in place to buttress the closure, the so called onlay jejunal patch.[5]

Recent data suggest that such reinforcement procedures add little more than time to the overall time of the operation.[6] Grade IV injuries without injury to ampulla and in grade III injuries with large defects not amenable to primary closure, reconstruction by Roux-en-Y duodenostomy[7] (Fig. 21.8) is recommended. Following debridement of duodenotomy, the distal (closed) end of a previously transected segment of jejunum is brought up in retrocolic fashion to injury site. Longitudinal antimesenteric jejunostomy is made to approximate

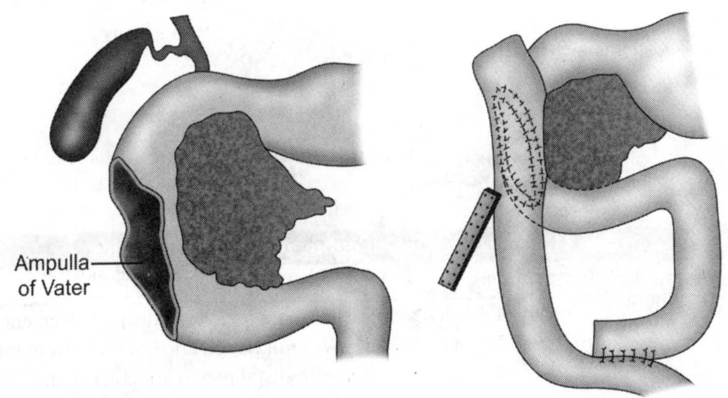

Fig. 21.8: Duodenojejunostomy using a Roux-en-Y loop for large defect in duodenum

the length of the duodenotomy, and standard two layer duodeno-jejunostomy is performed. A jejunojejunostomy 40 cm distal to the initial anastomosis restores the gastrointestinal continuity. External drainage devices, gastrotomy, and decompressive duodenostomy are recommended.[2] When there is extensive mural damage or coexistent injury to the head of the pancreas or the distal common bile duct (Grades IV and V injuries) the options available are:

Duodenum diverticulization: Standard components of this procedure include: closure of the duodenum injury, extensive drainage of the pancreatic injury, tube duodenostomy through uninjured duodenum wall, gastric antrectomy, and gastro-jejunostomy. A cholecystostomy should be established or a T-tube placed in the common duct, depending upon on size of the duct[8] (Fig. 21.9). Additional component of vagotomy is not favored by many. Drawback of the procedure is the complexity and time consuming nature of the technique in already critically ill patients.

Pyloric exclusion: Following repair of the duodenum injury, a greater curvature gastrotomy is positioned to accommodate a gastrojejunostomy. The pylorus is identified through the gastrotomy and closed with a running 2-0 absorbable suture, such as polyglycolic acid, polyglactin 910, polydioxanone. Side to side gastrojejunostomy is then performed to complete the procedure[9] (Fig. 21.10). Long-

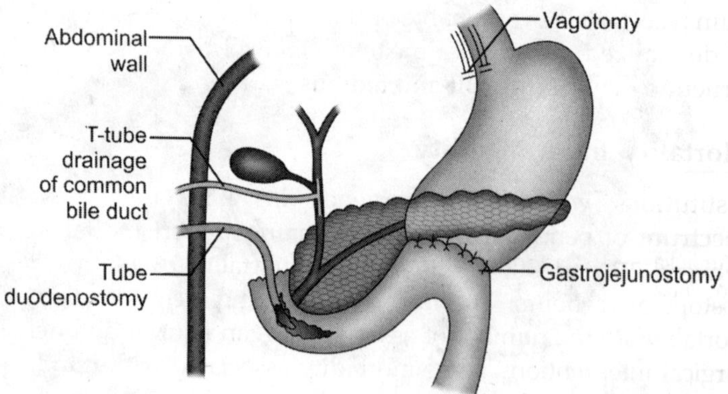

Fig. 21.9: Duodenum diverticulization-partial gastrectomy, gastrojejunostomy, closer of duodenum stump over a tube, closer of injured duodenum, drainage of CBD

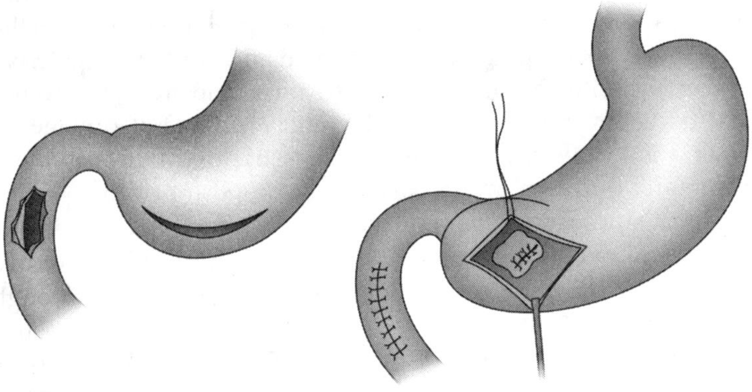

Fig. 21.10: Demonstration of pyloric exclusion technique

term follow-up obtained on many of these patients documented a return of normal physiologic function within months of the initial procedure. Usefulness of this procedure has been widely reviewd. Most of the studies conclude that the use of PEX in patients with severe duodenum injuries may contribute to longer hospital stay and confers no survival or outcome benefit.[9a-9c]

Pancreaticoduodenectomy: Grade V duodenum or pancreatico-duodenum injuries or a severe duodenum injury with the division of both pancreatic and the common bile duct pancreaticoduodenum resection is a reasonable option. It is in essence, debridement of devitalized parts and a means to control hemorrhage. Reconstruction may be difficult and tedious.

Mortality and Morbidity

Institutions with vast experience in managing the entire spectrum of penetrating and blunt injuries report mortality rates between 10 and 30%. Fifty percent mortality occurs within 48 postoperative hours. The major contributing factors to this early mortality are the number of associated organ injuries and delay in surgical interventions.[10] The morbidity associated with duodenum injury is primarily due to leakage. If the drains had been placed the diagnosis is obvious. There is sudden increase in drainage output. If the drain had not been instituted or removed earlier, a clinical pattern of hemodynamic instability, consistent with septic shock that suddenly interrupts what was a fairly smooth course, should alert the surgeon to the possibility of anastomotic leak. Emergency laparotomy is indicated and most often one have to content with thorough peritoneal toilet and multiple drains. The tissue are necrotic and friable and reclosure of duodenum wound is mostly unsuccessful. Nasogastric decompression and parenteral nutrition are important during postoperative period. Contrast studies may be performed to find out if it is end fistula or lateral duodenum fistula. End fistula have got tendency to heal while lateral fistula will need operative intervention. Procedures designated to convert lateral to end fistula have met with a considerable success. A two stage approach to the treatment of lateral fistula is recommended:[11]

i. Control the fistula and drain any surrounding septic foci
ii. Surgically convert a lateral to end-duodenum fistula.

REFERENCES

1. Moore EE, Cogbill TH, Malangoni MA, et al. Organ injury scaling II: Pancreas, duodenum, small bowel, colon, and rectum. J Trauma 1990;30:1427.
2. Ferrara JJ, Curreri PW. Gastrointestinal trauma. In Moyalon JA (ed): Trauma Surgery. Philadelphia, J B Lippincott & Co 1988;243-52.
3. Jones WR, Hardin WJ, Davis JT, Hardy JD. Intramural haematoma of the duodenum: Are view of the literature and case report. Ann Surg 1971;173:534-44.
3a. Pandey S, Niranjan A, Mishra S, et al. Retrospective analysis of duodenal injuries: A comprehensive overview. Saudi J Gastroenterol 2011;17(2):142-4.
4. Moore JB, Moore EE. Changing trends in management of combined pancreatoduodenum injuries. World J Surg 1984;8:791-7.
5. McInnis WD, Aust JB, Cruz AB, Root HD. Traumatic injuries of duodenum: A comparison of 10 closure and the serosal patch. J Trauma 1975;15:847-53.
6. Ivatury RR, Gaudino J, Ascer E, et al. Treatment of penetrating duodenum injuries: Primary vs repair with decompressive enterostomy/serosal patch. J Trauma 1985;25:337-41.
7. Jones SA, Joergenson EJ. Closure of duodenum wall defects. Surgery 1963;53:438-42.
8. Berne CJ, Donovon AJ, White EJ, et al. Duodenum "diverticulisation" for duodenum and pancreatic injury. Am J Surg 1974;127:503-7.

9. Vaughan GD, Frazier OH, Graham DY, et al. The use of pyloric exclusion in the management of severe duodenum injuries. Am J Surg 1977;134:785-90.
9a. Seamon MJ, Pieri PG, Fisher CA, Gaughan J, Santora TA, Pathak AS, Bradley KM, Goldberg AJ. A ten-year retrospective review: does pyloric exclusion improve clinical outcome after penetrating duodenum and combined pancreaticoduodenum injuries? J Trauma 2007;62(4):829-33.
9b. DuBose JJ, Inaba K, Teixeira PG, Shiflett A, Putty B, Green DJ, Plurad D, Demetriades D. Pyloric exclusion in the treatment of severe duodenum injuries: results from the National Trauma Data Bank. Am Surg. 2008;74(10):925-9.
9c. Velmahos GC, Constantinou C, Kasotakis G. Safety of repair for severe duodenum injuries. World J Surg. 2008;32(1):7-12.
10. Leviason MA, Petersen SR, Sheldon GF, Trunkey DD. Duodenum trauma: Experience of atrauma centre. J Trauma 1984;24:475-80.
11. Malangoni MA, Madura JA, Jesseph JE. Management of lateral duodenum fistulas: A study of fourteen cases. Surgery 1981;90:645-651.

Chapter

22 Injuries of Small Intestines

SK Kochar

Aristotle was the first to recognize that intestinal injury could occur as a result of blunt abdominal trauma, and Hippocrates was the first to report that intestinal perforation could result from penetrating wounds.[1] The modern use of exploratory laparotomy for suspected intestinal injury was not observed until late World War I. The incidence of small intestinal injury secondary to blunt abdominal trauma ranges anywhere from 5 to 15%.[2] The incidence of intestinal injury secondary to penetrating injury ranges from 30%[3] in stab injuries to 80%[4] in gunshot wounds in those patients where the peritoneum has been violated.

MECHANISM OF INJURY

The small intestines lies free in the abdomen and is relatively unprotected. Mobility of intestines around fixed points (ligament of Treitz, adhesions or cecum) predisposes the intestines at these points to avulsion injuries from shearing forces. The characteristic convolutions of small bowel predispose it to folding or kinking, creating a close loop on itself. The extensive series of anastomotic vascular arcades within the mesenteric folds serve to help preserve intestinal viability by carrying blood distally to damaged segmental vessels. Injury may be blunt or penetrating. Penetrating injuries are due to stab wounds or gunshot wounds and in rural set up due to bull horn injuries. Stab wound may be due to knife or various forms of sharp weapons used by many tribals in the rural set up. Small bowel rupture secondary to blunt abdominal trauma is uncommon[5] and the injury mechanism remains controversial. There are three proposed mechanisms of intestinal rupture following blunt abdominal trauma:

- Direct impact,
- Shearing force, and
- Pseudo-closed loop obstruction

Direct impact: The intestines may be crushed between the direct blow/impact/crushing force and the vertebral column. The characteristic injuries produced are large perforations, with frank disruptions and associated injuries to other organs.[6]

Shearing force: Shearing force applied to the small intestines at the ligament of Treitz and the cecum as it occurs during rapid deceleration in the lateral and horizontal plane during vehicle accidents may result in small intestinal injury. It may also occur following fall/jump from heights (vertical deceleration).[7] When intestines are held in a fixed position as in adhesions, groin hernias and terminal ileitis these segments are more prone to injuries thus giving credence to the theory of shearing force.

Pseudo-closed loop obstruction: Experimental data[8] has demonstrated that blunt abdominal forces transmitted to a given segment of small intestine were harmlessly channeled through the lumen of remaining small bowel. However, when a loop of small intestine filled with succus entericus, gas or food gets entrapped between an external force and a firm anatomical object, even small amounts of external force are able to generate the intraluminal bursting pressure of 140 mm Hg required to rupture the small intestine.[6]

Small intestinal perforations occurring as isolated injury are probably due to blow out of a pseudo-close loop while large perforations with mesenteric hematoma are due to direct impact as the sole etiology.

CLASSIFICATION

Small bowel injury scale[9] follows in Table 22.1.

Table 22.1: Classification of small bowel injury scale

Grades		*Injury descriptions*
I	Hematoma	Contusion or hematoma without devascularization
	Laceration	Partial thickness, no perforation
II	Laceration	Laceration < 50% of circumference
III	Laceration	Laceration >50% of circumference without transection
IV	Laceration	Transection of the small bowel
V	Laceration	Transection of the small bowel with segmental tissue loss
	Vascular	Devascularized segment

Advance one grade for multiple injuries up to grade III.

Diagnosis

The diagnosis of blunt injury to the small intestines is often difficult due to lack or late appearance of physical signs. It may take several hours before classic signs of peritonitis are evident,[10] given the typically slow leakage of intestinal contents, which are minimally irritant to the peritoneum. Impaired sensorium due to head injury may add to the difficulty. Pain abdomen following blunt injury, tenderness, guarding, rigidity of varying grade should arouse the suspicion of small gut injury till not proved otherwise by various diagnostic tests. An upright chest X-ray will demonstrate gas under the diaphragm in 20-50% of cases.[11] Diagnostic peritoneal lavage appears to offer a much higher diagnostic yield. This may be improved further by measuring alkaline phosphatase levels in the lavage fluid.[12] However, negative diagnostic lavage does not rule out intestinal injury.

CT Findings of Bowel or Mesenteric Injury[12a]

Bowel Discontinuity

Discontinuity of bowel is the primary finding of bowel injury. This findings are uncommon in the literature. Because direct visualization is unusual, one must generally rely on secondary findings.

EXTRALUMINAL

Oral Contrast Material

Free intraperitoneal oral contrast material is 100% specific for bowel perforation if concentrated intravenous contrast material from genitourinary tract perforation is not a confounding factor. The sensitivity of this CT finding is 12% or less in the literature.[12b]

Extraluminal Air

The finding of pneumoperitoneum has a sensitivity of 44–55%.[12b] Pneumoretroperitoneum in the setting of duodenal injury seems to be a more sensitive finding. Extraluminal intra- or retroperitoneal air is not diagnostic of bowel perforation. Although bowel perforation is a major source of this finding, barotrauma and mechanical ventilation can result in air below the diaphragm.

Intramural Air

Major bowel injuries (those requiring laparotomy, such as perforations) and minor bowel injuries (which can be treated conservatively, such as serosal abrasions) have findings of bowel-wall thickening and free fluid in common. CT does not appear to be able to readily help distinguish the two in all instances. Along with extraluminal air, the presence of intramural air will highlight a probable full-thickness rather than partial-thickness injury (Fig. 22.1).

Bowel-Wall Thickening

Bowel-wall thickening, seen in 75% of transmural injuries, is more sensitive for bowel-wall injury than is extravasation of oral contrast material or pneumoperitoneum (Fig. 22.2).[12b] Isolated mesenteric lacerations may also demonstrate this sign, probably as a result of interruption of the arterial supply or venous drainage. Disproportionate thickening compared with normal segments or bowel-wall thickness greater than 3 mm with adequate bowel distention is abnormal.

Bowel-Wall Enhancement

The proposed cause of enhancement of reduced perfusion and interstitial leak of contrast material fits into the categories of either

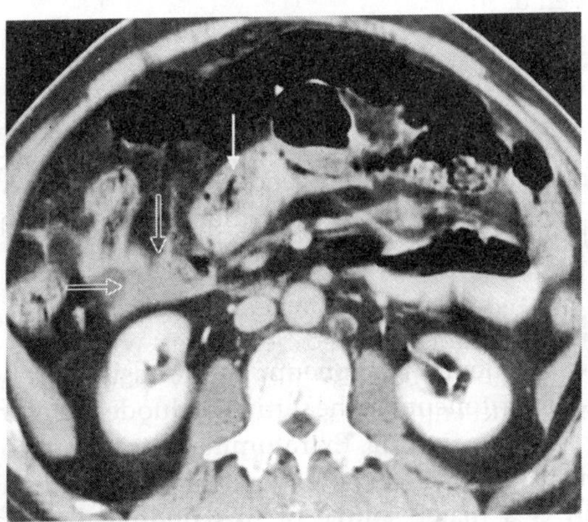

Fig. 22.1: Proximal ileum perforation and mesenteric hematoma. Abdominal CT scan demonstrates intramural air in the ileum (solid arrow) and adjacent interloop free fluid (open arrows)

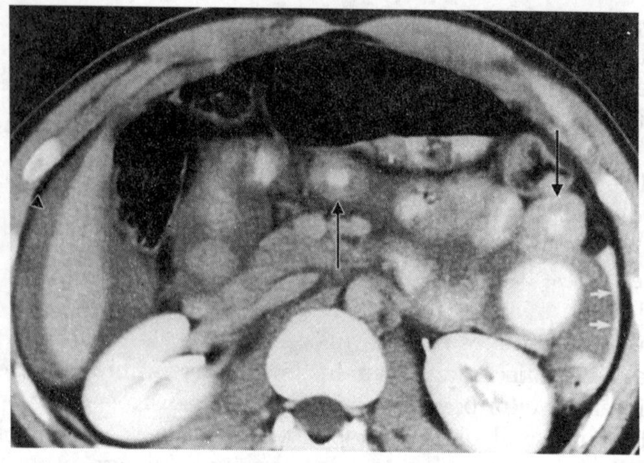

Fig. 22.2: A 10 cm long jejunal laceration and mesenteric avulsion of the descending colon. CT scan demonstrates thick-walled jejunal loops (black arrows), hemoperitoneum (arrowhead), and free intraperitoneal contrast material (white arrows)

local vascular damage related to bowel or mesenteric injury or the more systemic hypoperfusion complex.

The definition of bowel-wall enhancement is not uniform. Empiric assessment, enhancement greater than that of the psoas muscle, or enhancement equal to that of adjacent blood vessels have all been used.

Mesenteric Infiltration

Mesenteric infiltration or "stranding" can be associated with mesenteric injury with or without bowel perforation, but bowel-wall thickening associated with stranding is highly suggestive of significant bowel injury. Sensitivities and specificities of 69-77% and 44-100%, respectively, have been reported for this sign.[12c] Mesenteric findings are more common when bowel injury is along the mesenteric border. A localized hematoma within the mesentery in the absence of a bowel abnormality points to an isolated laceration of a mesenteric vessel.

Intraperitoneal and Retroperitoneal Fluids

Hematomas can occur in the peritoneal cavity, retroperitoneum, or both. Retroperitoneal hematoma along with wall thickening helps identification of duodenal trauma and is frequently present with this type of injury. Hemoperitoneum is a common finding in patients with intraperitoneal bowel or mesenteric laceration (88-100% of patients).[12b] Periduodenal hematoma is a fairly specific sign of duodenal injury because retroperitoneal blood tends to localize at the site of injury. This is in contrast with intraperitoneal blood for which the absence of restriction allows blood from solid organ injury to flow freely where it may be associated with normal bowel loops. It follows that hemoperitoneum in the absence of solid organ injury would imply bowel or mesenteric laceration as the source of bleeding. In this setting, free fluid on more than three contiguous 10 mm thick sections suggests the presence of a significant bowel or mesenteric injury.

There is a 5% frequency of major bowel injury with hepatic laceration and 4% with splenic trauma. In the absence of bowel-wall thickening, mesenteric stranding, or free air, a simultaneous injury to mesentery or bowel might not be suspected if free fluid is instead linked to solid organ damage. However, fluid location may be helpful. Interloop fluid specifies fluid between the folds of mesentery and bowel. These usually polygonal collections are uncommonly associated with solid organ injury and more likely to be related to bowel or mesenteric injury.

Intraparenchymal contusion is also a solid organ injury, but it does not extend to cause capsular disruption and would not be expected to result in hemoperitoneum. Bowel or mesenteric injury should be suspected in this instance.

Fluid in the intra- or extraperitoneal compartments may not be from hemorrhage but rather may be due to leakage of bowel contents, urine, bile, or pancreatic juice, or the introduction of diagnostic peritoneal lavage fluid. Of these fluids, opacified intraperitoneal urine would most completely mask the presence of intraperitoneal blood or bowel contents. Hemorrhage from damage to other organs in the same anatomic space can also be misleading.

Serial physical examination preferably by the same surgeon seems to be the best bet. When in doubt exploratory laparotomy is the only faultless test for the diagnosis of intestinal injury. In penetrating trauma violation of peritoneum is the indication for surgery when patient has sustained gunshot wounds while in stab injury serial physical examination is an alternative, available under control conditions.

Management

There is no role of conservative management in small intestinal injury. Midline incision is preferred. The entire small intestine must be carefully examined from the ligament of Treitz to ileocecal valve, including all mural surfaces and mesenteric attachments. The rule that an odd number of hollow viscus perforation (gunshot wound) requires a search until another hole is found, is valid. Either a rare tangential injury or even rare intraluminal location of the missile are reasons for an exception to this rule.

Perforations

Most perforations are closed by primary repair. Edges are debrided till it bleed and two layers closure is done (Fig. 22.3), i.e. inner layer of absorbable and outer layer of silk. When there are multiple perforations in a close area or the closure of large laceration results in narrowing resection anastomosis is done. Resection anastomosis should not be performed in last 15 cm of ileum due to precarious blood supply. Rather end to side ileocolic anastomosis is preferred. Peritoneal cavity must be liberally irrigated with warm saline and particulate matter removed. Drains are optional. However, subcutaneous drains after fascial closer do decrease the septic complications. Some authors recommend secondary closure.[13]

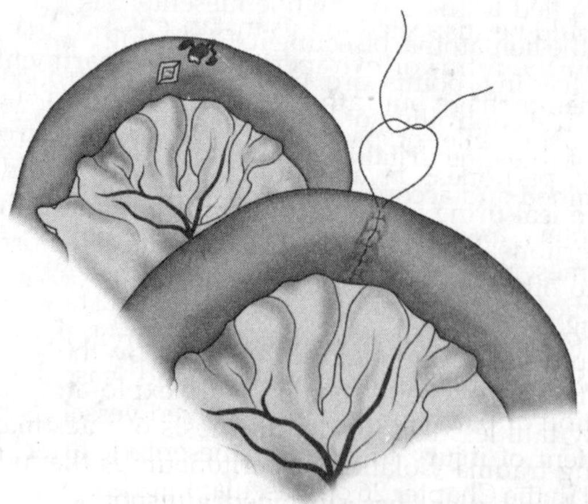

Fig. 22.3: Repair of injury to small intestine

Mural Damage without Perforation

The management of contusions and intramural hematomas of the small intestines require assessment for consideration of resection anastomosis verses leaving the intestines *in situ* and opting for observation and second look surgery. Doppler ultrasound probe over the site of injury and intravenous fluorescein[14] have been used to clarify questionable areas that appear ischemic but not frankly necrotic. These methods have not become popular and clinical judgment by observing the involved segment for signs of intestinal viability such as active peristalsis and color throughout the procedure are of paramount importance. Small mucosal hematoma (< 1 cm), nonexpanding may be turned in by a series of interrupted sutures. For larger mucosal hematoma, transmural debridement/segmental resection should be done whenever there is doubt regarding viability.

Mesenteric Hematoma

Assessment should be done to define the size, stability, i.e. is it expanding or nonexpanding, contained or it has ruptured the mesenteric folds. Exploration is required for large, expanding and uncontained hematomas. At exploration, the involved mesentery proximal to the hematoma (towards the base) should be examined and if possible site of vascular control defined. Manual compression is then applied to that point while mesentery is incised over the length of the hematoma, bisecting it. Following careful evacuation of clot, bleeding points are individually controlled with silk sutures. Once controlling of hemorrhage has been accomplished, viability of intestine distal to the area of vascular damaged must be determined and accordingly dealt with. Injuries to the base of the mesentery associated with large hematoma are suspect for superior mesenteric artery or vein injury and may cause severe bowel ischemia to the entire length of small bowel. Collateral flow is often inadequate to maintain viability.[15] Resection under these circumstances is unsuccessful, and vascular repair by interposition or patch graft of the involved vessels is mandatory. Management of injury to superior mesenteric artery have been discussed in the Chapter 26 on Vascular injuries. When large areas of ischemic bowel are in question one may opt for second look surgery/relaparotomy. In cases requiring relaparotomy certain guidelines[16] have been found to be useful. These guidelines are briefed in Table 22.2. Laparotomy is performed between 24 and 48 hours after first surgery.

COMPLICATIONS

Postoperative complications are missed injury, bleeding, suture line leak, anastomotic disruption, fistula formation, obstruction, and abscess.[17] If one is careful and screened the whole intestine from ligament of Treitz to ileocecal junction, missed injuries are rare. One should be careful towards the mesenteric border of the intestines where small perforation may be missed.

Hemorrhage: Intraluminal blood loss may occur at suture lines, anastomosis, or areas of bowel contusion. Hemoglobin may fall, tachycardia may be present and patient may have melena or haematochezia depending on the amount of blood loss. If the patient does not respond to conservative treatment re-exploration should not be delayed.

Suture line disruption and fistula: Diagnosis is often difficult in postoperative period. Patient who was progressing well and develop pain abdomen, distention, absent or decreased bowel sounds, tachycardia, and fever is the candidate where suture line leak/disruption has taken placed. At times it occur as catastrophic event. Prompt recognition is mandatory and treatment consists of re-exploration after resuscitation. Edges are debrided and anastomosis performed. At times intra-abdominal

Table 22.2: Guidelines for relaparotomy

Condition	*Repair*
The entire small intestine is necrotic	No procedure are performed and the patients incision expeditiously closed, and patient returned to ICU where supportive care can be resumed
Areas of patchy necrosis are encountered throughout the length of small bowel	Expeditious closure, parenteral hyper-alimentation and supportive care
Isolated segment of necrotic bowel identified	Local resection and primary anastomosis performed

sepsis is far advanced and the bowel loops are adherent and friable. Temporary jejunostomy/ileostomy may be life saving. Fortunately, such situations are rare if one have been meticulous at primary surgery. Fistula formation is rare and if there is no distal obstruction these heal spontaneously. However, if there is obstruction due to adhesions, bands, operative repair after assessment will be required.

REFERENCES

1. Loria FL. Historical aspects of penetrating wounds of the abdomen. Int Abstr Surg 1948;89:521.
2. Di Vincenti FC, Rives JD, Laborde EJ, et al. Blunt abdominal trauma. J Trauma 1968;8:1004.
3. Lowe RJ, Boyed DR, Folk FA, et al. The negative laparotomy for abdominal trauma. J Trauma 1972;12:853.
4. Nance FC, Wennar MH, Johnson LW, et al. Surgical judgement in the management of penetrating wounds of the abdomen: Experience with 2112 patients. Ann Surg 1974;179:639.
5. Pontius GV, Kilborne BC, Paul EG. Nonpenetrating abdominal trauma. AMA Arch Surg 1956;72:800.
6. GeoghenT, Brush B. The mechanism of intestinal perforation from nonpenetrating abdominal trauma. AMA Arch Surg 1957;73:455.
7. Lukas GM, Hutton JE, Lim RC, et al. Injuries sustained from high velocity impact from water: An experience from the Golden bridge. J Trauma 1981;21:612.
8. Williams RD, Sargent FT. The mechanism of intestinal injury in trauma. J Trauma 1963;3:288-94.
9. Moore EE, Cogbill TH, Malangoni MA, et al. Organ injury scaling II: Pancreas, duodenum, small bowel, colon, and rectum. J Trauma 1990;30:1427.
10. Phillips TF, Brotman S. Perforating injuries of the small bowel from blunt abdominal trauma. Ann Emerg Med 1983;12:75-8.
11. Maull KI, Reath DB. Impact of early recognition on outcome in nonpenetrating wounds of the small bowel. South Med J 1984;77:1075-77.
12. Marx JA, Bar-Or D, Moore EE, et al. Utility of lavage alkaline phosphatase in detection of isolated small intestinal injury. Ann Emerg Med 1985;14:10-14.

12a. Jeffrey M Brody, Danielle B Leighton, Brian L Murphy, et al. CT of blunt trauma bowel and mesenteric Injury: Typical Findings and Pitfalls in Diagnosis November Radiographics, 2000;20:1525-36.

12b. Levine CD, Gonzales RN, Wachsberg RH. CT findings in bowel and mesenteric injury. J Comput Assist Tomogr 1997;21:974-9.

12c. Breen DJ, Janzen DL, Zwirewich CV, et al. Blunt bowel and mesenteric injury: diagnostic performance of CT signs. J Comput Assist Tomogr 1997;21:706-12.

13. Robbs Jv, Moore SW, Pillay SP. Blunt abdominal trauma with jejunal injury: A review. J Trauma 1980;20:308-11.

14. Marzella L, Brotman S, Mayer J, et al. Evaluation of injured intestine with the aid of fluorescein. Am surg 1984;50:599-602.

15. Lucas AE, Richardson JD, Flint LM, et al. Traumatic injury of the proximal superior mesenteric artery. Ann Surg 1981;193:30.

16. Schwab CW, Shaikh KA, Talucci RC. Injury to the stomach and small bowel. In Moore EE, Feliciano DV, Mattox KL (Eds). Trauma. Norwalk, CT, Appleton & Lange, 1991;485-98.

17. Blaisdell FW, Trunkey DD (Eds). Trauma management, Vol I: Abdominal trauma. New York, Thieme-Stratton, 1982.

Chapter

23 Injuries of Colon and Rectum

SK Kochar

COLONIC INJURIES

Colonic injuries are common among patients who have sustained penetrating injuries. The incidence of colonic injuries range between 25 and 30 in patients who sustain gunshot wounds of the abdomen and stab wounds are responsible for 5% of incidence. Colorectal injury due to blunt trauma to the abdomen is rare. Blunt trauma may occur following road traffic accidents, and may be as a result of misapplied lap belt riding too high over the iliac crest. Other causes of injuries to colon are: Over enthusiastic bowel insufflation during sigmoidoscopy or colonoscopy; during rigid sigmoidoscopy; faulty administration of enema, perforation due to rectal thermometer and occasionally due to deep biopsies. Rectal impalement injury occurs due to any sharp object like a stick, handle of the broomstick or a pitchfork, striking the perianal region. Crush injury may damage the colon or rectum in two ways. Pelvic fracture may produce perforation of the rectum by bone spicules, and occasionally, an implosion injury associated with Valsalva at the time of crush may occur. Mortality rate ranges from 3 to 10% but morbidity and its potential to increase the mortality and morbidity rate of other abdominal organs justifies the concern for colon and rectal injuries.

Pathophysiology

When the colon is perforated, bowel may leak from the lumen contaminating the peritoneum or retroperitoneal tissues. Bacterial flora is extensive. *E. coli*, *Enterococcus*, and *Bacteroides* predominate in the flora. Stab wounds generally produce clean incised wounds of the colon. Shot gun injuries not only destroy the colon but massively macerate and contaminate the adjacent organs and tissues predisposing to myonecrosis and sepsis. In blunt trauma it is usually a blow out resulting from sudden compression of the air filled bowel. Occasional patients develop colonic hematomas that may perforate days or weeks after the injury.[1]

Classification

Organ injury scale approved by the American Association for the Surgery of Trauma has been accepted by most of the trauma surgeons which is given in Tables 23.1 and 23.2.

Diagnosis

History of penetrating injury, blunt injury or having undergone some rectal procedures may be available. In psychiatric patients this may not be forthcoming. Following injury varying intensity of pain in abdomen is present. Tenderness, guarding and rigidity may or may not be present. Shock is due to blood loss as a result of other associated injuries and not due to colonic injuries. Occasionally, symptoms of peritonism may take few

Table 23.1: Colon injury scale

Grades		*Injury descriptions*
I	Hematoma	Contusion or hematoma without devascularization
	Laceration	Partial thickness, no perforation
II	Laceration	Laceration < 50% of circumference
III	Laceration	Laceration > 50% of circumference without transection
IV	Laceration	Transection of the colon
V	Laceration	Transection of the colon with tissue loss

Advance one grade for multiple injuries up to grade III.

Table 23.2: Rectum injury scale

Grades		*Injury descriptions*
I	Hematoma	Contusion or hematoma without devascularization
	Laceration	Partial thickness laceration
II	Laceration	Laceration less than 50% of circumference
III	Laceration	Laceration > than 50% of circumference
IV	Laceration	Full thickness with extension into the perineum
V	Vascular	Devascularized segment

Advance one grade for multiple injuries up to grade III.

hours or days to develop. There may be blood on finger stall on per rectal examination or tenderness in pelvic peritoneum may be noticed. When bleeding is present, per rectal examination should be followed up with proctoscopy and rigid sigmoidoscopic examinations. Plane X-ray abdomen rarely shows gas under the diaphragm but in those patients who sustain injury following colonoscopy or sigmoidoscopy or insufflation injury, it is mostly present. Diagnostic peritoneal lavage, when positive for intestinal contents, bacteria, bile it indicates perforation of the hollow viscus. USG abdomen may not contribute much. Enema with water soluble contrast CT scan in selected cases may be done where the symptoms are minimal and the diagnosis is doubtful. High index of suspicion and repeated clinical examination is mostly rewarding. Clinical deterioration in the patient's status, increased abdominal tenderness, an evolving pattern of sepsis, and development of paralytic ileus or mechanical obstruction are common findings in patients with either a missed injury or delayed perforation.

CT findings in bowel injury include the following (Figs 23.1 to 23.3):

- Bowel injury is suggested by free intraperitoneal air, free intraperitoneal or retroperitoneal fluid, focal areas of bowel wall thickening, abnormal bowel wall enhancement, bowel wall hematoma (i.e. duodenal hematoma), and intramural air.
- The most specific finding is the visualization of oral contrast extravasation and bowel wall disruption.
- A pattern of more diffuse bowel wall thickening, abnormal enhancement, and mesenteric infiltration can suggest mesenteric vascular injury resulting in ischemic bowel.
- In intestinal vascular injury, evaluate the celiac axis, superior mesenteric artery, and superior mesenteric vein. A mesenteric hematoma or a focal area of higher density clotted blood (i.e. "sentinel clot") can suggest vascular injury.
- Focal contrast extravasation can indicate active hemorrhage.

Management

Historical Perspective

During World War I the average mortality rate was generally reported as 60%. Ogilvie, recounting the experience of the British

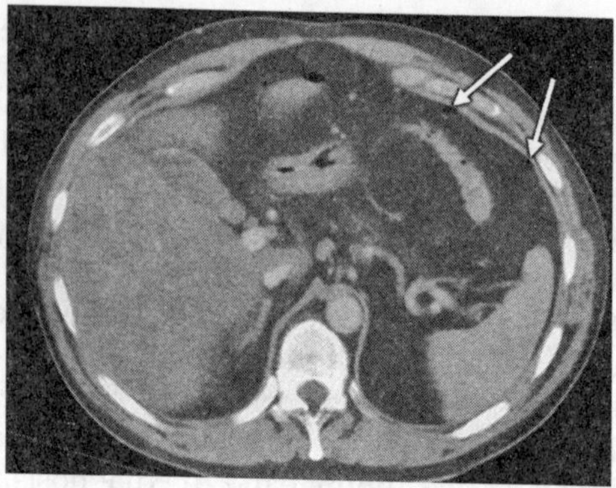

Fig. 23.1: Axial CT through upper abdomen reveals 2 spots of free intraperitoneal air (arrows)

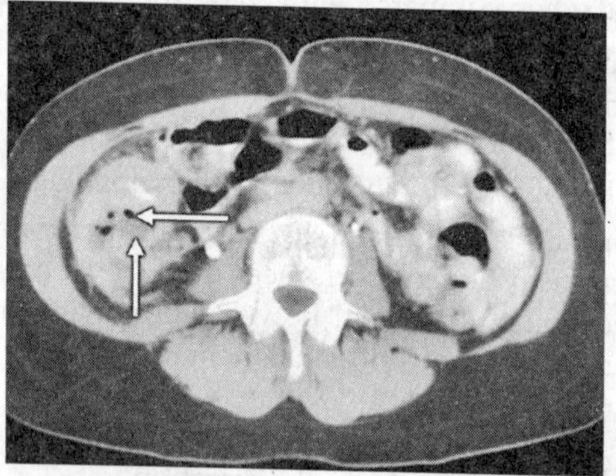

Fig. 23.2: Axial CT through the abdomen shows focal gas bubbles (white arrows) and an extraluminal fluid collection adjacent to the contrast-filled colon

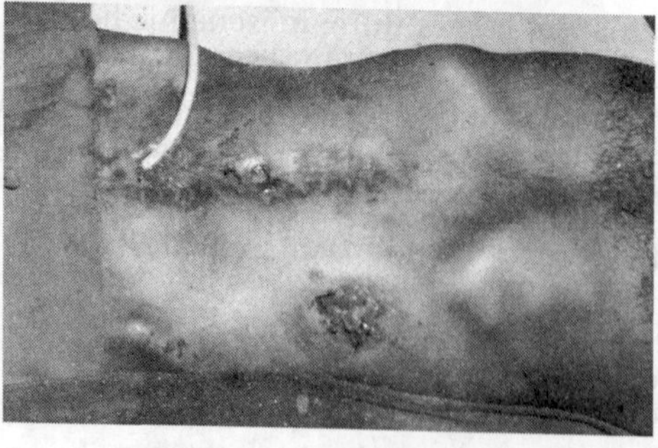

Fig. 23.3: Gunshot wound abdomen. Colonic injury treated with proximal colostomy *(For color version, see Plate 6)*

surgical team in the North African Desert Compaign of World War II, reported significant reductions in mortality attributed to the performance of colostomies in the treatment of colon injuries.[2] Based upon this philosophy and other improvements in medical care, mortality rate fell to 30% during World War II. Further reduction in mortality rate to 10-15% was noted during Korean and Vietnam conflicts. This was attributed to improvements in antibiotics; resuscitation; rapid evacuation, allowing early operation; blood availability; and better overall supportive care. Woodhall and Ochsner in 1951 suggested[3] the safety of primary repair in selected cases with civilian colon injury. Diversion remained the standard of care during the period from 1950 to 1980. However, Stone and Fabian,[4] in a 1979 prospective randomized study of perforating colon injuries, clearly demonstrated that, in selected cases, primary repair was effective when compared with colostomy. In the last 10 years, primary repair has assumed an increasing role in the treatment of colon injuries.[5,6] Inspite of reduction of mortality over the years to below 10%, one is still plagued with major complications in 15-50% of cases. Surgical options are:

- Primary closure without colostomy
- Primary closure with defunctioning colostomy
- Resection and anastomosis
- Exteriorization of injured colon/colostomy
- Exteriorized repair.

Over the years, a number of factors have been identified that were thought to contributing to postoperative complications (Table 23.3) and had influenced the choice of procedure.

Shock

Shock has been a relative contraindication to primary repair for many years. During periods of even transient hypotension, blood flows to the bowel is reduced and may be a factor in the development of anastomotic leaks.[7] Although shock prior to surgery and during intraoperative period does influences the mortality rate, the presence of shock does not significantly contribute to increase postoperative sepsis and is not a significant factor in the complication rate of patients undergoing primary repair when compared to those treated with a colostomy.[8-10] Inspite of these findings, it is well known fact that prolonged shock state contributes to increase mortality and in case colostomy saves time, this should be preferred procedure over primary repair.

Table 23.3: Risk factors

- Shock
- Fecal contamination
- Associated injuries
- Interval from injury to repair
- Mechanism of injury
- Severity of colon injury
- Location of injury

Fecal Contamination

Faecal contamination has been defined as mild if the spillage is confined to the immediate area around the injury; moderate if a somewhat larger amount of spill was confined to a single quadrant and major, if a large volume of feces was found in more than one quadrant.[10] Although most authors agree that minimal contamination poses less of a risk, there is still a healthy respect for the patient who has gross contamination as these patients have higher complications rate.

Associated Injuries

Associated injuries, both in numbers and complexity reflect the seriousness of the patient's condition and play an integral part both in the type of management selected and the ultimate patient outcome. The penetrating abdominal trauma index (PATI) is a score derived by combining the values of each injured organ as determined by operation. A sharp increase in morbidity and mortality has been observed in patients having associated injuries in more than two organs/PATI score more than 25. A very healthy respect for such injured organs as the duodenum and ureter can strongly motivate conversion of a colon injury to colostomy.

Interval from Injury to Repair

The increase in fecal contamination, coupled with blood loss provides a milieu for significant infectious potential. The time period is not absolute but probably all patients arriving later than 6-8 hours are not the candidates for primary repair.

Mechanism of Injury

Stab wounds generally produce less severe injury and are mostly amenable to primary repair. In gunshot wound the damage is much beyond what is clinically discernible and colostomy is preferred by most of the surgeons.

Severity of Colon Injury

Colon injury scale of 3 or 4 seems to be reliable predictor of septic complications and becomes a risk factor for primary closure.

Anatomical Location

There was some initial evidence that primary repair might best be reserved for right sided colon injury because of its favorable characteristics of liquid contents with both fewer and less variety of microorganisms, better blood supply, and larger luminal diameter. However, it has since been demonstrated that despite such differences, penetrating trauma to the right and left hemicolon can be managed in similar fashion.[11]

Exposure and Exploration

When the diagnosis is not definite midline incision should be employed. An attempt to control hemorrhage should be made first. Once the bleeding has been controlled and hemodynamic stability established a brief exploration should be made looking for obvious perforations. A systemic search for the colonic injury should accompany the exploration. In the absence of a suspicious missile track, careful inspection of the colon, mesentery, and retroperitoneum will usually suffice. The vascular supply to the colon should be assured and the mesenteric attachments confirmed. Examination of the colon is competed by systematically tracking the entire colon from the ileocecal valve to the rectum.

Methods of Repair

Primary repair: Relative contraindications for primary closure have been the followings:

- Prolonged or persistence hypotension
- Greater than 6-hour delay between injury and surgical intervention
- Gross fecal spillage
- Extensive damage to abdominal or retroperitoneal muscle

- Significant hemoperitoneum
- Multiple coexistence visceral injuries
- Devitalization of more than one-fourth of the colon wall
- Impairment of the blood supply to the injured segment
- Colon injury grade 3 or more.

Most of these risk factors may not affect the outcome individually but collectively it merits consideration. Primary repair is appropriate for colonic and intraperitoneal rectal injuries and that extraperitoneal rectal injuries require diverting colostomy. Shock on admission, increased blood transfusion requirements, associated organ injury and severity of the injury were associated with high mortality.[11a] Primary repair is a safe procedure for treatment of colon injuries. Patients with primary repair had lower morbidity ($p < 0.009$). Surgery during the first 6 h ($p < 0.006$) and in hemodynamically stable patients ($p < 0.014$) had a lower risk of complications.[11b]

In a recent landmark prospective multicenter study of 297 patients, Demetriaides et al compared primary anastomosis with diversion.[11c] There were 197 patients in the primary anastomosis group as compared to the 100 in the diversion group. There was no difference in colon-related complications between the two groups (22% vs. 27%, $p < 0.313$ for primary anastomosis and diversion, respectively). Multivariate analysis including all potential risk factors with p values < 0.2 identified three independent risk factors for abdominal complications: severe fecal contamination, transfusion of > 3 units of blood within the first 24 hours, and single-agent antibiotic prophylaxis. The type of colon management was not found to be a risk factor. The authors concluded that in severe colon injuries requiring resection, the method of colon management does not influence the incidence of colon-related abdominal complications, irrespective of the presence or absence of any risk factors. The intensive care unit and hospital stays were shorter in the primary repair group, although not statistically significantly. In view of these findings and the fact that colon diversion is associated with worse quality of life and requires an additional operation for closure, colon injuries requiring resection should be managed by primary repair, irrespective of risk factors. More prudent approach will be that treatment of traumatic colon injury should be case specific, taking into account the mechanism of the lesion, its severity and associated injuries.[11d]

The technique involves thorough and meticulous debridement of the wound edges followed by a standard two-layer closure (an inner layer of running or interrupted absorbable sutures followed by an outer layer of interrupted silk Lembert sutures). Wide debridement of any tract created by a missile after it exits the colon is uniformly indicated. Prior to facial closure the abdomen is liberally irrigated with saline and all particulate matter is removed. Drains are normally not indicated. The skin and subcutaneous tissues may be closed primarily with or without a subcutaneous drain/or by delayed primary method.

Primary resection and anastomosis: This procedure is ideal when there is extensive wounds of the right colon. Right hemicolectomy with ileocolic anastomosis can be accomplished with reasonable dispatch and an acceptable rate in the majority of patients. Hemodynamically unstable patients should have an ileostomy if taking time for anastomosis will jeopardize their survival. Primary anastomosis may be performed in the left colon following resection of extensively damaged portion but it should be protected by a proximal colostomy.

Colostomy

Indications for colostomy are: When the condition of the patient precludes taking the time to make a repair or anastomosis; when a distal anastomosis may be tenuous, when extensive distal destruction of the colon would require a low rectal anastomosis.[12] It may be accomplished by: (i) Exteriorization, (ii) Defunctioning colostomy, and (iii) End colostomy and Hartmann procedure.

Exteriorization of the colon: It is the most rapid method available for managing a colon injury. Even in the fixed portions of the colon, mobilization can be accomplished quickly. If exteriorization is elected as an option, a small lateral incision is made, and the two limbs of the mobilized colon are brought out as a double barreled colostomy.

Defunctioning colostomy: It is performed by separating the limbs and bringing each out as a single stoma. This option provides complete fecal diversion and leaves the patient a single stoma colostomy that is far easier to manage. It has the disadvantage of being more difficult to close than a loop or double barrel colostomy. Complete diversion by end diversion may be indicated for various reasons. Resection of devitalized bowel may lead to loss of considerable length and primary repair be deemed inadvisable. A loop colostomy at the site of injury may not reach the skin surface, particularly in an obese patient. The injury to the bowel may be circumferential or almost so and thus not amenable to a loop colostomy. Whenever possible, the distal defunctionalized colon should be attached to the peritoneum adjacent to the end colostomy to simplify closure.

Closure of colostomy: Colostomy closure at 1 to 2 postoperative months is associated with a lower morbidity compared to that which occurs when the operation is performed between 2-12 months. Prior to closure, endoscopy and barium enema should be employed to assure an adequate lumen and complete healing. The skin is carefully incised around the entire mucocutaneous junction. Blunt dissection will usually serve to mobilize the subcutaneous portion of the colostomy but sharp dissection is required to free the colostomy from the fascia. If the posterior wall is intact, the colostomy is closed by interrupted sutures, otherwise suture anastomosis is performed. If stapler is available staple anastomosis may be performed. The colon is gently pushed below the fascia and the fascia closed.

Exteriorized repair: There was a brief period of interest in closure of the colonic wound that was exteriorized.[13] The rod under the colostomy was removed after a week and the colon allowed to float back into the abdomen, or a second procedure was performed to replace the colon in the abdomen. Breakdown of the colonic suture line was common; a fascial defect and hernia resulted with the float technique. With increasing use of repair without diversion, this procedure has become essentially obsolete.

Nonoperative Management

Mucosal tears produced by enema tips or thermometers confined within the bowel wall may be evaluated by proctoscopy and cautiously observed. There are reports in the literature of colonic perforation following colonoscopy having been successfully managed conservatively.[14] The surgeon/physician who elects this course of management bears the heavy responsibility of insuring that the patient does not deteriorate or become septic.[12]

RECTAL INJURIES

Anorectal injuries may follow blunt or penetrating trauma. Blunt injury is typically a crushing or compressive force applied to the pelvis or lower abdomen, as would occur when the victim has been struck or run over by a motor vehicle. Causes of penetrating injuries are gunshot wound, stab injury, injury from bicycle seats, enema tips, rectal thermometers, fall on a sharp object and unusual attempt at sexual gratification.

Diagnosis

The diagnosis of anorectal injury alone or in concert with a perineal laceration should be entertained whenever there is clinical or X-ray evidence of fracture pelvis. In these cases, examination of the skin overlying the lower abdomen and perineum for ecchymosis may further raise the suspicion of fracture pelvis. The presence of missile wounds in the thighs, perineum, buttocks, or lower abdomen should alert the surgeon of the injury to the rectum. Per rectal examination followed by proctosigmoidoscopy is essential for assessment of the injury. X-ray of the abdomen including pelvis will not only demonstrate fracture pelvis but it may also reveal the presence of the missile lodged there. An assessment must be made of the followings:

- Injury to other organs, particularly intra-abdominal viscera, that mandates urgent surgical intervention.
- Presence and extent of pelvic fracture.
- Perineal injury that has converted a closed pelvic fracture to an open one.
- Violation of the closed retroperitoneal space by a deep perineal laceration.
- Presence or suspicion of anorectal injury.

Management

Management of rectal injury rests on the three Ds: Diversion, Debridement and Drainage. Early definitive surgical management is indicated in any patient with following condition:[14]

1. Endoscopically visualized anorectal injury, regardless of associated injuries.
2. A possible anorectal injury, clinically suspected but not identified.

3. Open pelvic fracture, whether or not anorectal injury has been identified.

If anorectal injury is readily accessible to transanal approach, wound approximation using a single layer of running 3/0 absorbable suture may be attempted. If the sphincter mechanism has been injured, muscle approximation is performed using interrupted horizontal mattress 3/0 absorbable sutures. The anal mucocutaneous junction is left open for drainage purposes. Primary closure of anorectal wound does not obviate the need of defunctioning colostomy. Presacral retrorectal drains are inserted.

Rectal injuries can be closed relatively easily through the abdominal incision by opening the peritoneum and freeing the upper rectum as is done in elective rectal resection. These wounds should be closed if the situation is favorable. A two layer closure with an inner layer of absorbable suture and outer layer of 3/0 interrupted silk suture is preferred, but one layer is acceptable. It is not necessary to expend excessive effort to debride and close a defect lying deep in the pelvis. Establishment of adequate drainage and fecal diversion are key to success. A sigmoid loop colostomy with or without staple closure of the distal limb or end sigmoid colostomy with Hartman closure should be performed. Drains are placed in retrorectal space and brought out just anterior to the coccyx. Some authors prefer suction drains. Rectal dilatation to three or four fingers is a useful adjunctive measure after completion of operation. Distal washout or rectal wash has fallen out of favor with most of the surgeons. If no significant leak is apparent at the end of 5 days, the drain may be removed safely. Primary closure of intraperitoneal rectal injuries has been advocated.[11a]

REFERENCES

1. Nance FC, Shpitz B, Zager M, et al. Intramural haematoma of the colon following blunt trauma to the abdomen. Am Surg 1968;34:85.
2. Ogilvie WH. Abdominal wounds in the Western Desert. Surg Gynecol Obstet 1944;78:225-38.
3. Woodhall JP, Ochsner A. The management of perforating injuries of the colon and rectum in civilian practice. Surg 1951;29:305-20.
4. Stone HH, Fabian TC. Management of perforating colon trauma: randomisation between primary closure and exteriorisation. Ann Surg 1979;190:430-33.
5. Chappuis Cw, Frey DJ, Dietzen CD, et al. Management of penetrating colon injuries. Ann Surg 1991;231:492-8.

6. Saski LS, Allaben RD, Golwala RL, et al. Primary repair of colon injuries: A prospective randomised study. J Trauma 1995;39:895-901.
7. Shannon FL, Moore EE. Primary repair of the colon: When is it safe a safe alternative? Surg 1985;98:851-60.
8. Burch JM, Brock JC, Gevirtzman L, et al. The injured colon. Ann Surg 1986;203:701-11.
9. Nelkin N, Lewis F. The influence of injury severity on complication rates after primary closure or colostomy for penetrating colon trauma. Ann Surg 1989;209:439-47.
10. George SM Jr, Fabian TC, Voeller GR, et al. Primary repair of colon wounds. Ann Surg 1989;209:728-34.
11. Thompson JS, Moore EE, Moore JB. Comparison of penetrating injuries of the right and left colon. Ann Surg 1981;193:414-8.
11a Govender M, Madiba TE. Current management of large bowel injuries and factors influencing outcome. Injury 2010;41(1):58-63.
11b. Salinas-Aragón LE, Guevara-Torres L, Vaca-Pérez E, et al. Primary closure in colon trauma. Cir 2009;77(5):359 64.
11c. Demetriaides D, Murray JA, Chan L, Ordoñez C, et al. Committee on Multicenter Clinical Trials. American Association for the Surgery of Trauma. Penetrating colon injuries requiring resection: diversion or primary anastomosis? An AAST prospective multicenter study. J Trauma 2001;50:765-75.
11d. Robles-Castillo J, Murillo-Zolezzi A, Murakami PD, Silva-Velasco J. Primary repair vs. colostomy in colon injuries. Cir 2009;77(5):365-8.
12. Nance FC. Injuries to the colon and rectum. In Mattox Kl, Moore EE, Feliciano DV, Eds. Trauma 2nd ed. Norwalk: Appleton and Lange. 1991;521-32.
13. Okies EJ, Bricker DL, Jordan GL, et al. Exteriorised repair of colon injuries. Am J Surg 1972;124:807.
14. Ferrara JJ, Curreri PW. Gastrointestinal trauma. In Moylan JA, ed. Trauma Surgery Philadelphia: JB Lippincott & Co. 1988;270-5.

Chapter

24 Renal, Ureter and Bladder Injuries

Subhash Kotwal, Alok Kumar Jha

RENAL INJURIES

Introduction

Renal trauma occurs in 5% of all abdominal trauma cases.[1] Majority of theses injuries can be managed conservatively. Minority of cases may require exploration with an aim of preventing life-threatening hemorrhage and retain enough functioning renal tissue. Increased use of CECT scanning has improved. Staging and better patient selection for operative management.

Etiology

Most closed injuries or blunt injuries occur as a result of high speed automobile accidents, fall from motorcycle/bicycle, pedestrian struck by a car or a blow/assault to the loin compressing the kidney between the 12th rib and lumbar vertebra. Hydronephrotic kidney is more prone to get injured even following trivial trauma.[2] Penetrating injuries are generally caused due to gunshot wounds and stab wounds. In most trauma centers the rate of blunt renal trauma to penetrating injury is in the ratio of 8 to 9 blunt to one penetrating injury. Renal pedicle injury accounts for approximately 3-5% of all renal trauma.

Pathology

Following trauma the renal parenchyma is split leading to hematuria. Minor trauma generally results in contusion with microhematuria and blood loss is minimal and there is no shock. In severe cases, blood loss may be considerable giving rise to hemodynamic instability and shock. Large volume blood loss can be unpredictable as the Gerota's fascia envelops the kidney and exerts tamponade effects to stop bleeding. Massive deceleration also causes severe injury to renal parenchyma or to the pedicles leading to immediate and immense quantity of blood loss thereby making the kidney anoxic. These cases need urgent exploration with no loss of time even for IVU/CT evaluation. Tear in the collecting system leads to extravasation of urine and urinoma formation.

Classification

The American Association for the Surgery of Trauma has created a scale[3] which correlates with patient outcomes and allows for appropriate management to be undertaken (Table 24.1).

Diagnosis

History is highly contributory in cases with trauma. The mechanism of trauma should always be elicited. Obvious history of trauma, blow, fall or compression resulting from road accidents

Table 24.1: Injury severity scale for the kidney

Grades		*Injury descriptions*
I	Contusion	Microscopic or gross hematuria, urologic studies normal
	Hematoma	Subcapsular, nonexpanding without parenchymal laceration
II	Hematoma	Nonexpanding perirenal hematoma confined to renal retroperitoneum
	Laceration	<1. 0 cm parenchymal depth of renal cortex without urinary extravasation
III	Laceration	> 1 cm parenchymal depth of renal cortex without collecting system rupture or urinary extravasation
IV	Laceration	Parenchymal laceration extending through the renal cortex, medulla and collecting system
	Vascular	Main renal artery or vein injury with contained hemorrhage
V	Laceration	Completely shattered kidney
	Vascular	Avulsion of renal hilum which devascularizes kidney

Advance one grade for bilateral injuries up to grade III.

is forthcoming. In cases with blunt trauma to abdomen or to the flank, exclusion of urinary tract injury is essential. Absence of hematuria does not exclude renal injury. 20% of patients with significant injury to the upper urinary tract do not have hematuria. Presence of microhematuria only does not exclude a severe renal injury.[4,5] Onset of loin pain, fullness over renal area, increasing abdominal girth, ileus, ecchymosis over flanks due to associated intra-abdominal injury or hematuria and unexplained hemodynamic instability or fracture of 10, 11, 12 ribs following blunt abdominal trauma need to be investigated.

Investigations are done with two main purposes. Firstly, to stage the injury, and secondly, to see for the presence and functional status of kidney on the other side. Urinalysis and ultrasonography are useful preliminary screening procedures.

Contrast enhanced CT scanning with delayed images has replaced the excretory urogram as the imaging modality of choice (Fig. 24.1). Imaging should be done in all patients with penetrating injuries, blunt trauma with gross hematuria, blunt trauma with microscopic hematuria if shock present. In pediatric patients one should keep a low threshold for imaging. CECT will reveal size and location function of kidney of hematoma, degree of lacerations, devitalized tissue, extravasation, function of kidneys and associated injuries (Fig. 24.2). In contrast enhanced CT, renal infarcts are classically described as cortical rim sign. It represents a thin peripheral region of cortical enhancement that is thought to be due to intact subcapsular cortex, perfused by perirenal capsular circulation. The cortical rim sign is reported to be present in 50% of focal or global infarct. It is seen as a 2-4 mm high density subcapsular rim with smooth margins.[6,7]

If CECT scan is not available: Intravenous urography (IVU) with high dose infusion nephrotomography demarcates renal outlines with or without extravasation or renal laceration. Parenchymal defects are easily visualized as negative shadows in otherwise well opacified renal parenchyma during the nephrographic phase. Urinary extravasation is seen during the excretory phase (Fig. 24.1). Angiography is seldom indicated in Figure 24.3. It is more commonly used therapeutically to stent thrombosed renal artery or to angioinfarct a bleeding artery.

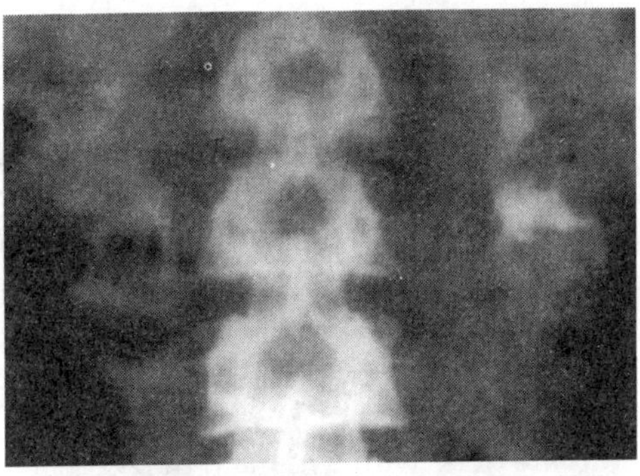

Fig. 24.1: IVU showing extravasation of contrast

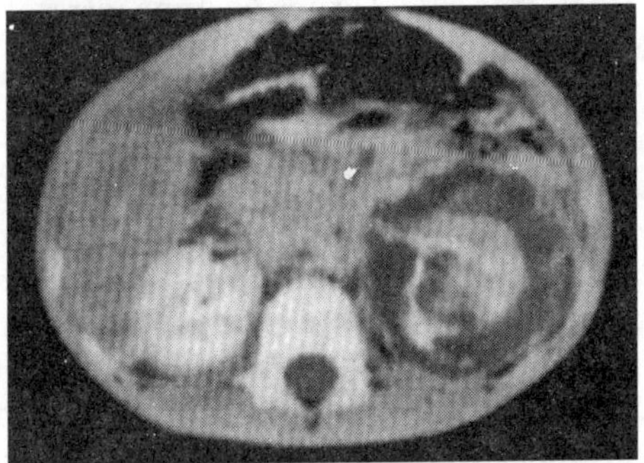

Fig. 24.2: CT scan showing type III renal injury (left) kidney and perirenal hematoma

Management

Renal contusions and lacerations (types I and II) make up 85% of blunt injuries and are to be treated conservatively with bed rest, broad spectrum antibiotics, and later restricted activity for 2-3 weeks with no significant sequelae. Regular measurements of pulse rate, blood pressure, abdominal girth and urine examination to see if the bleeding is reduced. The remaining 15% which contribute to major (types III and IV) renal injuries need surgical intervention. Vascular injuries make 2-5% of renal injuries and need immediate resuscitation and exploration in view of the deteriorating condition and hypovolemic shock. Penetrating injuries need exploration and debridement and control of bleeding vessels. Algorithm for management protocol of renal injury is depicted in Flow chart 24.1.

It is the type III injuries which roughly constitute 10-12% that have been a subject of controversy whether to manage them conservatively. To apply wait and watch policy with close surveillance and subsequently subject them to delayed operative intervention as and when indicated or whether to go in for early surgery. It must be remembered that only 2% of bluntly injured

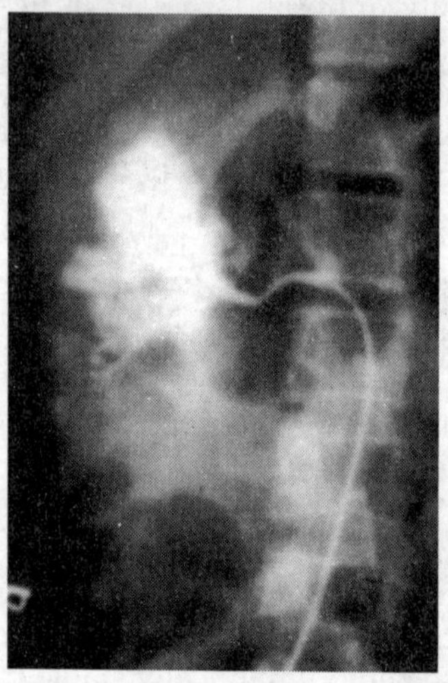

Fig. 24.3: Renal angiography demonstrating contrast extravasation and nonperfusion of lower pole (R) kidney

Flow chart 24.1: Management protocol for renal injury

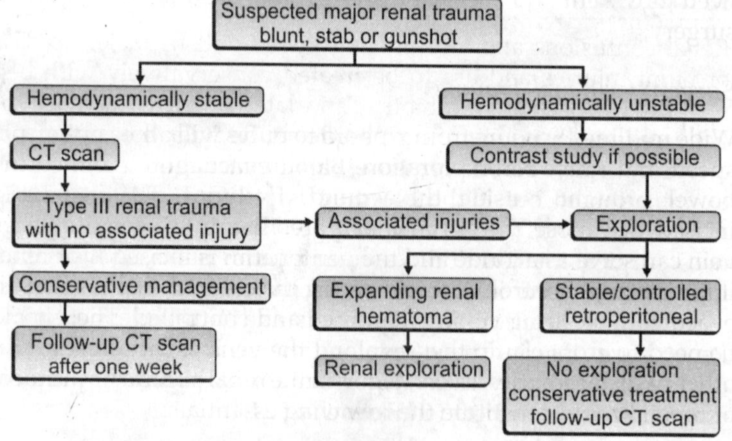

kidneys require exploration while 55% of penetrating injuries require exploration.

Thall et al in their study have suggested that type III penetrating trauma may be successfully managed conservatively with similar outcome to those patients with type III blunt injuries. Initial surgical intervention may only be necessary in those with associated intra-abdominal injuries or hemodynamic instability. In his series 67% of type III were successfully managed conservatively. The remaining 33% required surgery.[1] Kristjanson indicated that patients with significant extrarenal leakage on urography, CT or angiography did best with immediate surgical management. Seven out of 18 of his patients failed conservative treatment and required delayed surgery.[8]

Patients presenting with trauma who have had gross hematuria, microhematuria and shock, rapidly dropping hematocrit and or peritoneal signs and those with penetrating injuries would be benefited using McAninch criteria. CT is preferred as an initial investigation to establish the treatment plan and thereafter a intraoperative IVU or arteriogram may be done to evaluate the extent of renal or pedicle injury. Those with penetrating or blunt type III trauma in whom associated injuries do not require immediate exploration, observation is the preferred management option in otherwise hemodynamically stable patients.

Urinary extravasation may be managed percutaneously if necessary as delayed intervention with excellent results.[9,10] It has been observed that 85% of renal trauma will only need conservative treatment and no surgery. 5-10% of cases will need judgment and surgical exploration and other 5% will need surgery.[11]

Surgery for Renal Trauma

Wide midline exposure from xiphoid to pubis will allow optimum speed and space for exploration. Blood evacuation is done and bowel brought outside the wound. Posterior peritoneum is incised to expose the aorta. If required the inferior mesenteric vein can serve as a guide and the peritoneum is incised medial to it for vascular control. After reflecting the colon the hematoma is evacuated, bleeding vessels identified and controlled. There may be need to cross clamp the aorta and the vena cava to assess the other vascular injuries associated with the renal pedicle. Principles of repair would constitute the following essentials:

i. Debridement of all devitalized renal parenchyma.
ii. Meticulous hemostasis.
iii. Water tight closure of the collecting system.
iv. Approximation of margins and obliteration of the dead space.

It is essential to secure the pedicle before exposing the kidney. Capsule is reflected to uncover the parenchymal defects. Collecting system is repaired using 4/0 or 5/0 absorbable sutures. Ureteropelvic junction disruption is repaired by spatulating the ureter over double J stents and suturing with 4/0 or 5/0 absorbable sutures. Simple lacerations of renal vein is repaired using 5/0 or 6/0 prolene sutures. Loss or narrowing of a segment of the vein is repaired using autologous vein graft. In case with renal arterial injury, thrombosis secondary to the intimal injury, the intima is repaired or excised. Autologous vein graft is ideal replacement for the injured segment. Reanastomosis of the renal artery may be undertaken where feasible. Autotransplantation has been undertaken with good results when vascular repair is not possible.

Maximum conservation of renal parenchyma is aimed. Wrapping of shattered kidney in a net of collagen or other synthetic suture material is useful. Limited or partial nephrectomy is done where essential during the debridement of devitalized parenchyma. If kidney is irrecoverable, nephrectomy is necessary (Fig. 24.4). If internal bleeding is present but the patient is in a

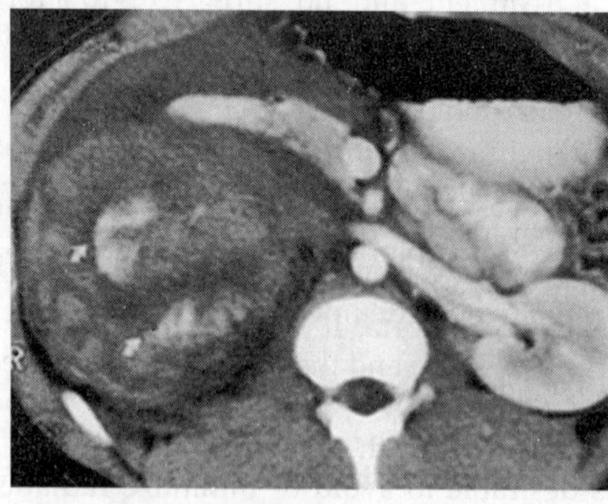

Fig. 24.4: Grade 5 renal parenchymal injury. CT scan demonstrates a shattered and partially devascularized right kidney (arrows), surrounded by a large hematoma

stable state, renal angiography is done to identify the bleeding vessel and plug it with gelfoam or small Gianturco coil. In severe hemorrhage, angiography is done and renal artery is blocked using angioplasty balloon. This will reduce the blood loss and enable to gain time for resuscitation and repair the damage. If tremendous bleed is present, it may be necessary to cross-clamp the aorta and the IVC. When facility for angiography is not available, patient is promptly shifted to the theater and explored.

Complications

a. Secondary hemorrhage occurs in a small percentage of the cases but poses potentially life-threatening problem. Careful watch has to be made for 10-14 days.
b. Late hypertension known to occur following:
   i. Renal artery damage resulting in stenosis. Excision of segment and reanastomosis of renal artery done using graft bypass.
   ii. Kidney is encased in fibrous tissue resulting from resolving perirenal hematoma. Excision and release of fibrous encasement is done.
c. Pseudocyst and urinoma are uncommon but pose dangerous complication. Extravasated urine is walled off by fibrous cyst which often communicates with the pelvis. The resulting cavity is lined by urothelium. Later stage calcification and heterotropic bone formation occurs and appears as "egg shell"(urinoma). Urinoma may get infected or cause absorption from granulation tissue leading to hyperchloremic acidosis. Drainage of cavity is seldom sufficient. It is advisable to dissect the cavity and also repair the renal and pelvic defects simultaneously.
d. AV fistula occurs following penetrating injury to parenchyma or following renal biopsy. Audible bruit is heard over kidney area. Angiography is useful to establish diagnosis. Great fistula can even destroy the entire kidney. Renal artery is occluded first when attempt at closure or repair is made.

Trauma in Pregnancy

Care of the mother's health takes priority over the fetus. It is nevertheless desirable to avoid or minimize radiation to fetus. Ultrasonography is ideal for monitoring both the fetus as well as for staging of the renal injury. Open surgery is indicated in penetrating trauma when peritoneal cavity is perforated or laceration of the renal artery is present or when the uterus is perforated. If period of gestation is more than 36 weeks, immediate cesarean is done. In case when pregnancy is 26-35 weeks, presence of fetal distress is an indication of cesarean section.[12]

URETERIC INJURIES

Introduction

Ureteric injuries though rare must be suspected in any patient with abdominal trauma. A high degree of suspicion of ureteric involvement in injuries occurring in close proximity to the ureter must be evaluated appropriately to exclude damage to the ureter so as to avoid disastrous complications at a later stage. The ureter may be injured during procedures involving obstetric and gynecological operations, general surgery, urology or vascular surgery. It is reported that two-thirds of such injuries occur during gynecological surgery.[13] 85% of all intraoperative ureteric injuries are usually to the distal end of the ureter.[14-16]

Causes

The common factors causing ureteral injuries are:
- Stab injuries
- Gunshot wounds, missile injuries
- Iatrogenic injuries following open and endoscopic surgery
- Post radiation.

Classification

Organ injury scale of the ureter[17] (Table 24.2).

Table 24.2: Organ injury scale of the ureter

Grades		*Injury descriptions*
I	Hematoma	Contusion/hematoma without devascularization
III	Laceration	>50% transection
IV	Laceration	Complete transection with 2 cm devascularization
V	Laceration	Avulsion with 2 cm of devascularization

Advance one grade if multiple injuries exist.

Mechanism of Injury

Other than intraoperative iatrogenic injuries, the ureter is rarely involved by itself. In association other intra-abdominal visceral injuries are usually present. Colon is the most common associated visceral injury (56%) and small bowel involvement occurs in 8% of cases.[18] Aorta and the common iliac artery are also known to be involved in penetrating injuries. Amongst children, acute hyperextension of the spine with blunt abdominal trauma commonly results in avulsion at the pelvic ureteric junction. High velocity missiles (2200 ft/sec) are known to cause significant coagulation necrosis in comparison to shotgun wounds. Iatrogenic injury is the commonly seen during pelvic surgery when the ureter is caught in the ligature for hemostatic sutures or is divided accidentally, mistakenly for the appendix or the fallopian tubes during laparoscopic surgery. Endoscopic urological procedures like ureteroscopy and endopyelotomy are known to produce ureteric injury. The ureter may be injured at its upper, middle or lower third.

Presentation

Shock may be the presenting feature when multiorgan injury is present in association with ureteral injury. Macroscopic hematuria was present in 82% of cases due to external trauma and in 18% a high index of suspicion was required to evaluate the ureteric injury in association with other intra-abdominal injuries.[18] Intraoperative injury to the ureter if missed at the time of surgery usually presents within 4-6 days with severe flank pain and high fever. The kidney is tender and may be palpable. Hematuria may or may not be present. Urine may show presence of infection. Urinary leak from vagina may occur. In case with bilateral ureteric injury, the patient may be totally anuric in the immediate postoperative period.

Evaluation

Ultrasonography is useful as a preliminary screening procedure to detect hydronephrosis and dilatation of the proximal ureter. Retroperitoneal collection of urinoma can be detected early. Intravenous urography will delineate the site of ureteric injury which is seen as a cut off or may show presence of extravasation

(Fig. 24.5). Back pressure changes and demonstration of forniceal leak seen along with the cut off sign are classical features of ureteric injury. Presence of urinary leak per vagina is confirmed by estimation of urea and creatinine values in the fluid and comparing with those of the plasma.

Management

Early recognition and correction of ureteric injury is associated with favorable results. Delayed open management was associated with success rate of 67% as compared to those treated immediately at the time of surgery with 100% success.[19,20] Management of associated injuries must take precedence in order of their severity like primary repair of large bowel injury or colostomy where indicated or vascular repair in the event of a vascular injury. The principles of management of ureteric injuries require correction of obstructive lesion or ureteric fistula management or ureteric anastomosis itself. The modalities of management include open surgical repair or endoscopic management of ureteric obstruction, stricture and fistula.

Percutaneous Nephrostomy (PCN)

In obstructive lesions, when the patient is not in a state to undergo major procedure, it is best to undertake percutaneous

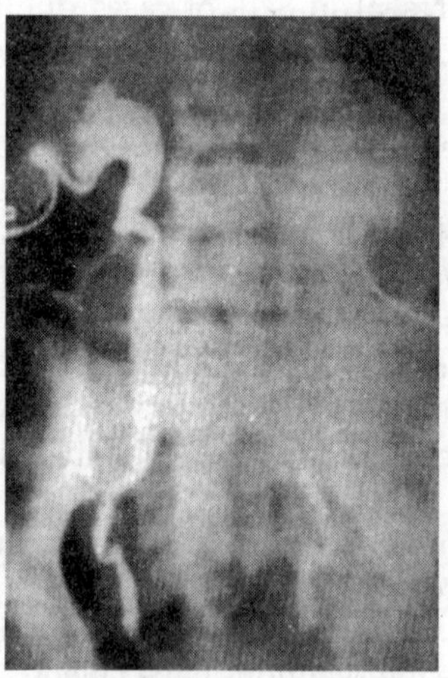

Fig. 24.5: Bilateral ureteral ligation during hysterectomy

nephrostomy till the condition of the patient stabilizes. Cases with penetrating ureteric injury do well by diverting the urine with PCN. It allows time for patients to stabilize, wound to heal and plan repair at later stage.

Intubation

A guidewire is passed either by antegrade or retrograde across the injury site and thereafter double J stent is passed over the guidewire and kept for 4-6 weeks till healing occurs with no stricture formation.

Endoscopic Dilatation

Endoscopic dilatation of strictures using ureteric dilators or balloon dilatation can be tried for short length of stricture. Alternatively, rigid endoscope can be used for ureteric dilatation and cold or hot knife incision is employed for cutting the stricture segment endoscopically. Stenting of the ureter is done following endoscopic procedure to prevent urinary leak and narrowing of the lumen.

Surgical Procedures

Open surgery for repair of defects includes:

a. Reimplantation of ureter (ureteroneocystostomy) for lower ureter or intramural defects. Politano-Leadbetter technique is preferred in reimplanting the ureter.
b. Boari-Okerblad bladder flap is reliable and is used for gaps more than 10 cm.
c. Bladder, ureter and kidney can be mobilized to gain about 7 cm of length. Bladder is hitched to the psoas muscle to prevent mobility of extramural ureter.
d. Ureteroureterostomy-spatulated, watertight tension free anastomosis is done. However, risk of damage to the good ureter is present. The procedure is suitable for upper and middle ureteric injuries.
e. Ileal substitute is used in case when there is total destruction of the ureteric length.
f. Autotransplantation is also carried out in situation where total loss of ureter is present.
g. Nephrostomy is done as a last resort as a life saving measure when multiple interventions have failed.

BLADDER INJURIES

Introduction

Classically described as intraperitoneal and extraperitoneal injury depending on the site of injury. Bladder trauma commonly occurs following application of blunt external force to a fully distended bladder, gunshot wounds, penetrating injuries, fracture pelvis, iatrogenic intraoperative accidents during pelvic surgery and hernia repairs and during transuretheral resection procedures. Extraperitoneal injuries occur in 75% of the cases and are generally in association with fractures of the pelvis. 8-10% of pelvis fractures cause bladder injury due to laceration by the bony fragments. Intraperitoneal injury to the bladder occurs in about 25% of cases and follows application of blunt force to a fully distended bladder or in motorcycle accidents, fall from height and in penetrating missile injuries or may be associated with fracture pelvis also.[21]

Classification

Organ injury scale of the American Association for Surgery for Trauma[16] (Table 24.3).

Clinical Features

Bruising over lower abdomen with nonlocalized tenderness is commonly seen. Extravasation of urine and inability to void urine or hematuria may be present (95% of blunt bladder ruptures have gross hematuria while 50% of penetrating bladder injuries have gross hematuria. The remaining have microscopic hematuria).

Table 24.3: Bladder injuries

Grades	*Injury type*	*Descriptions of injuries*
I	Hematoma	Contusion, intramural hematoma
	Laceration	Partial thickness
II	Laceration	Extraperitoneal bladder wall laceration < 2 cm
III	Laceration	Extraperitoneal (>2 cm) or intraperitoneal (< 2 cm)
IV	Laceration	Intraperitoneal bladder wall laceration >2 cm
V	Laceration	Intra- or extraperitoneal bladder wall laceration extending into the bladder neck or ureteral orifice (trigone)

Advance one grade if multiple lesions exist.

Later on abdominal distention with absent bowel sounds and decreased urine output will be seen.

Rectal examination will reveal high riding prostate which may be difficult to feel if significant pelvic hematoma is present. Also the anal tone will give a clue about spinal function. One should always look for associated injuries.

Diagnosis

Plane X-ray pelvis confirms presence of fracture pelvis and the position of the fracture fragments. Cystogram is diagnostic (Fig. 24. 6). 300 ml of sterile contrast material is used to distend the bladder. Intraperitoneal rupture is diagnosed by contrast extravasation with accentuation of bowel loops (Fig. 24.7). Most of the contrast lies above the superior margin of the acetabulum. Extraperitoneal rupture has the classical 'Flame'like appearance (Fig. 24.8). Bladder contusion and laceration can be diagnosed by alterations in the outline. 'Tear Drop' appearance may be seen in case of large pelvic hematoma. CT cystography with retrograde instillation of contrast is not only accurate but can assess other associated injuries.

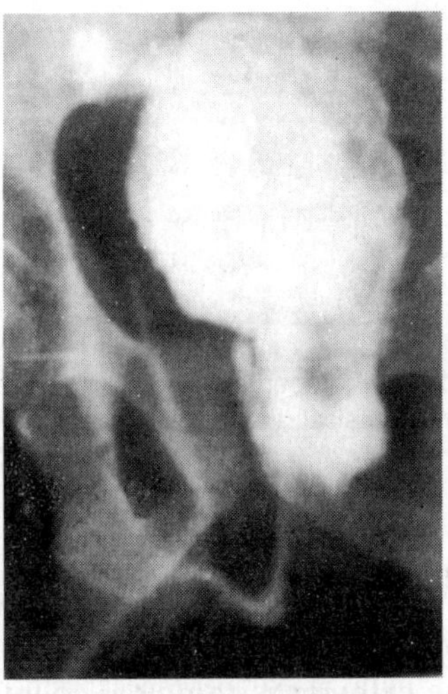

Fig. 24.6: Cystogram showing extravasation in extraperitoneal rupture bladder

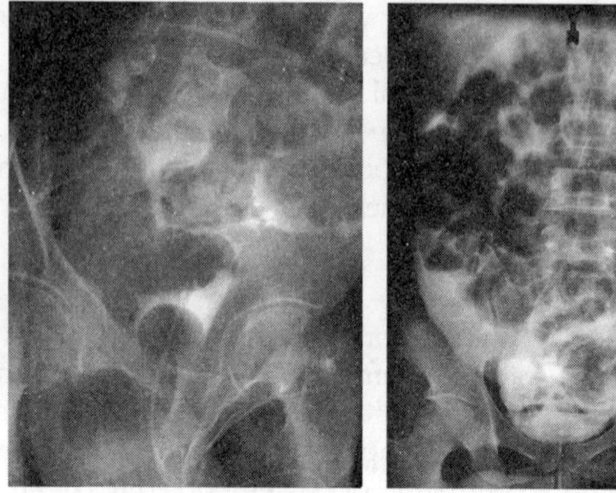

Fig. 24.7: Intraperitoneal rupture of bladder showing accentuation of bowel loops

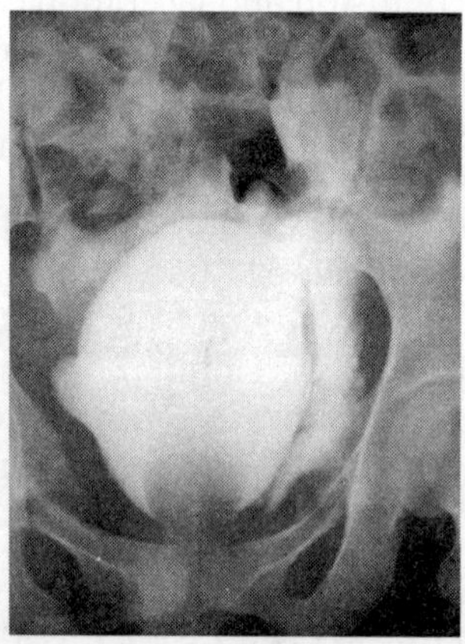

Fig. 24.8: Extraperitoneal rupture of bladder showing classical 'flame shaped extravasation'

Management

Extraperitoneal Rupture

Ideally managed by keeping a per urethral or suprapubic catheter for 10-14 days. The catheter is removed following cystogram to confirm healing. 11-13% cases may require prolonged catheterization for 2-13 weeks for complete healing.

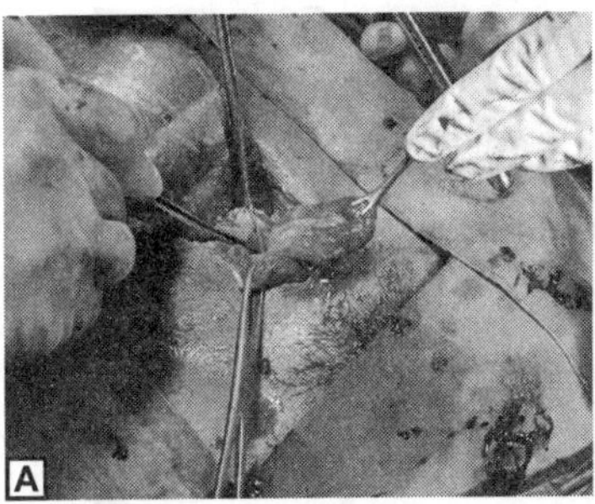
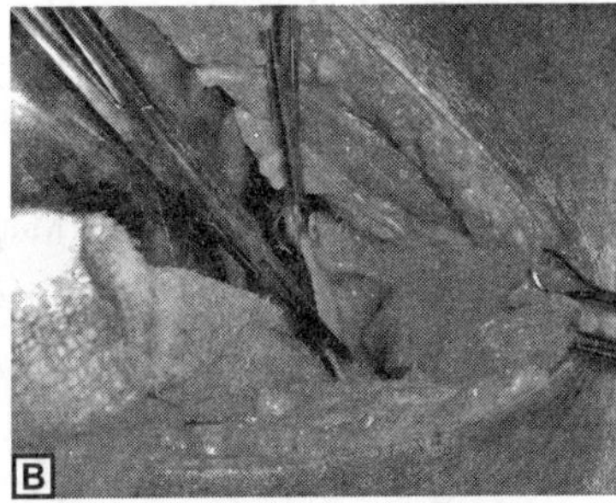

Figs. 24.9A and B: Repair of intraperitoneal rupture of bladder
(For color version, see Plate 6)

Repair of rupture can be contemplated if exploration is being done for other injuries. The rent is closed from inside the bladder.

Intraperitoneal Rupture

Open repair of the bladder is preferable (Figs 24.9A and B). It allows for inspection of the abdominal viscera for associated injuries which can also be taken care of. The bladder neck must also be sutured to prevent incontinence. The ureteric orifices must be examined for clear efflux. Suprapubic bladder catheter is kept and perivesical space is drained. 10 to 14 days later a cystogram is done to look for any leak following which the catheter is removed. (see also Chapter 27 on Pelvic Trauma).

Laparoscopic repair of intraperitoneal bladder injury has also been described.

REFERENCES

1. Thall EH, Stone NN, Chang DL, et al. Conservative management of penetrating and blunt type III renal injuries. Br J Urol 1996;77:512-7.
2. Peters PC, Sagalowsky AI. Genitourinary trauma in Walsh PE, Retik AB, Stamey TA, Vaughan ED (Eds) Campbells Urology 6th edition Philadelphia, WB Saunders Company, 1992;2571-94.
3. Moore EE, Shackford SR, Pachter HL, et al. Organ injury scaling; Spleen, liver and kidney. J Trauma 1989;29:1664.
4. Scott R Jr, Carlton CE Jr, Ashmore AJ, et al. Initial management of nonpenetrating renal injuries: Clinical review of 111 cases. J Urol 1963;90:535.
5. Hellier WPL, Higgs B. Severe renal laceration from blunt trauma presenting with microhaematuria and a normal intravenous urogram. Case report. Br J Urol 1996;78:309-10.

6. Karmel IR, Berkowitz JF. Assessment of cortical rim sign in post-traumatic renal infarction. J Comp Ass Tomog 1996;20(5):803-6.
7. Carroll PR, McAninch JW. Staging of renal trauma. Urol Clin of North Amer 1989;16:193.
8. Kristjanson A, Pedersen J. Management of blunt renal trauma. Br J Urol 1993;72:692-6.
9. McAninch JW. Indications for radiological assessment in suspected renal trauma. Urol Clin North Amer 1989;16:187-92.
10. Robert M, Drianno N, Muir G, Delbos, Guiter J. Management of major blunt renal lacerations: Surgical or nonoperative approach? Eur Eurl 1996;30:335-9.
11. Carlton CE Jr. Injuries of the kidney and ureter. In Harrison JH, Glitters RF, Perlmitter AD, Stamey TA and Walsh PC (Eds) Cambell Urology, 4th edition. Philadelphia, WB Saunders Co 1978.
12. Sakala EP, Kort DD. Management of stab wounds to the pregnant uterus; A case report and a review of the literature. Obst Gynae Sem 1988;43:319.
13. Giberti C, Germinale F, Lillo M, et al. Obstetric and Gynaecological ureteric injuries treatment and results. Br J Urol 1996;77:21-6.
14. Lezim MA, Stoller ML. Surgical ureteral injuries. Urol 1991;38:497-506.
15. Zinman LM, Libertino JA, Roth RA. Management of operative ureteral injuries. Urol 1978;12:290-303.
16. Mann WL, Arato M, Patsner B, Stone ML. Ureteral injuries in an Obstetric and Gynaecology training programme: Etiology and management. Obst Gynecol 1988;72:82-5.
17. Moore EE, Cogbill TH, Jurkowich GJ, et al. Organ injury scalling III. Chest wall, abdominal vascular, ureter, bladder and urethra. J Trauma 1992;33:337-9.
18. George CVelmachos, Elias Degiannis, Mike Eai Wells, Irene Souter. Penetrating ureteral injuries: The impact of associated injuries on management. The American Surgeon 1996;6:461-8.
19. Blandy JP, Badenoch DF, Fowler CG, Jenkin BJ, Thomal NWM. Early repair of iatrogenic injury to the ureter or bladder after gynaecological surgery. J Urol 1991;146:761-5.
20. Mendez R, Mc Gintry DM. The management of delayed recognised ureteral injuries. J Urol 1978;119:192-3.
21. Corriere Jn Jr, Sandler EN. Management of the ruptured bladder; 7 years of experience with 111 cases. J Trauma 1986;26:830.

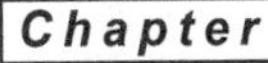

Genital Injuries

PM Deka, DK Sarma

INTRODUCTION

Incidence of genitourinary tract injury in all trauma admission vary from 2.2 to 10.3%.[1] Trauma to the external genitalia comprises about 27.8 to 68.1% amongst these urological injuries.[2-7] Penetrating injuries of the penis in civilians are uncommon, accounting for 6-26% of all genital injuries.[8,9] During war time the incidence of injury to external genitalia varies from 30.8 to 41.6% amongst the genitourinary injuries.[10,11] Most of the genital injuries during war are due to explosions and sometimes, by shooting gunshot wounds (GSW).

Though the voilence in civil life is gaining momentum in the past few decades, GSW to the external genitalia is relaively uncommon.[2-5,12] Genital injuries comprise of injury to the penis, scrotum and the testicles (Table 25.1). Penetrating injury due to sharp weapon or GSW may lead to urethral injury.

Table 25.1: Incidence of trauma to external genitalia

Author	*Penis*	*Scrotum*	*Urethra*
Civilian			
Brandes et al[1]	12.2	41.0	2.8
Waterhouse & Gross[3]	12.7	16.7	3.6
Vietnam War			
Busch et al[5]	25.0	35.4	6.3
Salvatierra et al[2]	16.2	25.4	3.6
Crotian War			
Tucak et al[15]	8.0	17.3	2.5

Investigations

Steven B Brandes et al suggested that in absence of major associated injuries, genital GSW required only two diagnostic studies: (i) retrograde urography (RGU) for suspected urethral injury and (ii) a routine abdominal radiography.[1] RGU positive for contrast extravasation indicates urethral injury and also locates the site of rupture and delineates the urethral anatomy. However, the amount of extravasation does not correlate with the severity of injury.[13] To prevent further extravasation, the patient is to be discourged from voiding prior to retrograde urethrography. Flexible cystoscopy is another examination for evaluation of urethral injury. In case of GSW of scrotum, scrotal ultrasonography can be used to evaluate the integrity of the tunica albuginea in equivocal cases of scrotal swelling.[9,14] The role of scrotal USG for this study has been debated. For diagnosing other assiociated injuries, arteriograms, intravenous pyelography, cystography and sigmoidoscopy may be necessary.

Management

Management of genital injuries should be as restricted as possible, and as conservative as feasible as injury to the sex organ can lead to permanent psychological trauma besides somatic and functional disorders.[16,17] One should be very much cautious in the approach for retaining maximum function with minimum loss of organs. The general management of wounds follow the general surgical principles. It comprises of vigorous saline wash of the part with removal of foreign bodies, careful debridement of the devitalized tissues, hematoma evacuation, proper hemostasis, repair of the associated injuries and then, the primary closure.[1]

Injury to the Penis

Injury to the penis may be either penetrating, resulting from GSW and stab wounds or blunt, following vehicular accident, assault or sexual intercourse. Rupture of the Buck's fascia leads to extravasation of blood or urine limited to the attachment of Colles' fascia. Penile injury involving the skin only is managed by wound debridement and primary closure of the wound. Minor tear in the Buck's fascia can be repaired with non-absorbable sutures under local or general anesthesia. Most of the gunshot injuries of the penis present with bleeding which can be managed by stitching of the Buck's fascia. If the deficiency of the Buck's fascia is large, it can be closed by using the fascia of rectus abdominis muscle. Penile injuries involving the corporal bodies and corpus spongiosum should be considered as wounds of vasculature. Debridement should be limited but thorough. Closure should be done with absorbabale sutures after good hemostasis.

Degloving Injuries of the Penis

Degloving injuries of the penis may be caused by machinery used for gardening or farming. This happens when the penis and the clothings are caught in the machine while working. The degloved portion of the skin is reflected up to the coronal sulcus and the wound is thoroughly cleaned and debrided. If there is considerable gap between the two edges of the skin of the penis for easy suturing, one should use split thickness skin graft. This usually gives satisfactory functional result.

Penile Amputation

Penile amputation is not a rare event nowadays in the fast growing voilent world. Of late, several reports of amputation of penis due to assault or self-infliction has come into notice. This can happen by accident also. It may be partial or complete. Reimplantation of the penis may be tried if the patient presents within 8 hours. A tourniquet should be applied to the proximal penile segment as early as possible to prevent life-threatening hemorrhage. The amputated part should be cleaned with sterile normal saline and it should be preserved in normal saline in a container surrounded by ice. The primary aim is to keep the dismembered part vital. The patient, along with the container should be transported to the nearest center equipped with microsurgical facilities. If microsurgical surgery cannot be performed for arterial repair, venous reanastomosis should be tried. If venous anastomosis is successful, usually the amputated segment survives. The corpus cavernosum can be approximated easily. The urethra should be repaired over an indwelling catheter.

Strangulating Injury of the Penis

This lesion can be caused by introduction of metal rings and use of strings, ropes, etc. around the circumference of the penis. These objects are used very often for erotic pleasure or as a part of abnormal sexual behavior. Lubricants can be tried for the offending objects. A ligature can be fastened off. If it fails, the ring, string or rope may have to be removed by metal cutting instruments. If the strangulation is of some duration, edema of the distal part of the penis occurs and it can lead to urethral fistula.

Problems of erection, penile curvature and stricture of urethra are the common residual effects of penile trauma. The main goal of treatment of penile injury is to prevent penile deformity or dysfunction.[1] After limited debridement and primary surgical repair potency rates are reported as 87 to 100%.[9] Results of management may not be satisfactory if corporal injuries are not repaired promptly. Gunshot injuries of the penis are usually extensive, requiring prolonged recovery. Hence, there might be significant physical as well as functional inadequacies.

Injuries to the Scrotum

Gunshot wounds of genitals involves scrotum in 91.1% of patients with an equal frequency in each hemiscrotum.[1] In civilains, the scrotal injury range from 16.7 to 41% amongst the genitourinary injuries (Figs 25.1 and 25.2).[3] If there is only involvement of the skin over the scrotum, wound debridement with primary closure of the wound is sufficient. A significant scrotal skin deficit can be dealt with scrotal wall debridement and loose primary repair. The elastic property of the scrotal skin will commonly allow primary closure of even a large defect. If the skin loss of the scrotum is significant, the testes can be covered by mobilizing skin flap from the perineum. If there is severe laceration with multiple injuries with contamination, the testes should be cleaned thoroughly and regularly. Granulation tissue will gradually cover up the testes facilitating skin grafting later on. If placement of the testes becomes necessary, they should be put to the adjacent thighs, preferably in the subcutaneous space. When there is physical evidence that the wound is deep to the dartos fascia or the depth of the penetrating wound is undetermined, or there is scrotal hematoma, exploration of scrotum is mandatory. This can be achieved by a transverse mid-scrotal incision which is helpful in finding out the extent of injuries in both the scrotal cavities. Unilateral longitudinal incision over one scrotal cavity can be considered if there is no involvement of the other scrotal cavity. In soft tissue damage, wound debridement will suffice. A hematocele is to be drained.

Testicular Trauma

In surgery of scrotal cavity, testes preservation is the goal in order to maintain androgen production and cosmesis.[1] Early exploration of scrotal cavity maintains a higher salvage rate, when compared to delayed exploration.[18] The principle of management of a lacerated testes with exposure of testicular tissue is thorough debridement using normal saline, meticulous removal of foreign particles and devitalized tissue. The tunica albuginea should be closed by absorbable sutures. Most of the studies reveal that testes reconstruction does not maintain fertility but some studies claim it following reconstruction (Fig. 25.3).[19]

Orchiectomy: A devastated and non-viable testes need orchiectomy. It is much more common in military high velocity missile injuries.[12] In civilian practice orchiectomy is rare. However, reimplantation of amputated testes and cord is tried. If the patient presents within 6-8 hours with the testes well preserved in cold saline microvascular surgery can be performed.

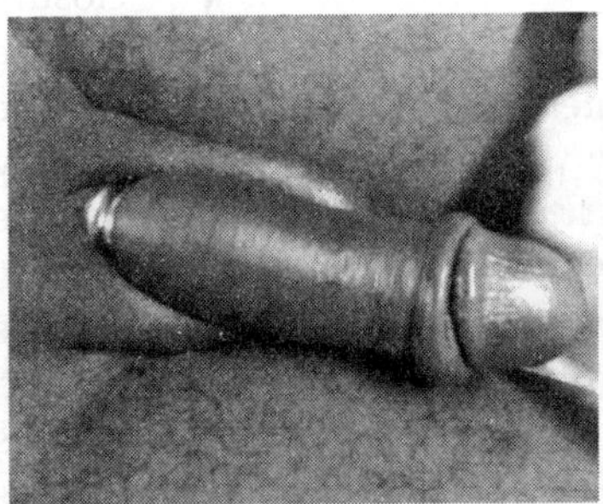

Fig. 25.1: Metal ring around root of penis (strangulation injury of penis) *(For color version, see Plate 6)*

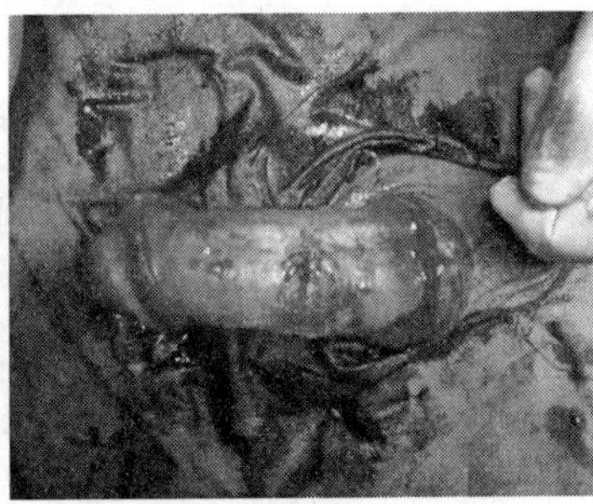

Fig. 25.2: Degloving injury of penis *(For color version, see Plate 7)*

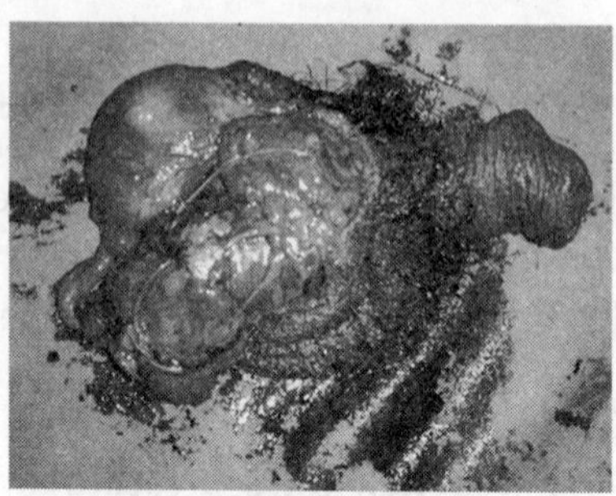

Fig. 25.3: Machine tool injury of penis
(For color version, see Plate 7)

Epididymis Injury

Injury to the epididymis is managed conservatively as far as possible with wound debridement and primary closure. A running closure with absorbable suture maintaining the cavity is to be used.

Vas deferens Injuries

Injury to vas deferens is relatively uncommon. Steven B Brandes et al observed bilateral transection of vas deferens by a single gunshot wound in one patient.[1] A vasovasostomy, if possible, is to be tried. In unhealthy wounds, a delayed vasovasostomy is preferred. Hemostasis is obtained by ligating the vasa with metal clips for future recognition of the ends of the vasa for vasovasostomy.

Urethral Injuries

Penile urethral trauma is encountered in civilian as well in the military practice. It may present as an associated injury following blunt trauma. In penetrating injuries, e.g. sharp cutting weapon wounds, gunshot wounds, etc. anterior urethra may be injured. The injury may be partial or complete. If the urethral trauma is confirmed within the Buck's fascia, the extravasation of urine and blood will be limited to the shaft of the penis within the confines of the Buck's fascia. If the Buck's fascia is ruptured, the extravasation of blood and urine is limited to the attachment of the Colles' fascia. In these cases, local drainage and urinary diversion by suprapubic cystostomy are necessary. Delayed repair of the urethra is carried out as and when necessary. Penetrating injuries of the penile urethra should be managed by suprapubic urinary diversion, debridement of the wound and primary spatulated repair of the urethra over a Foley's catheter. Controversy exists regarding results of primary repair verses delayed repair of penetrating injury of urethra.

Female Genital Injuries

Causes:

- Foreign body placed in the vagina particularly in young girls
- Assault
- Rape
- Sexual abuse
- Trauma

Genital injuries may be extremely painful and can bleed heavily. Common symptoms are bleeding, bruising, object embedded in a body opening, genital pain, swelling, difficulty in urination, foul smelling vaginal discharge, etc. Internal bleeding should not be overlooked.[20]

Management of female genital trauma is complex and should be undertaken by a team of well trained health care professionals. Many female genital injuries lead to significant psychological and emotional distress apart from physical injury. As some of these injuries are due to criminal acts proper documentation is extremely important.

Animal Bites of the Male External Genitalia

Animal bites comprise 1% of all genital injuries. 60-70% of them are boys aged about 15 years.[21] Therapy depends upon the type of injuries. Smaller superficial wounds may be treated by cleaning the wound and dressing or suturing of the wound. Extensive wounds should be treated conservatively initially. If the wound remains uninfected, reconstruction should be attempted. In case of partial amputation of the penis or in the rare events of unilateral or bilateral testicular loss, primary reconstruction should be attempted. The long-term follow-up of urethral injuries from animal bites shows the worst results.

The main problem in animal bite wounds is the risk of infection, which usually occurs in the first 48 hours. A broad spectrum antibiotic should be started after cleaning the wound. In addition the vaccination status of the individual should be ascertained. If such protection is lacking then vaccination against tetanus or rabis should be immediately started. In case of human bites, there is the additional risk of transmitting diseases like syphilis, tetanus, hepatitis, HIV, herpes and *Actinomycosis* or tuberculosis.

REFERENCES

1. Brandes SB, Buckman RF, Chelsky MJ, et al. External genitalia gunshot wounds. A ten years experience with fifty six cases. J Trauma 1995;39:266-72.
2. Salvatierra G, Ringdon WO, Norris DM, et al. Vietnam experience with 252 urologic war injuries. J Urol 1969;101:615.
3. Waterhouse K, Gross M. Trauma to the genitourinary tract: A 5 years experience with 251 cases. J Urol 1969;101:241.
4. Dehsner TG, Busch FM, Clarke BG. Urogenital wounds in Vietnam. J Urol 1969;101:224.
5. Busch FM, Chenault OW, Zinner NR, et al. Urologic aspects of Vietnam war injuries. J Urol 1967;97:763.
6. Archbold JAA, Barros D'sa AAB, Morrison E. Genitourinary tract injuries of civil hostilities. Br J Surg 1981;68:625.
7. Selkowitz SM. Penetrating high velocity genitourinary injuries. Urol 1977;9:371.
8. McAninch JW, Kahn RI, Jeffry RB, et al. Major traumatic and septic genital injuries. J Trauma 1984;24:291.
9. Berfini JE, Corriere JN. The aetiology and management of genital injuries. J Trauma 1988;28:1278.
10. Vuckovic J, Tucak A, Gotovac J, et al. Crotian experience: the treatment of 629 urogenital war injuries. J Trauma 1995;39:733.
11. Hardeway RM. Vietnam wound analysis. J Trauma 1978;18:635.
12. Selkowitz SM. Penetrating high velocity genitourinary injuries: part 2, urethral. Lower tract and genital wounds. Urol 1977;9:493.
13. Milas BJ, Poffenberger RJ, Farah RN, et al. Management of penile gunshot wounds. Urol 1990;150:1147.
14. Gomez RG, Castenheira AC, McAninch JW. Gunshot wounds to the male external genitalia. J Urol 1993;150:1147.
15. Tucak A, Lukacevic T, Kuvezdic H, et al. Urogenital wounds during the war in crotia in 1991/1992. J Urol 1995;153:121.
16. Berini JE Jr, Corriera Jn Jr. The aetiology and management of genital injuries. J Trauma 1988;28:1278.
17. Cendron M, Whitmere KE, Carpinielo V, et al. Traumatic rupture of the corpus cavernosum. Evaluation and management. J Urol 1990;144:987.
18. Cass As. Testicular trauma. J Trauma Urol 1983;129:299.
19. Cass As, Ferrarao L, Wolpert J, et al. Bilateral testicular injury from testicular trauma. J Urol 1988;140:1435.

20. Gerber GS, Brendler CB. Evaluation of the urologic patient: History, physical examination, and the urinalysis. In: Wein AJ, Ed. Campbell-Walsh Urology. Philadelphia, Pa: Saunders Elsevier; 2007, Chapter 3.
21. Van Der Horst, et al. Male genital injury: diagnosis and treatment. BJU International 2004;93:927-30.

Vascular Injuries

Kumud Rai

INTRODUCTION

Vascular injuries are present in less than 10% of polytrauma patients.[1] However, major vascular injuries demand urgent treatment as death may result from rapid exsanguination if bleeding is not promptly controlled. In addition, arterial injuries of extremity require prompt revascularization, otherwise a major amputation is often inevitable. This was confirmed by the fact that amputation rate after major arterial injury fell from 50% in World War II[2] to 13% in Korean war[3] and about 10% in Vietnam War[4] after adoption of the policy of repairing arterial injuries. Several civilian series have reported low mortality and an amputation rate of 1-3% with a policy of aggressive resuscitation, speedy evacuation and prompt definitive reconstructive surgery.[5-7] Patients with associated vascular injuries tend to have higher injury severity scores (14 vs 10), longer hospital stay (15 days vs 10 days), doubling of hospital expenses (22,500 vs 12,300 USD), and an increased overall mortality (13% vs 6%).[8]

HISTORICAL BACKGROUND

The first repair of an injured artery was performed by Hallowel in 1761 when he repaired a small defect in the brachial artery by a small steel pin which everted the lips of arterial wound; a ligature around its ends held the pin in place. The first permanent union of blood vessels was performed by Niolai Von Eck in 1871 when he performed the porta caval shunt. Jassinowsky (1891) described repair of arterial wounds using a suture that he tried to keep entering the lumen of the vessel. Murphy (1897) performed successful end-to-end anastomosis using invagination of the proximal into distal artery. Alexis Carrel established the basic techniques of modern vascular anastomosis in a series of experiments between 1900 to 1907; he was awarded with the Noble prize for this seminal contribution in 1912. Moniz (1927), dos Santos (1929) and Seldinger (1953) developed and refined the technique of modern arteriography. Even though techniques of arterial surgery were perfected by 1908, even in World war II only 3% of arterial injuries were repaired and the rest were ligated. The availability of antibiotics, monofilament suture material, understanding of pathophysiology and management of hemorrhagic shock, and speedy evacuation of battle casualties, etc. all contributed towards the trend to repair arterial injuries. Synthetic grafts was used first by Voorhees in 1952, and widely employed by Hughes (1954) and Spencer (1955) who also initiated the trend to primary repair of arterial injuries during the Korean war. Fogarty introduced his versatile balloon catheter in 1963; this was used not only for thromboembolectomy but also for control of arterial bleeding.[9] Last two decades have seen the use of catheter based (endovascular) techniques to control bleeding by embolization,[10] for hemostasis by percutaneously placed intra-arterial balloons,[11] and for placement of covered stents (stent-grafts) in inaccessible arteries.[12]

ETIOLOGY

Injuries may be direct due to **blunt trauma** (automobile accident) or **penetrating trauma** (missile, bullets, shrapnel, etc.). Indirect injuries are due to a bony fragment impinging on a vessel, classically seen in fracture shaft femur or humerus fractures. **Iatrogenic injuries** constitute the third group; these are being increasingly encountered after invasive procedures like arteriography or percutaneous trans-luminal angioplasty. Arterial thrombosis following accidental intra-arterial drug injection is a rare iatrogenic injury.

ANATOMICAL CLASSIFICATION

Arterial injuries may be classified into the following anatomic types (Fig. 26.1):

i. Contusion (this may lead to local thrombosis)
ii. Puncture (leading to hemorrhage)
iii. Laceration
iv. Intimal damage (causing intimal dissection or vessel thrombosis)

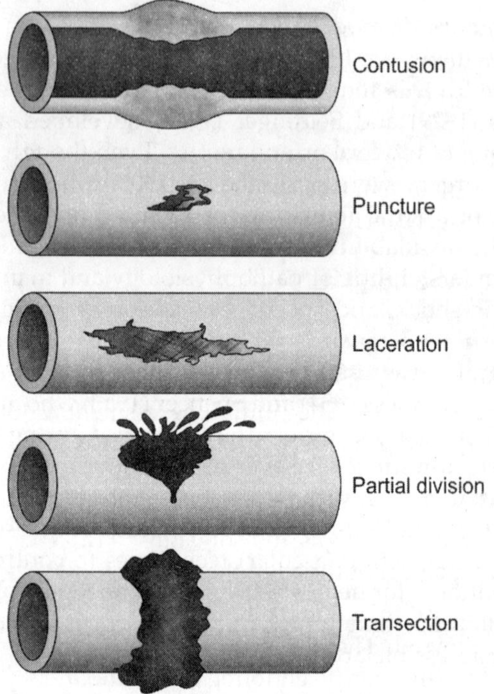

Fig. 26.1: Types of arterial injuries

v. Partial division
vi. Compete transaction
vii. False aneurysm (due to continuing bleeding which gets localized)
viii. Arteriovenous fistula (when there has been simultaneous injury to both artery and a neighboring vein).

SEQUELAE OF VASCULAR INJURIES

The classical feature of arterial injuries is hemorrhage which may be open with profuse external bleeding, or closed which manifest as a rapidly expanding hematoma or unexplained hypotension. Sequelae of vascular injuries include:

i. Acute hemorrhage
 Overt (external)
 Contained (e.g. in a muscle compartment)
 Concealed (e.g. in pleural cavity)

ii. Shock (hypovolemic)
iii. Hematoma
iv. Delayed bleeding/rebleeding
v. Thrombosis—acute or delayed
vi. Organ ischemia—acute or delayed
vii. False aneurysm (see above)
viii. Arteriovenous fistula (see above).

CLINICAL ASSESSMENT

History: This should be directed to the mechanism of injury, blood loss prior to admission, and presence of any co-morbidities.

Clinical examination: The initial assessment should follow ATLS (advanced trauma life support) guidelines. Life-threatening conditions should be addressed immediately. The injuries should be documented and prioritized. The signs of arterial injury have been classified as hard signs and soft signs[13] (Table 26.1). Detailed clinical assessment is outlined in the regional sections.

Resuscitation and initial management: The ABC of trauma care should be followed. The airway should be secured promptly, if necessary, by emergency endotracheal intubation. It is useful to remember that resuscitation of an unstable patient in need of urgent surgery is probably best conducted in the operating room. In severe hemorrhagic shock, where bleeding has temporarily stopped due to hypotension, vasoconstriction, and thrombus formation, aggressive fluid resuscitation may lead to dislodgement of hemostatic plug, with increased bleeding and mortality.[14] Hypotensive resuscitation (permissive hypotension) which aims to keep a systolic blood pressure between 70-90 mm Hg (to maintain cerebral and renal perfusion) should be practiced.

Table 26.1: Signs of vascular injury

	Hard signs	*Soft signs*
1.	Pulsatile bleeding	History of significant bleeding
2.	Shock with ongoing bleeding	Injury of anatomically related structure (e.g. nerve)
3.	Expanding or pulsating hematoma	Small hematoma
4.	Bruit over the artery	Wound near a major vessel
5.	Absent distal pulses	Diminished distal pulse
6.	Signs/symptoms of acute ischemia	Multiple fractures/extensive soft tissue injury

Active bleeding should be controlled with direct pressure/ pressure bandage. Tourniquets over extremities should be avoided as far as possible. Blind clamping of vessel is to be depreciated except in "in extremis" where bleeding persists despite all other measures, and it is felt that patient may exsanguinate to death before he reaches hospital.

Fractures should be stabilized by splints; this relieves pain and reduces ongoing blood loss. Evacuation to a center geared to treating vascular injuries should be arranged by fastest available means.

Special Investigations

If the diagnosis of arterial injury is evident (e.g. external hemorrhage, or limb ischemia), no further investigation is required and patient is taken for operative treatment straightway. The importance and accuracy of a thorough clinical examination in diagnosing vascular injury has been documented in many studies.[15] Blood should be sent for urgent grouping and a few units of crossmatched blood should be considered. The following investigations may be helpful.

Plain radiography: They are taken for associated fractures/ dislocations. Chest X-rays are useful in patients with chest injuries.

Doppler pressure studies: This useful noninvasive test can be used to record the pressure in a distal (extremity) artery. If the pressure is significantly lower than that in contralateral limb vessel, this is diagnostic of arterial injury. A pressure difference of more than 20 mm Hg is significant. The ankle/arm index, if lower than 0.9, is also diagnostic in absence of previous peripheral vascular disease.[16]

Color Doppler (Duplex scan): This is useful in diagnosing false aneurysm, arteriovenous fistula and arterial thrombosis, but may not be of much use in an emergency situation. Meissner et al reported their experience in 93 patients.[17] Four of the 60 scans were positive in patients where proximity to a major vessel was the sole indication for imaging. There were 4 false negative results; however, no major injury was missed. Ultrasound is also useful in assessment of neck and abdominal injuries.

Angiography: The role of angiography in initial assessment of arterial injuries is controversial. If unequivocal signs of arterial injury are present it should not be done as valuable time may be lost in trying to localize the site of injury and irreversible distal ischemia may result. Similarly, arteriography is contraindicated in a hemodynamically unstable patient. An on-table angiogram in the operation theater is acceptable for most limb injuries. In doubtful situations (soft signs) it has been recommended by some authors, even though, the pickup rate of arterial injury is low.[18,19] A recent good study has recommended against the use of arteriography for excluding vascular injury in the absence of hard clinical signs, especially in extremity trauma.[20] Arteriography is however very useful in patients with suspected injury of thoracic aorta. The indications for arteriography in vascular injuries are mentioned in Table 26.2. Angiographic signs of arterial injury are listed in Table 26.3, and shown in Figures 26.2 to 26.6.

Computed tomography angiography (CTA): This test is useful in blunt cervical, thoracic and abdominal trauma. It is also being increasingly used in suspected extremity vascular injury. The recent CT machines (64 slice and above) offer excellent resolution and image quality, and the test can be performed rapidly (10-15 minutes). CT angiography has a much wider availability than conventional angiography, and has the potential to replace the latter in assessment of vascular trauma.

Table 26.2: Indications for angiography in vascular injury

Preoperative

i. Suspected thoracic aorta injury
ii. Fracture pelvis with suspected retroperitoneal pelvic vascular injury
iii. "Soft signs" of vascular injury
iv. Abnormal Doppler study in suspected vascular injury

Operative

i. Before exploration: Injuries distal to axillary and femoral arteries
ii. After vascular repair to detect unsuspected technical errors

Table 26.3: Angiographic signs of arterial injury

Lumen obstruction	Arterial wall irregularity
Filling defects in lumen	Leakage of contrast outside the artery
AV fistula	False aneurysm

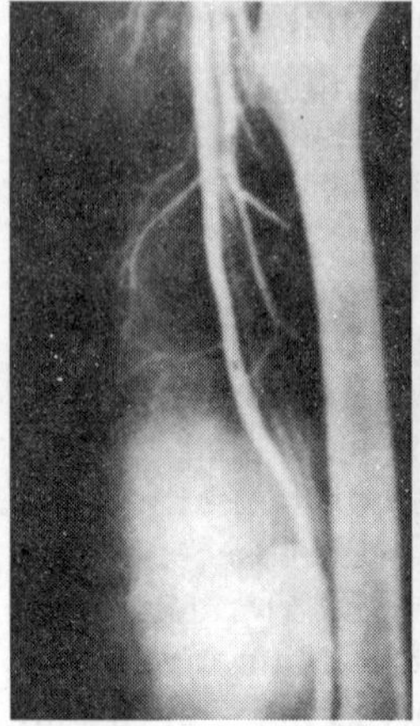

Fig. 26.2: Angiogram showing extravasation of contrast in femoral artery injury

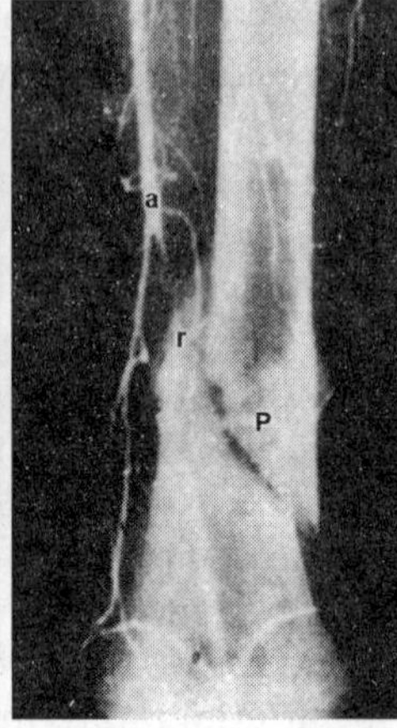

Fig. 26.3: Traumatic arteriovenous fistula

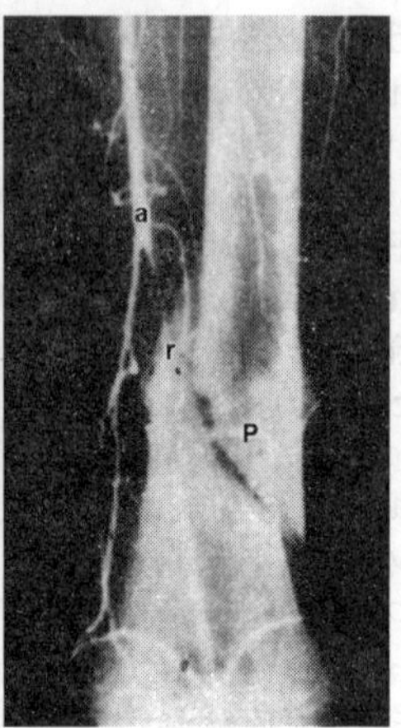

Fig. 26.4: Abrupt cutoff of dye in arterial injury. The missile is also seen

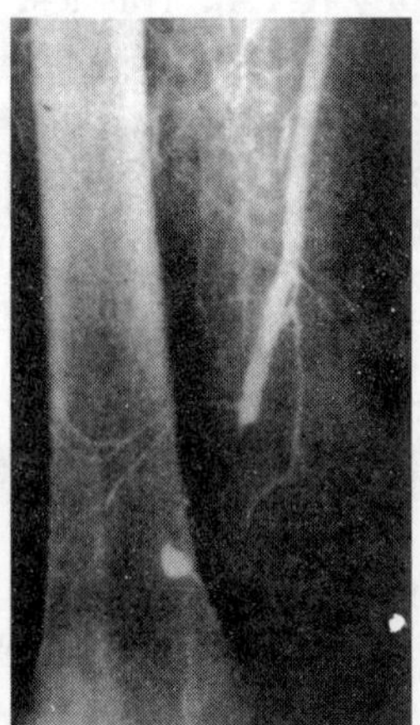

Fig. 26.5: Femoral artery injury in a case of fracture femur

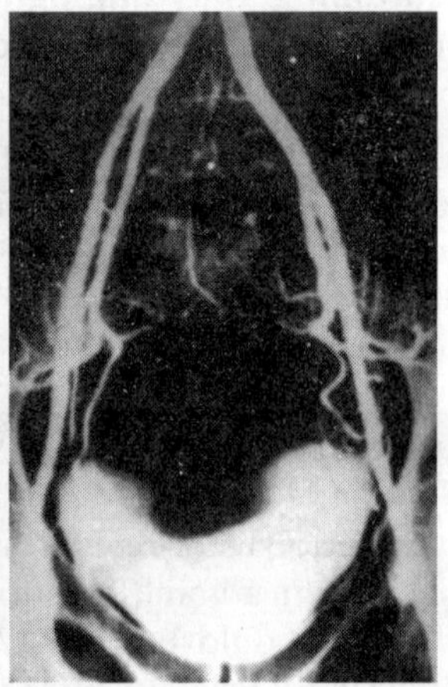

Fig. 26.6: Wall-irregularity (more marked on right side) and hold-up of dye indicated arterial injury

GENERAL PRINCIPLES OF VASCULAR REPAIR

Vascular repairs need a modern sterile operation theater with facilities for perioperative angiography, good illumination, an assortment of atraumatic vascular clamps, fine prolene sutures, Fogarty balloon catheters, blood and blood products, and a fair degree of surgical expertise. Autotransfusion facilities (cell savers) are of great help while managing major vascular trauma. The patient should be kept warm during the operation.

The operation should be performed under strict asepsis. Preoperative antibiotics are administered and continued for at least 5 days. A temporary pneumatic tourniquet may be used for extremity injuries; this should be removed once the vessel is controlled proximally and distally.

Adequate exposure is vital; this requires preparation of adjacent anatomical areas (e.g. preparation of thorax in cervical vascular injuries and vice versa). An uninjured leg is prepped for possible harvesting of saphenous vein, should this be required.

Wide exposure (a generous incision) should be made to rapidly expose and control the proximal and distal portions of the artery before approaching the actual injured area. Artery should be controlled by bulldog or other suitable atraumatic vascular clamps. If these are not available, a Rumel's tourniquet can easily be made by passing umbilical tape or no 2 silk around the vessel and threading the two ends through a piece of plastic intravenous tubing and "snugging" it on the artery. In blunt and high velocity trauma there is often extensive intimal damage, and debridement of vessel may be required till the normal appearing intima appears. Heparin 5000 IU should be administered intravenous at this stage, unless specifically contraindicated (e.g. massive blood loss, or head injury). Repair should be carried out by 3/0, 4/0 or 5/0 prolene.

Several methods are available for repair of vascular injuries (Fig. 26.7). A small laceration may be repaired by simple suture or a lateral continuous suture. However, if this causes narrowing of the arterial lumen, a vein patch, harvested from any neighboring superficial vein should be used. Alternatively a Dacron or PTFE patch may be used. Primary end-to-end anastomosis of a transacted artery is usually possible if the distance between two ends is less than 1.25 cm. Otherwise a reversed saphenous vein interposition graft (harvested from opposite limb) or rarely a PTFE or Dacron tube graft should be used to bridge the vascular defect (especially in infected wounds).[21] When there is considerable mismatch between the diameters of the injured vessel and the available vein, a 'panelled' or 'spiral' vein graft technique can be used to enlarge the diameter of saphenous vein. Two anchoring ("stay")

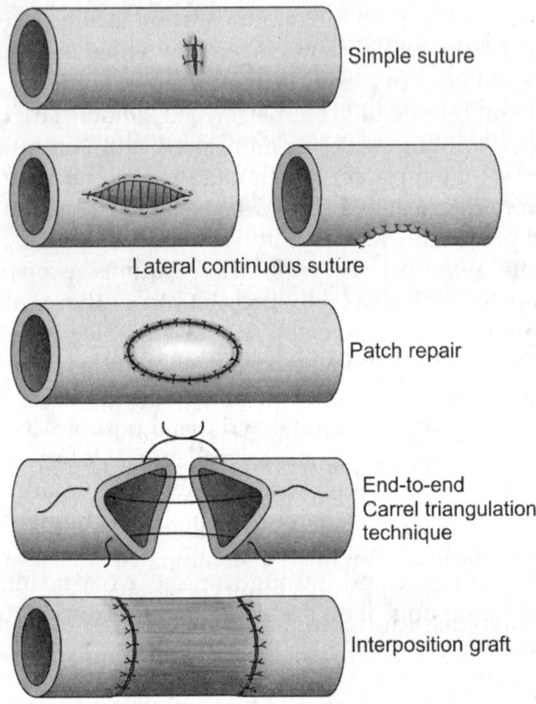

Fig. 26.7: Methods of repairing arterial injuries

sutures are placed first at 180 degrees on the vessel to be repaired. Continuous prolene suture is used for anastomosis taking 1 mm bites at 1 mm distance. Distal back-bleeding should be confirmed prior to distal anastomosis. If this is absent, gentle distal thrombectomy is performed using a 3F or 4F Fogarty catheter. Completion angiogram should ideally be performed to exclude any unsuspected technical faults. After completion of anastomosis clamps are removed, starting with the distal clamp. Gentle sponge pressure is maintained at the anastomosis site for 5 minutes to facilitate hemostasis. If major suture line leak still persists it should be under run by additional stitch. Persistent arterial spasm may be relieved by local instillation of 1% lignocaine, or 5% papaverine, or 20% magnesium sulfate solution. Intra-arterial tolazoline (an alpha-adrenergic blocker) has also been tried.

After repair the site should be covered by a neighboring muscle. In dirty, contaminated wounds appropriate local debridement of soft tissues should be done. If generalized ooze persists from raw areas, a suction drain should be used. A concomitant fracture, if present, should be properly stabilized before undertaking vascular repair as abnormal movements may jeopardize the arterial repair. However, if the ischemia is prolonged an "indwelling shunt" (commonly a length of sterile intravenous tubing) should be inserted from proximal to distal artery to maintain distal perfusion during the time taken for fixation of fracture.[22,23]

Endovascular Treatment of Vascular Injuries

Percutaneous catheter based (endovascular) (techniques are increasingly being used to treat vascular injuries. These offer several potential advantages: surgical trauma with its attendant effects (blood loss, hypothermia, etc.) is avoided; general anesthesia is not required; arteries do not require cross-clamping (thereby avoiding ischemia–reperfusion injuries); contained hematoma at injury site is not opened (its tamponading effect is not suddenly released and fresh bleeding is avoided); and complex lesions in challenging locations (subclavian, thoracic aorta) can be accessed from a remote artery (usually femoral). Limitations of endovascular techniques are that they require cath lab/hybrid OT suite with hardware (guidewires, catheters, etc.) and requisite skills; they cannot be used in unstable patients or those with ongoing bleeding, end-organ ischemia or where concomitant injuries require open exploration; and there may be technical limitations (inability to cross the lesion with the guidewire). Endovascular techniques have been used to manage vascular trauma in the following three situations.

Control of hemorrhage: Injured vessels (both arteries as well as veins) can be embolized using a variety of agents: coils, gel foam, alcohol, and balloons. These have been widely used in management of bleeding associated with pelvic fractures.[24] They have also been used to control bleeding from splenic and hepatic vessels.[25]

Obtaining temporary vascular control: A balloon can be positioned in the damaged artery (or just proximal to it) and inflated to control hemorrhage. This is especially useful in inaccessible vessels like proximal subclavian artery and the carotid arteries (Zones 1 and 3 of the neck).[11]

Definitive vascular repair. Stent grafts (stents covered with fabric) can be placed intraluminally across the damaged segment of an artery; this provides definitive treatment. They have been extensively utilized in managing trauma of deep seated inaccessible vessels where surgical exposure can be extremely difficult: thoracic aorta, thoracic outlet vessels, carotid and vertebral arteries.[26,27]

EXTREMITY VASCULAR INJURIES

Introduction

Vascular injuries of the extremity are the most common form of vascular trauma encountered both in war as well as in civilian practice. These accounted for 96.1% of all vascular injuries in World War II,[2] 91% in Vietnam War,[3] 87% in the report from Dallas[5] and 84% in the report from New Orleans.[13] Blunt trauma accounted for only 1% of war injuries[4] whereas it accounts for 10% or more of vascular injuries in civilian trauma.[7,13] Improved survival and low amputation rate has been reported from most of the reports in 80's and 90's, and the trend has continued in the 21st century. The chances of limb loss are high after blunt injury, high velocity missile injury, or shotgun injury.

Clinical Features

Open (overt) arterial injuries declare themselves by appearance of bright red, pulsatile blood. Closed injuries with contained or concealed bleeding may be difficult to detect, and the presenting feature may be low BP in an otherwise conscious patient. In both types of injuries there may be distal circulatory deficit. However, the six classical P's of acute limb ischemia (pain, pallor, paresis, pulselessness, paresthesia and poikilothermia) may be difficult to assess in a severely injured patient. The signs of extremity arterial injury have been classified as hard signs and soft signs (Table 26.1). Absence of distal limb pulses is the most specific sign, especially if the contralateral pulses are well felt. However, this sign may be fallacious in an hypotensive patient. Moreover, presence of distal pulse does not exclude arterial injury, as sometimes the adequate collateral circulation may ensure presence of distal pulse beyond an injured artery. Presence of one or more hard sign is sufficient to diagnose arterial injury confidently.

Associated fractures/dislocation, and injury to the nerve and soft tissues should be documented. Occasionally reduction of dislocation leads to return of extremity pulse.

Investigations

If the diagnosis of arterial injury is evident (e.g. external hemorrhage, unexplained hypotension or limb ischemia), no further investigation is required and patient is taken for operative treatment straightway. Absence of hard signs means there is no significant vascular injury, and diagnostic arteriography is not indicated. The patient with soft signs should be observed for 24 hours, as delayed thrombosis following arterial injury is well documented. Duplex scan may play an important role in this group of patients.[28]

Management

First Aid

Measures as detailed in the previous section should be followed. Hemorrhage should be controlled by direct pressure/pressure bandage. Tourniquets over extremities should be avoided as far as possible; these should be released periodically if at all used. Military antishock trousers (MAST) have been tried in extremity trauma, but their efficacy remains unproven.

Operative Principles

General principles of vascular repair as mentioned previously should be adhered to. Every attempt should be made to revascularize the limb within 6 hours of injury. However, this time limit is not absolute; revascularization should be attempted as long as the limb is viable.

Reperfusion injury and its sequelae including kidney damage can occur following limb revascularization if there has been prolonged period of ischemia. This can be minimized by: (i) adequate hydration ensuring good urinary output (1-2 ml/kg/min), (ii) IV mannitol and soda bicarb prior to release of arterial clamps. Patient should be monitored for hyperkalemia, acidosis and myoglobinuria in the postoperative period.

Four compartment open fasciotomy of calf is strongly recommended after lower limb revascularization when the period of ischemia has been more than 6-8 hours or when signs of acute limb ischemia are present; when there is a concomitant venous injury; if there is prolonged hypotension, severe soft tissue trauma or distal limb swelling; or if the compartment pressure is raised.[29] This should be of "open" type using two or more incisions or alternatively by resecting a piece of fibula. If fasciotomy has not been performed, monitoring of intercompartmental pressure is recommended. Fasciotomy should be performed if the pressure is above 20 cm of water.[30] Compartment syndrome due to swelling of muscle is inevitable and failure to perform a fasciotomy may lead to muscle necrosis with subsequent gangrene or a functionless limb due to ischemic contracture.

In limb trauma vascular repair takes precedence over nerve, orthopedic and reconstructive repairs.

Primary amputation should be considered if there is extensive soft tissue/orthopedic injury or injury to a major nerve (e.g. sciatic). Mangled extremity severity score (MESS) has been developed to predict limb salvage.[31] A score of 7 or more has an amputation rate of almost 100%. In such situations, rather than embarking on complicated repairs, patient can be observed for 24-48 hours, and a decision made in consultation with patient and his family.

Complications

Complications after proper repair of vascular injuries are not uncommon; these are listed in Table 26.4.

Thrombosis of repaired artery necessitates prompt re-exploration and proximal and distal thrombectomy using Fogarty balloon catheters. If a technical fault is present this should be corrected. Persistent hemorrhage, usually from suture line also needs re-exploration and control of bleeding by additional

Table 26.4: Complications after repair of vascular injuries

Local	*General*
Thrombosis	Acute renal failure
Hemorrhage	Metabolic acidosis
False aneurysm	Hypothermia
Hematoma	Coagulopathy
Infection	ARDS
Compartment syndrome	Multisystem organ failure
Distal gangrene	
Ischemic contracture	

sutures. Occasionally, slow persistent ooze may result in a false aneurysm at the anastomotic site. A small local hematoma may not require evacuation, but large ones specially those causing neurovascular complications should be surgically evacuated. Infection at the operation site leading to disruption of vascular anastomosis ("blow out") may lead to massive hemorrhage which may prove fatal. This dangerous and difficult complication is treated by proximal and distal ligation of the artery and an extra-anatomical bypass (e. g. axillofemoral bypass) through uninfected areas. Compartment syndrome may develop if extremity revascularization was delayed beyond 8 hours. Limb gangrene and ischemic contracture may occur if there was prolonged ischemia prior to revascularisation or due to undiagnosed postoperative thrombosis.

Outcomc

The outcome after extremity injury depends on several factors. Shah et al[32] reported no amputation in 151 patients with single missile/sharp instrument vascular injury whereas 10 of their 35 patients with blunt/shotgun injury underwent an amputation. The artery involved is also important. Popliteal injuries are notoriously difficult to treat. The chance of gangrene after ligation of common femoral and popliteal artery approaches 80%. A concomitant venous injury also worsens the prognosis. Gregory et al have devised a Mangled Extremity Syndrome Index[33] which takes into account the following factors: Injury severity score, integument, nerve, vascular and bony injuries, lag time before treatment, age of the patient, pre-existing disease and shock (systolic BP <90 mm Hg). Points are awarded for each of these parameters and they found that an MESI of less than 20 was associated with limb salvage approaching 100% whereas if the score was more than 20 amputation was certain. A recent publication has reviewed the outcomes after lower limb arterial injuries.[34]

THORACIC VASCULAR INJURIES

Thoracic vascular injuries account for 1.1-4.1%[5,32] of all vascular injuries, and are more frequently encountered in civilian practice. Penetrating injuries account for 15-20% of vascular injuries in civil trauma,[7] blunt injuries accounting for the remainder. These injuries are associated with a high mortality. They may be conveniently classified as penetrating injuries and blunt injuries.

Penetrating Thoracic Trauma

These injuries present as one of the three following ways:

1. Asymptomatic patient with wounds of thoracic inlet or superior mediastinum, normal BP and chest X-ray with proximity of stab wound or missile track near a major vessel.
2. Slightly hypotensive patient with evidence of contained hematoma (e.g. mediastinum widening on chest X-ray).
3. Profoundly hypotensive patient with large mediastinum mass or massive hemothorax.

Diagnosis is usually suspected in view of evidence of penetrating trauma. An emergency chest X-ray in emergency room is the initial investigation. In group 1 (stable) patients an angiogram is usually required to confirm or exclude vascular injury. Group 2 patients also require an emergency angiogram in order to plan appropriate treatment. Transesophageal echography is a promising investigative modality in this group and may replace angiography for this group of patients. Group 3 patients require aggressive resuscitation and emergency thoracotomy if necessary in the casualty department itself.[35]

Emergency treatment in unstable patients consists of inserting large bore (10-gauge) cannulas through which infusion rate of 1.5 l/min can be achieved. Blood is sent for crossmatching. Emergency intubation may be performed in casualty and the patient is wheeled into the OT. During surgery it is of vital importance to avoid hypothermia in these patients. One or more of the following measures may be employed. The head of the patient is covered with a turban; the patient is placed on a rewarming blankets during surgery; one or both lower limbs are covered with thermal blankets or large plastic bags; all intravenous fluids are infused through a rapid rewarming system; the cascade on anesthesia machine is turned to a high temperature mode; and warm saline is placed over heart/pleural cavity during thoracotomy.

Standard anterolateral thoracotomy through 3rd-5th intercostal space is employed for majority of cases. For a right sided wound a transverse sternotomy extended as a left anterolateral thoracotomy is useful for cross-clamping of ascending and descending aorta. Alternatively, a median sternotomy with lateral extension (supraclavicular, with or without removal of clavicle) may be used especially in case of innominate artery or right subclavian injury. Left subclavian artery injury is usually accessible by a high anterolateral thoracotomy. Common carotid artery injury is tackled by an incision along the anterior border of sternomastoid, extended proximally as median sternotomy if required. These incisions are depicted in Figure 26.8. Most of the penetrating injuries can be treated by simple suture or by a (Dacron) patch closure. Rarely an appropriate size Dacron/PTFE bypass graft is required to restore circulation. Innominate artery injury usually requires proximal and distal ligation and a bypass from ascending aorta to beyond the site of injury.

Blunt Thoracic Trauma

Motor vehicle accidents account for the vast majority of blunt thoracic vascular injuries. 15% of patients, dying of motor vehicle accidents, have rupture of descending aorta (DTA) on autopsy.[36]

The tear is classically located at the isthmus of aorta just distal to left subclavian artery (site of attachment of ligamentum arteriosum). Rarely the distal thoracic aorta is injured; this is often associated with fracture (dislocation of thoracic spine). Innominate and intercostal arteries may be injured in this trauma. Frontal deceleration is the mechanism of injury in most blunt injuries; however side-impact collisions are also responsible.[37] Several features in history may point to injury of thoracic vessels.

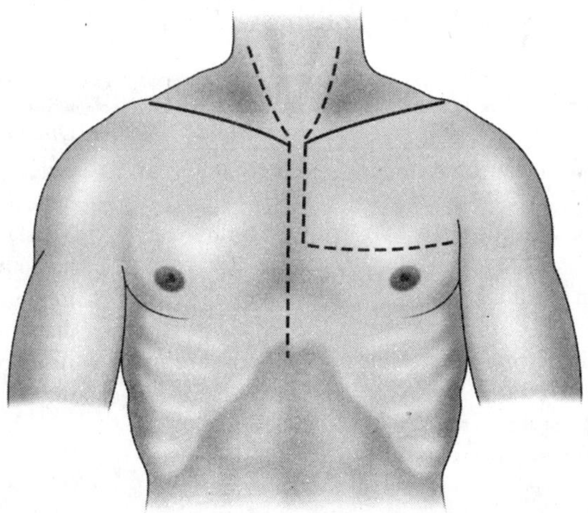

Fig. 26.8: Operative incisions for exposure of thoracic vessels

These are:
1. History of vehicle accident with speed more than 60 kmph
2. History of sudden deceleration
3. Death of another victim in same accident
4. History of wearing seat belt.

Similarly the following clues on examination may point to these injuries:
1. Presternal contusion/palpable sternal fracture
2. Fracture 1st/2nd rib
3. Multiple rib fractures or flail chest
4. Decreased femoral pulses
5. Difference in BP of the two upper extremities
6. Upper extremity hypertension (pseudocoarctation syndrome)
7. Interscapular/precordial murmur
8. Hoarseness or voice change without thoracic injury
9. Tenderness/fracture thoracic spine
10. Paraplegia/paraparesis.

Chest X-ray often reveals tell-tale signs of vascular injury (Table 26.5). Mediastinal widening is seen in more than 90% of thoracic aortic injuries. Other investigative modalities employed in haemodynamically stable patients are CT scan, TEE, digital substraction angiography (DSA) or conventional angiography. Angiography has an advantage that it avoids unnecessary thoracotomy, accurately localizes the site of tear in aorta and identifies a second tear (not uncommon). Helical CT and CT

Table 26.5: Radiological findings of traumatic rupture of thoracic aorta[38]

Mediastinal findings	*Fractures*	*Other findings*
Mediastinal widening > 8 cm	Sternum	Apical pleural hematoma
Obliteration of aortic knob	First rib	Massive left hemothorax
Depression of left main bronchus > 140 deg	Second rib	Ruptured diaphragm
Loss of paravertebral pleural line	Thoracic spine	Anterior tracheal displacement
Tracheal deviation to right	Scapula	
Deviation of esophagus (NG tube) to right	Clavicle	
Obliteration of aortopulmonary window		

angiography have practically replaced conventional angiography as the definitive diagnostic procedure for suspected thoracic aortic injury.[39] CT angio is also vital for planning endovascular repair of traumatic aortic disruptions.

Emergency treatment is the same as for penetrating injuries. Operative treatment can be one by the following methods: cross-clamping of DTA with rapid repair by running suture; cross-clamping with insertion of sutureless aortic prosthesis; use of external heparin coated shunt during cross-clamping; use of left heart (atriofemoral) bypass; or use of left atrium-left femoral artery cannula with centrifugal pump.[40] Nonoperative treatment as vigorous antihypertensive therapy is recommended in following situations: Severe CNS injury; established sepsis or badly contaminated wounds/burns; severe respiratory insufficiency; hemodynamic instability or metabolic failure due to other concomitant injuries; and nonthreatening lesion (e.g. intimal defects) on angiography.[41] The overall mortality rate in thoracic vascular injuries is between 7-25% in good centers. Innominate artery injury mortality is 15% while subclavian injury mortality is less than 4%. Mortality after carotid injuries is high if the patient is comatose or has presented with neurological deficit on admission. Injuries of DTA have a high mortality approaching 100%.[40]

Endovascular repair. Traumatic aortic injuries have been successfully treated with endovascular stent grafts, with significantly lower mortality and morbidity compared to open surgery. The Percutaneous minimally invasive nature of these procedures which avoid thoracotomy in a critically ill patient makes them an attractive option. Longer term results are required to confirm whether EVAR can be accepted as a definitive treatment.[42]

ABDOMINAL VASCULAR INJURIES

Abdominal vascular injuries include injury to abdominal aorta/IVC/celiac axis/superior mesenteric artery or vein/hepatic artery or vein/portal vein/iliac artery or vein. The incidence varies from 3.9% in battle condition[4] to 34% in civilian trauma.[7] Gunshot wounds to abdomen causing injury to abdominal vessels forms the highest incidence (24.6%).[43] Blunt abdominal trauma is a rare cause and is associated with a vascular injury in only 5-10% of cases.[44] Penetrating stab wounds are also associated with abdominal vascular injury in only about 10% of cases. Iatrogenic injuries (retroperitoneal lymph node dissection, spinal disc removal, angiography) complete the remainder of causes. The diagnosis is suspected by the presence of one or more of the following clinical features/investigations:

1. Penetrating trauma between nipple and upper thigh
2. Moderate hypotension—other causes excluded
3. Peritoneal perforation of stab wound on digital exploration
4. Worsening of abdominal signs on repeated physical examination
5. Haziness on plain X-ray abdomen
6. Fluid seen on abdominal ultrasonography
7. Positive diagnostic peritoneal lavage
8. Severe hypotension with absent femoral pulses
9. Non-visualization of one kidney on single-shot IVP
10. Pelvic fracture with negative supraumbilical DPL. This indicates retroperitoneal hemorrhage.

Patients with abdominal vascular injury should undergo emergency laparotomy. In moribund patients emergency room left thoracotomy with cross clamping of distal thoracic aorta has been described. However, survival is low (3-5%) with this maneuver. This may be of use in hospitals where there is considerable distance between casualty department and the operation theater. A generous vertical midline laparotomy incision is employed and all clots and blood removed by suction or manual evacuation. The blood pressure may "crash" on opening the abdomen (due to loss of abdominal tamponade) and the anesthetist should be warned so that rapid infusion can be given at this stage. A rapid inspection of abdomen is made and hemorrhage from solid organs controlled by four quadrant packin/clips/resection (e.g. splenectomy). In face of massive hemorrhage, aorta should be clamped at the diaphragmatic crus level. Proximal and distal control of the affected vessel is obtained by judicious use of clamps/aortic compression device/sponge sticks/balloon catheters inserted intraluminally. Rapid single layer closure of gastrointestinal perforations is then performed. The abdomen is irrigated with copious amounts of saline or antibiotic solution, gloves and drapes changed and attention now directed to repair of vascular injuries. The general principles for repair of vascular injuries are already enunciated in the section on extremity injuries.

The retroperitoneum has been divided into 3 anatomical zones for treatment purposes. Zone 1 (Central retroperitoneal hematomas are always explored as they are due to associated vascular, duodenal or pancreatic injuries. Zone 2 (flank hematomas) caused by penetrating injuries should also be explored (possible iliac injury) while those due to blunt trauma are managed conservatively. Zone 3 (pelvic hematomas) are classically associated with pelvic fractures and are traditionally managed conservatively. However, Zone 3 injuries associated with penetrating trauma should be explored. The operative strategy for hemorrhage encountered at different intra-abdominal sites is detailed below.

Midline Supramesocolic Hematoma/Hemorrhage

In case of active bleeding the aortic compression device is employed below the diaphragmatic aortic hiatus. Alternatively, the lesser omentum is divided, esophagus retracted to left and a cross-clamp applied to aorta in the supraceliac region. If a large hematoma is present medial rotation of all left side viscera is performed (Fig. 26.9). The left colon, spleen, tail of pancreas, kidney and fundus of stomach is freed from retroperitoneal

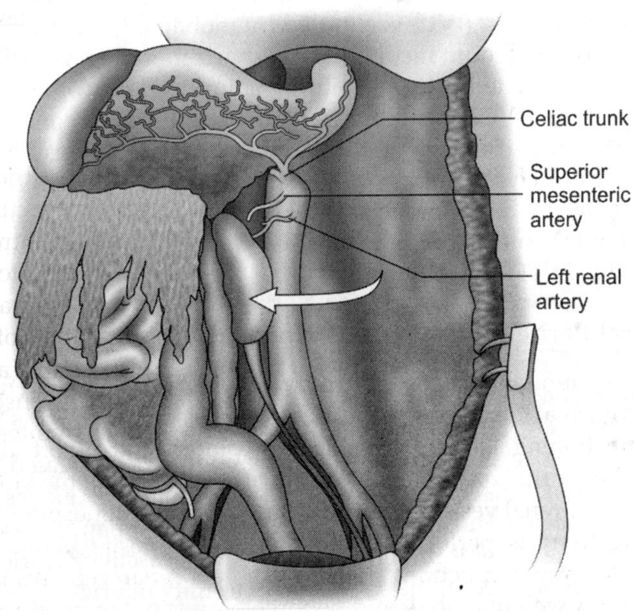

Fig. 26.9: Medial rotation of left side viscera

attachments by blunt and sharp dissection and the entire viscera rotated medially. The entire abdominal aorta is now visible and can be cross-clamped and its tear treated by simple suture or with Dacron patch. If the patient is critically ill, 'Damage control' can be done by placing a temporary intraluminal shunt (sterile thoracostomy tube); definitive repair is done once the patient is stable and physiological parameters have returned to normal.[45] If there is severe peritoneal contamination, aorta can be ligated and an extra-anatomical bypass (axillobifemoral) is performed.[46] Celiac axis injury is treated by ligation. Superior mesenteric artery (SMA) tears should be treated by simple suture by 5/0 prolene or interposition vein graft. Superior mesenteric vein (SMV) is approached by transaction of pancreatic neck. A tear should be ideally repaired by 5/0 or 6/0 prolene; however in desperate situation ligation of the vein is acceptable.

Midline Inframesocolic Hematoma/Hemorrhage

The aorta can be approached directly by incising the retroperitoneum and it should be cross-clamped below the left renal vein. It is then repaired in the manner described above. The inferior vena cava (IVC) is exposed by mobilizing the ascending colon and duodenum medially by kocherization (Fig. 26.10). The tear can be isolated by a side biting (Satinsky) clamp or by cross-clamping the IVC. IVC cross-clamping should be accompanied by aortic cross-clamping to reduce precipitate hypotension. The IVC tear is then repaired by running 5/0 prolene stitch. In case of missile injuries, a second tear in the posterior wall of IVC should be excluded and if present, repaired through the lumen of the vein (Fig. 26.11).

Lateral Perirenal Hematoma/Hemorrhage

This is commonly due to renal artery or vein injury. If preoperative IVP is normal the hematoma should not be disturbed. If IVP shows nonfunctioning kidney the area is explored and a soft clamp placed over the renal artery and vein after mobilizing the kidney. If repair of renal vessels is feasible this should be done; otherwise nephrectomy is performed (provided the opposite kidney has proven normal function). Ligation of left renal vein near the midline is well tolerated, and nephrectomy is not mandatory for isolated injury of the renal vein.

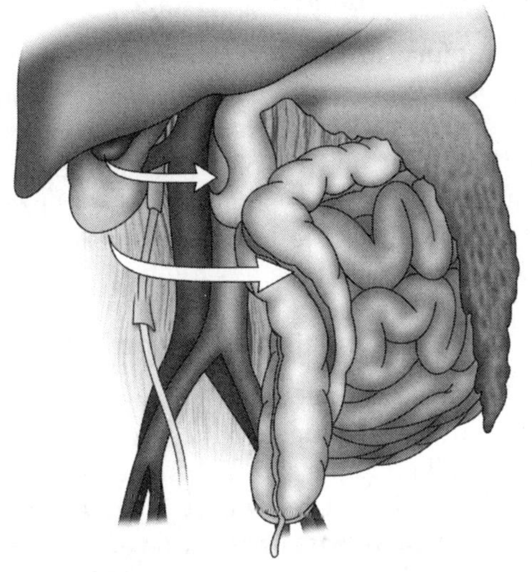

Fig. 26.10: Medial rotation of right side viscera

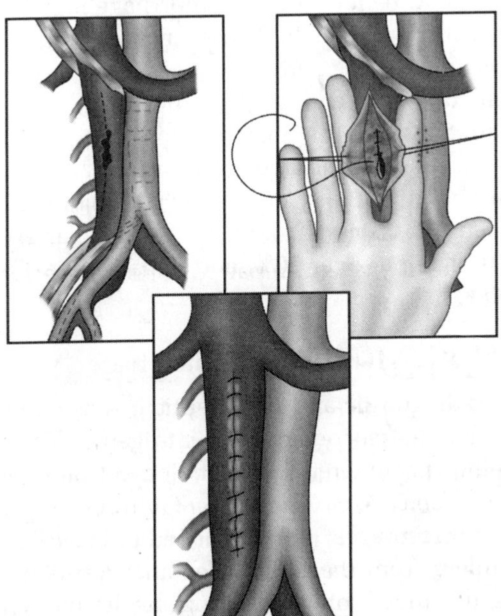

Fig. 26.11: Repair of posterior vena cava injury by deliberate enlargement of anterior injury

Lateral Pelvic Hematoma/Hemorrhage

This is due to injury to the iliac artery or vein. Proximal and distal control of these vessels by silastic loops is fairly straightforward and the injury is then repaired by simple suture or 8 mm interposition graft. In case of associated bowel injury with gross contamination the artery should be ligated proximally and distally and the circulation to lower limb restored by an extra-anatomic (axillofemoral) bypass.

Portal/Retrohepatic Hematoma/Hemorrhage

Hemorrhage from hepatoduodenal ligament can be controlled by Pringle maneuver. Proximal hepatic artery injury is treated by ligation whereas all attempts should be made to repair the distal hepatic artery injury. Portal vein injury may be treated by lateral repair, saphenous vein bypass or rarely an emergency portacaval shunt. Injury to hepatic veins/retrohepatic IVC are one of the most difficult injuries to treat and are frequently lethal. A hematoma in this region should be left intact. Hemorrhage may be controlled by a perihepatic packing. If this is unsuccessful, total hepatic vascular isolation is done and atriocaval shunt inserted using F36 thoracotomy tube or F8 endotracheal tube (Fig. 26.12). The injury is then repaired by simple suture or patch graft.

The overall mortality in abdominal vascular trauma is high. Aortic injury has a mortality of 55-65%; IVC injury 25-40%; Renal artery or vein 13%; SMA 42%; SMV 28%; Iliac artery 39%; Iliac vein 27%; Portal vein over 50%, and hepatic veins/retrohepatic IVC over 80%.[44]

IATROGENIC INJURIES

In this era of diagnostic and therapeutic interventional vascular procedures it is not surprising that iatrogenic injuries are increasingly being encountered.[47] The etiology of iatrogenic injuries are listed in Table 26.6. The type of iatrogenic injuries with approximate percentages[48] are mentioned in Table 26.7.

As is evident from the table, false aneurysms (pseudoaneurysms) are the most common iatrogenic lesions encountered.

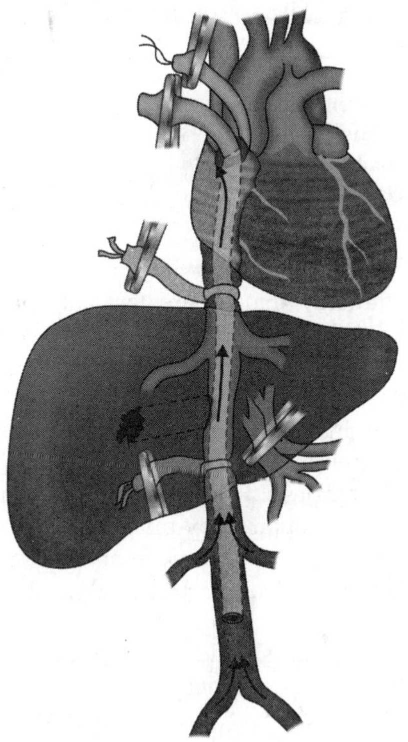

Fig. 26.12: Use of intracaval shunt inserted via atrial appendage for injury to retrohepatic IVC/hepatic veins

Table 26.6: Etiology of iatrogenic vascular injuries
• Diagnostic angiography • Angioplasty • Cardiac catheterization • Cardiac angioplasty • Intra-aortic balloon pump devices • Arterial cannulation for hemodialysis procedures • Accidental intra-arterial drug injection

Table 26.7: Types of iatrogenic vascular injuries

Types	*Percentage*
False aneurysm	53
Arteriovenous fistula	04
Dissection	13
Thrombosis	10
Laceration	10
Rupture	05
Hematoma	05

The arteries commonly injured are femoral, iliac, brachial and axillary. Diagnosis is by physical findings: absence of distal pulses, localized thrill or bruit, spreading hematoma, pulsatile mass or features of acute blood loss. Confirmation can be obtained by color Doppler examination. If the angiography catheter is *in situ*, contrast extravasation may be seen. Prompt surgical treatment is required for such injuries.[49] False aneurysms should be explored and the rent in artery repaired by underrunning stitch or lateral arteriorrhaphy. Recently, cure of such aneurysm by continuous pressure by ultrasound (colour Doppler) probe has also been described.

Arteriovenous fistulas should be disconnected under vision though they have been occasionally treated by coil embolization. Dissection usually requires local exploration and is repaired by interposition graft, though lately stents have been placed across the dissected area with good results. Thrombosis is managed by balloon catheter thrombectomy. Laceration are treated by simple repair or more commonly by replacement of the injured segment by a suitable graft. Arterial rupture is more commonly encountered in atherosclerotic arteries during angioplasty. If detected, the inflated angioplasty balloon should be left *in situ* while the patient is shifted to OT. Interposition graft should be placed across the ruptured artery; occasionally, patch angioplasty may suffice.[48]

Local arterial complications are encountered in 4-43% of cases of aortic balloon counterpulsation device.[50] The large size of the device and long periods of use predisposes to the complications, the most common of which is limb ischemia which is usually encountered on the first day itself. The incidence of complications is more in females, patients with atherosclerotic peripheral vascular disease, diabetes and hypertensives. It has been claimed that the complications are less if the device is placed by open method rather percutaneously. Two-third cases resolve by removal of balloon while remainder need exploration and repair.

VENOUS INJURIES

Whenever possible venous injuries should be repaired at the same time as arterial ones, and it was evident from the injuries in the Vietnam War that this was an important part of limb salvage.[51] The principles of repair of venous injuries are the same as outlined above for arterial injuries. However, repair of venous injuries is technically much more demanding. If the surgeon is not skilled in this he should not hesitate to ligate the bleeding vein using fine non-absorbable sutures.

REFERENCES

1. Herberer G, Becker HM, Ditmer H, et al. Vascular injuries in polytrauma. World J Surg 1983;7:68-79.
2. Debakey ME, Simeone FA. Battle injuries of arteries in World War II: An analysis of 2471 cases. Am J Surg 1946;123:534.
3. Hughes CW. Acute vascular trauma in Korean war casualties: An analysis of 180 cases. Surg Gyn Obs 1954;99:91.
4. Rich NM, Baugh JH, Hughs CW. Acute arterial injuries in Vietnam: 1000 cases. J Trauma 1970;10:359.
5. Perry MO, Thal ER, Shires GT. Management of arterial injuries. Ann Surg 1971;173:403.
6. Feliciano DV, Bitondo CG, Mattox KL, et al. Civilian injuries in the 1980: An experience with 456 vascular and cardiac injuries. Ann Surg 1984;199:717.
7. Mattox KL, Feliciano DV, Burch J, et al. Five thousand seven hundred and six cardiovascular injuries in 4,459 patients: Epidemiologic evolution 1958-1987. Ann Surg 1989;209:698.
8. Ollier DW, et al. J Trauma 1992;32:740.
9. Barker FW. A history of arterial and venous surgery. In, Bell PRF, Jamieson CW, Ruckley CV (Eds). Surgical management of vascular disease. WB Saunders Company Ltd London, 1992;1-19.
10. Coldwell DM, Stokes KR, Jakes WF. Embolotherapy: agents, clinical applications and techniques. Radiogra 1994;14:623.
11. Scalea TM, Sclafani SJ. Angiographically placed balloons for arterial control: a description of technique. J Trauma 1991;31:1671.
12. DuToit DF, Strauss DC, Blaszyck M, et al. Endovascular treatment of penetrating thoracic injuries. Eur J Vasc Endovasc Surg 2000;19:489.

13. Rowe VL, Yellin AE, Weaver FA. Vascular injuries of the extremities. In, Rutherford RB (Ed). Vascular Surgery 6th edn, Elsevier Saunders, Philadelphia, 2005;1044.
14. Bickell WH, Wall MJ, Pepe PE, et al. Immediate vs delayed fluid resuscitation for Hypotensive patients with penetrating torso injuries. N Eng J Med 1994;331:1105.
15. Dennis JW, Frykberg ER, Veldenz HC, et al. Validation of non-operative management of occult vascular injuries and accuracy of physical examination alone in penetrating extremity trauma: 5-10 years follow-up. J Trauma 1998;44:243.
16. Johansen K, Lynch K, Paun M, et al. Noninvasive vascular tests reliability exclude occult arterial trauma in injured extremities. J Trauma 1991;31:515.
17. Meissner M, Paun M, Johansen K. Duplex scanning for arterial trauma. Am J Surg 1991;161:522.
18. Reids JDS, Weighlt JA, Thal, et al. Assessment of proximity of a wound to major vascular structures as an indication for arteriography. Arch Surg 1988;123:942.
19. Anderson RJ, Hobson RW, Lee BC, et al. Reduced dependency on arteriography for penetrating extremity trauma: Influence of wound lovation and non-invasive vascular studies. J Trauma 1990;30:1059.
20. Weaver FA, Yellin AE. Is arterial proximity a valid indication for arteriography in penetrating extremity trauma? A prospective study. Arch Surg 1990;125:1256.
21. Shah DM, Leather RP, Carson JD, et al. Polytetrafluoroethylene grafts in the rapid reconstruction of acute contaminated peripheral vascular injuries. Am J Surg 1984;148:229.
22. Khalil IM, Livingstone DH. Intravascular shunts in complex lower limb trauma. J Vasc Surg 1986;4:582.
23. Barros D'Sa AAB. Complex vascular and orthopaedic injuries. J Bone Joint Surg 1992;74:116.
24. Panetta T, Sclafani SJA, Goldstein AS, et al. Percutaneous transcatheter embolization for massive bleeding from pelvic fractures. J Trauma 1985;25:1021.
25. Carrilo EH, Spain DA, Wohltman D, et al. Interventional techniques are useful adjuncts in non-operative management of hepatic injuries. J Trauma 1999;46:619.
26. Lachat M, Phammmater T, Witzke H, et al. Acute traumatic aortic rupture: early stent-graft repair. Eur J Cardiothorac Surg 2002;21:956.
27. Gomez CR, May AK, Terry JB, et al. Endovascular therapy of traumatic injuries of the extracranial cerebral arteries. Crit Care Clin 1999;15:789.

28. Schwartz M, Weaver F, Yellin A, et al. The utility of colour flow Doppler examination in penetrating extremity arterial trauma. Am Surg 1993;59:375.
29. Mubarak SJ, Hargens AR. Acute compartment syndromes. Surg Clin North Am 1983;63:539.
30. Mabee JR, Botswick TL. Pathophysiology and mechanisms of compartment syndrome. Orthop Rev 1993;22:175.
31. Johansen K, Daines M, Howey T, et al. Objective criteria accurately predict amputation following lower extremity trauma. J Trauma 1990;30:568.
32. Shah PM, Ivatury RR, Babu SC. Is limb loss avoidable in civilian vascular injuries? Am J Surg 1987;154:202.
33. Gregory TR, Gould RJ, Peclet M, et al. The Mangled extremity syndrome (M>E>S): A severity grading system for multisystem injury of the extremity. J Trauma 1985;25:1147.
34. Hafez HM, Woolgar J, Robbs JV. Lower extremity arterial injury: results of 550 cases and review of risk factors associated with limb loss. J Vasc Surg 2001;33:212.
35. Feliciano DV, Bitondo CG, Cruse PA, et al. Liberal use of emergency centre thoracotomy. AM J Surg 1986;152:654.
36. Williams JS, Graff JA, Uku JM, et al. Aortic injury in the vehicular trauma. Ann Thorac Surg 1994;57:726.
37. Katyal D, McLellan BA, Brenneman FD, et al. Lateral impact motor vehicle collisions: significant cause for blunt traumatic rupture of the thoracic aorta. J Trauma 1997;42:769.
38. Patel NH, Stephens KE, Mirvis SE, et al. Imaging of acute thoracic aortic injury due to blunt traima: a review. Radiol 1995;197:125.
39. Gavant ML, Menke PG, Fabian T, et al. Blunt traumatic aortic rupture: detection with helical CT of Chest. Radiol 1995;197:125.
40. Wilson RF. Thoracic vascular trauma. In Bongard F, Wilson SE, Perry MO (Eds). Vascular injuries in surgical practice. Appleton and Lange, Norwalk 1991;107.
41. Fisher RG, Oria RA, Mattox KL, et al. Conservative management of aortic laceration due to blunt trauma. J Trauma 1990;30:1562.
42. Arnofsky AG, Moll FL, Verhagen HJM. Thoracic endovascular aneurysm repair (TEVAR) for traumatic injuries. In: Greenhalgh RM (Ed.). More vascular and endovascular challenges. London: BIBA Publishing 2007;266.
43. Feliciano DV, Burch JM, Spjut-Patrinely, et al. Abdominal gunshot wounds: An urban trauma centre experince with 300 consecutive patients. Ann Surg 1988;208:362.
44. Cox CF. Blunt abdominal trauma. A 5 years analysis of 870 patients requiring coeliotomy. Ann Surg 1084;199:467.

45. Aucar JA, Hirschberg A. Damage control for vascular injuries. Surg Clin North Am 1997;77:853.
46. Asensio JA. Abdominal vascular injuries. Surg Clin North Am 2001;81:1395.
47. Qweid SW, Roubin GS, Smith RB, Salam AF. Post catheterisation vascular complications associated with percutaneous transluminal coronary angioplasty. J Vasc Surg 1990;12:310.
48. Franco CD, Goldsmith J, Veith FJ, et al. Management of arterial injuries produced by percutaneous femoral procedures. Surg 1993;113:419.
49. Rich NM, Hobson RW II, Collins GJ Jr. Traumatic arteriovenous fistulas and false aneurysms: A review of 558 lesions. Surg 1975;78:817.
50. Iverson HG, Herfindahl G, Ecker RR, et al. Vascular complications of intra-aortic balloon counterpulsation. Am J Surg 1987;154:99.
51. Rich NM, Hobson RW II, Collins GJ Jr, Anderson CA. The effect of acute popliteal venous interruption. Ann Surg 1976;183:365.

Chapter

27 Pelvic Trauma

VK Sinha

INTRODUCTION

Pelvic fracture carries a 4-10% mortality[1] as a group primarily because of the severity of trauma necessary to fracture these rugged flat bones. Such severe injuries are associated with injuries to the vessels leading to severe, and, at times, life-threatening hemorrhage. In addition, there is release of inflammatory mediators resulting in systemic inflammatory response syndrome which may lead to organ dysfunction, failure and ultimately death. Prompt diagnosis and treatment of the usually present associated injuries (over 60%) are essential to diminish morbidity and mortality.[2,3] Particularly at risk are those patients with pelvic trauma who have got head injuries or intra-abdominal lesions. The great majority of pelvic fractures are rather simple, straightforward problems.[4] Great majority represent minor injuries, regardless of the severity of trauma. The ones with significant disruption of the pelvic ring carry mortality between 10-20%.[5]

Basic Issues

The understanding of pelvic fractures revolves around three basic issues:

a. The pelvic stability
b. The associated hemorrhage
c. The visceral injuries.

Pelvic Stability

The pelvic ring is composed of two hip bones joined anteriorly at pubic symphysis and articulated posteriorly with sacrum. These articulations *per se* are not inherently stable but together with the strong ligaments and the muscles of the pelvic floor they become highly stable. As is true of any ring, a disruption in the ring is not an event taking place at one place only. The so called isolated fractures of the ring are a myth. It is now universally acknowledged that in so called only anterior injury there is invariable a hidden posterior injury as well. It has been demonstrated with technetium studies and by postmortem examinations that if an anterior ring injury was identified, a posterior ring injury also would be found. With the increased use of X-ray and CT examinations, this concept has been well documented by numerous investigators. Whether this translates into a clinical instability is a different issue. A stable pelvis can withstand normal physiologic forces without abnormal deformation. An injured pelvis which is unstable can lead to deformation either in transverse plane or vertically.

Mechanical Forces

Simple falls from standing heights or direct blow to vulnerable bony prominences such as the anterosuperior or inferior iliac spines, ischial tuberosities, or the superior pubic rami account for the majority of simple fractures.

The forces causing disruption of pelvic ring can be of the following type (Figs 27.1 to 27.4):[6]

a. *Lateral compression (LC) injuries*: Direct lateral impact with inward axial compression when the ilia are struck from the side or direct anterior impact with external rotation of the ilia in conjunction with springing of the posterior sacroiliac joint. This is most common and results in impaction of cancellous bone through the sacroiliac joint and sacrum. The injury pattern depends on location of force application. If forces act

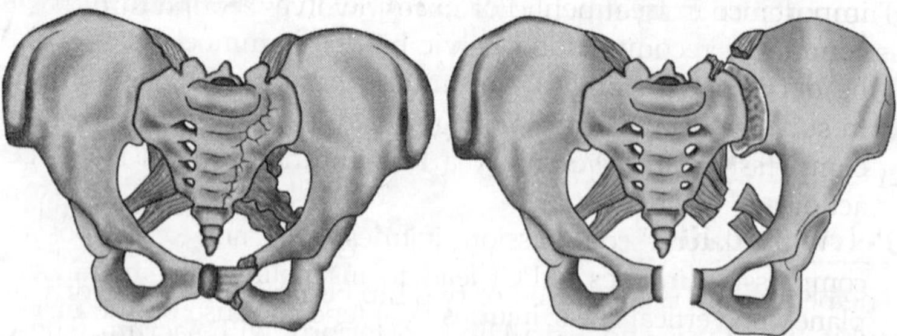

Fig. 27.1: Lateral compression injury **Fig. 27.2:** AP compression injury

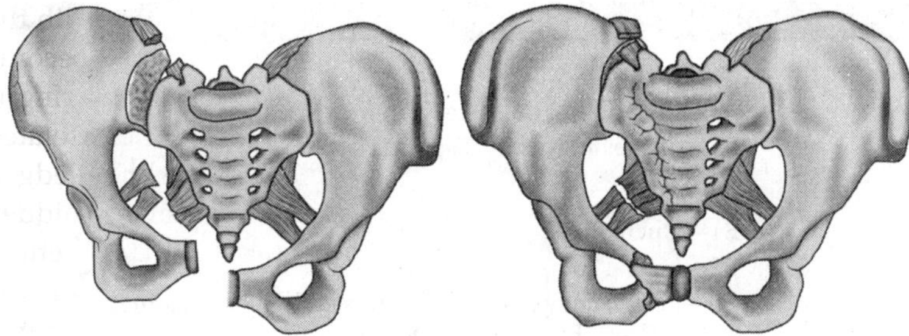

Fig. 27.3: Vertical shear injury **Fig. 27.4:** Combined mechanical injury

directly over greater trochanteric region: may be associated with a transverse acetabular fracture.

b. *Anteroposterior compression (APC) injuries*: These results in external rotation of the hemipelvis. The pelvis springs open, the anterior ligaments of the SI joints disrupts and the hemipelvis hinges on the intact posterior ligaments only. The pelvic vessels lie in front of the SI joint and they tend to get torn leading to hemorrhage.

c. *Vertical shear (VS) injuries*: The forces act in such a way so as to deform the pelvis in a manner that causes one hemipelvis to move up in relation to the other. This tends to cause a vertical separation made possible by either a fracture anteriorly as well as posteriorly or by a complete disruption of the SI joint posteriorly. In the elderly individual, bone strength will be less than ligamentous strength and will fail first.

   In a young individual, bone strength is greater, and thus ligamentous disruptions are likely.

d. *Combined mechanical (CM)*: Combination of injuries often resulting from crush mechanisms. The most common are VS and LC.

Understanding the mechanism of injury is of paramount importance in treatment. For example, in a case of LC injury the commonly recommended pelvic binder/hammock may actually be detrimental. Similarly an anteriorly applied external fixator in such a case will have to be applied in distraction rather than compression. In a VS injury a longitudinal traction is a logical action.

While lateral compression injuries (LC) and anteroposterior compression injuries (APC) lead to instability only in transverse plane, the vertical shear injuries (VS) tend to cause both transverse and vertical instability. This forms the basis of Tile's classification (Table 27.1).[7]

Table 27.1: Tile's classification of pelvic disruption

Type A	*Stable*
	A1—Fractures of the pelvis not involving the ring
	A2—Stable, minimally displaced fractures of the ring
Type B	*Rotationally stable, vertically stable*
	B1—Open book
	B2—Lateral compression: Ipsilateral
	B3—Lateral compression: Contralateral (bucket handle)
Type C	*Rotationally and vertically unstable*
	C1—Unilateral
	C2—Bilateral
	C3—Associated with acetabular fracture

Radiographic Evaluation

The key to pelvic fractures is SI joint. Any asymmetry or widening of SI joint denotes a posterior ring injury and is presumed to be a cause of hemodynamic instability. The aim of radiographic evaluation is not only to diagnose the injury, but also to understand and reconstruct the mechanical forces responsible for injury. Points to understand:

a. Anterior ring disruption (symphysis diastasis or a similarly separated fracture) suggests AP compression and if more than 2.5 cm, is usually associated with ipsilateral (or rarely contralateral) SI joint disruption (Fig. 27.5).
b. Anterior ring fractures (usually rami) oriented obliquely and if overlapping suggests lateral compression. Buckling or fracture of sacrum (detected by asymmetry of sacral foramina is post ring injury in such cases (Fig. 27.6).
c. Any vertical shift of one hemipelvis in relation to the other denotes VS injury. Comparison of the level of lesser trochanter or sciatic notch/ischial spine helps (Fig. 27.7).

Radiographic signs of instability include:

a. Sacroiliac displacement of 5 mm in any plane.
b. Posterior fracture gap (rather than impaction).
c. Avulsion of the fifth lumbar transverse process, the lateral border of the sacrum (sacrotuberous ligament), or the ischial spine (sacrospinous ligament).

Special views like inlet or outlet views help in better understanding but CT scan is more helpful. Advantages of CT scan are:

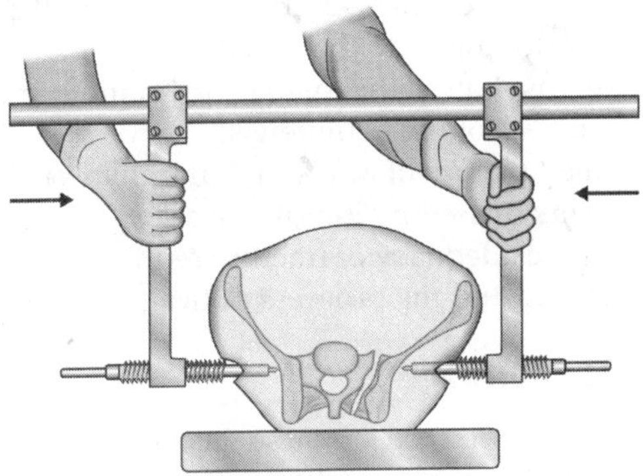

Fig. 27.5: Application of pelvic clamp

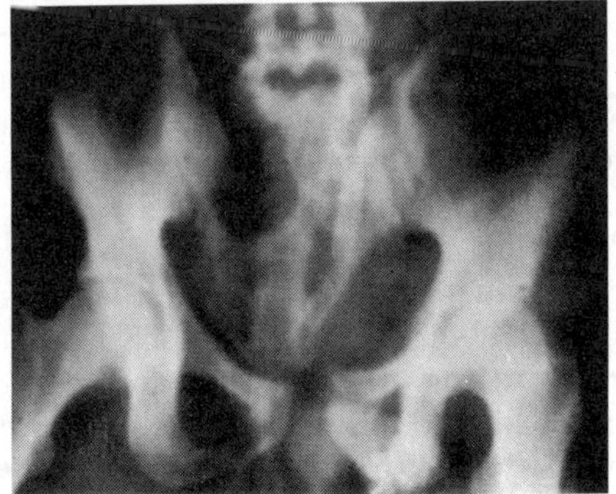

Fig. 27.6: Pubic symphysis disruption

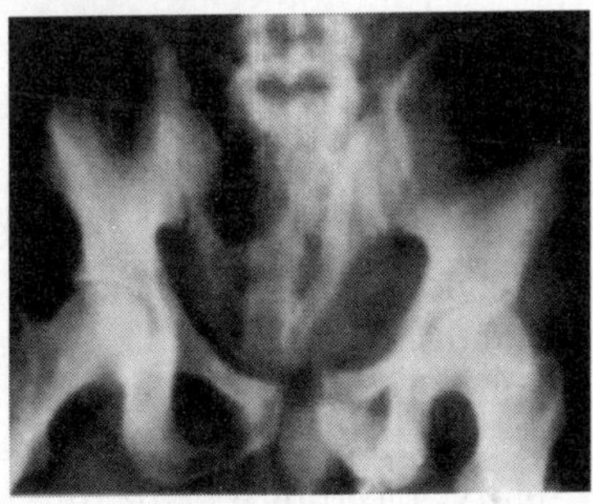

Fig. 27.7: Bilateral pubic rami fracture

a. An unobstructed cross-sectional image of the severity of the posterior injury to the pelvic ring.
b. A clear display of the spatial orientation and planes of displacement of the hemipelvis.
c. A detailed picture of any acetabular involvement.
d. In patients treated by internal fixation, an accurate evaluation of the adequacy of fracture reduction, the placement of implants, and the progress of healing of the fracture.

Associated Hemorrhage

The immediate importance of these injuries lies in their association with significant hemorrhage. The source of bleeding is commonly from the vessels that lie in the post wall of pelvis. In case of an open book injury (AP compression) or a vertical shear injury they tend to get disrupted. In the absence of any other source of bleeding as a cause of hypotension, the presumption of bleeding is from pelvis. Additionally visceral injury can also be a cause of bleeding. If the bleed is arterial in nature, therapeutic embolization or a surgical ligation helps. For a venous bleed surgical control is difficult and not advisable. The insult arising from the shock together with release of inflammatory mediators like interleukin-6, TNF-alpha, neutrophil elastase, etc. may results in systemic inflammatory response syndrome and coagulation failure which may lead to multiple organ system dysfunction or failure. Alternatively there may be singular lack of inflammatory response leading to complete anergy and vulnerability to sepsis and resulting consequences.

Diagnosis

History and details of accidents often suggest fracture pelvis. It should always be presumed to be present in a polytrauma patient with hypovolemic shock till not ruled out. Careful physical examination of the pelvis is mandatory in a case of polytrauma. Palpation of the iliac crests, anterior pubis, along with bilateral inward manual compression of the iliac wings, can elicit findings of underlying injury even in a semiconscious patient. History of lower abdominal injury, bleeding per rectum, inability to pass urine, blood at urinary meatus, distention of abdomen, and clinical signs of hypovolemic shock should raise the suspicion of intra-abdominal visceral injury. Tenderness, guarding in the lower abdomen may be difficult to assess due to fracture pelvis and anterior wall hematoma. Radiological evidence of free gas under the diaphragm may not be forthcoming, and occasionally, intraperitoneal rupture of the bladder does not give rise to signs of peritonism.[8] Rectal examination, sigmoidoscopy, hematocrit, urinary examination, cystogram and diagnostic peritoneal lavage normally clinch the diagnosis. Diagnostic peritoneal lavage should be done above the umbilicus to avoid entering fracture hematoma. Visceral injury should be suspected with Malgaigne and bilateral pubic ramus fracture.[9] A unique rectal injury characteristically results from a run over crush injury from an autopedestrian accident.[10] In these patients the pelvic contents have exploded following a severe compression force. The horrifying picture is pathognomonic. Inevitably there is explosive laceration of the buttocks, sacral areas or thighs. Major arterial disruption is mostly present. The anus is torn lose from skin and the anorectum rides isolated in the infraperitoneal region. Deep bladder, urethral, vaginal lacerations are usual accompaniments.

With fractures of femur pelvic fractures may be missed and in all cases of fracture femur, it is a sound practice to take radiograph of pelvis as a part of the protocol. It also reduces the chance of missing a fracture neck of femur.

Management

Pelvic fracture has been recognized for decades as serious injury associated with high mortality rates.

Factors increasing mortality are:

a. Type of pelvic ring injury (Posterior disruption is associated with higher mortality)
b. High injury severity score
c. Associated injuries (Head and abdominal, 50% mortality)
d. Hemorrhagic shock on admission
e. Open fractures
f. Increased age.

The considerable force that is required to fracture the pelvis also involves other areas of the body resulting in many associated injuries. The severity of injuries to these areas determine the outcome from injury to most patients,[5] unless the patient is clearly bleeding from the pelvis and not from other site, these must take priority over the pelvic fractures.[11] Thus order of priority in fracture pelvis management consist of:

1. Attention to life-threatening hemorrhage
2. Total body evaluation with special emphasis on those injuries directly related to the pelvis
3. Management of fracture pelvis *per se.*

Control of Hemorrhage

Over 60% of hemodynamically unstable pelvic fracture patients can be stabilized by usual basic modalities of resuscitation.[12] Although remaining third of the patients who remain hemodynamically unstable in spite of appropriate resuscitative efforts account for less than 5% of all patients with pelvic fractures (Flow chart 27.1).

In all cases of open book injury, the closure of the ring structure decreases significantly the volume of the retroperitoneum and speeds tamponade. An emergency room application of pelvic binder, belt, clamp; and if nothing else is available a bed sheet held by a towel clip may be life saving (Fig. 27.8).

Flow chart 27.1: Management protocol for hemorrhage

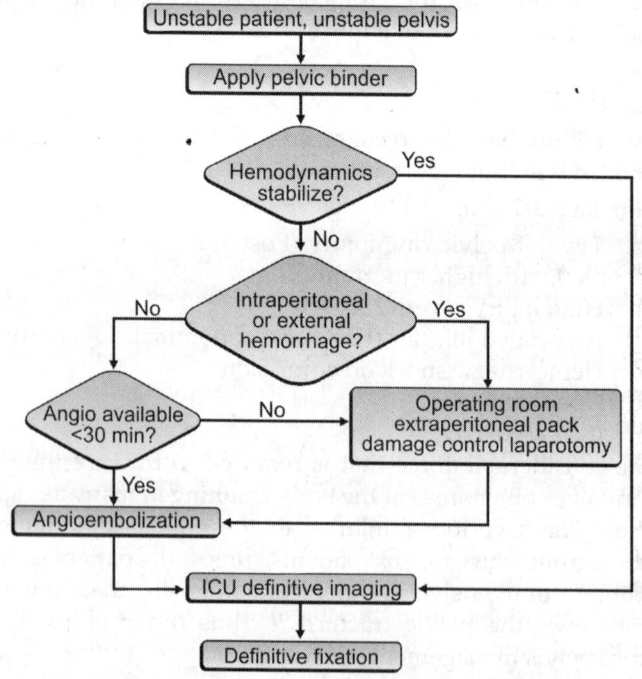

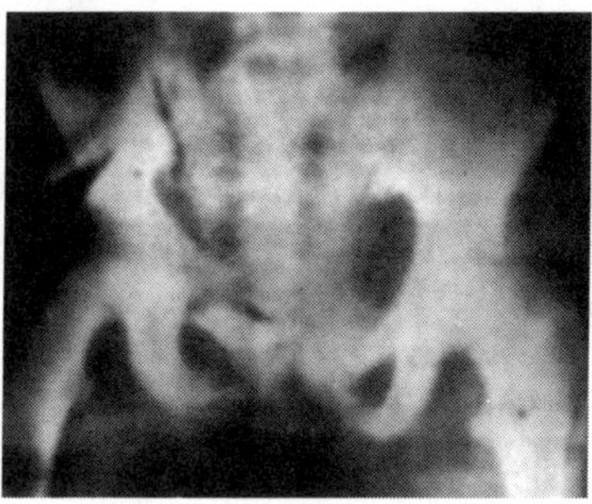

Fig. 27.8: Verticle disruption

Application of external fixation follows. Application of skeletal traction in a vertical shear injury is similarly helpful pending definitive fixation if considered necessary.

If hemorrhage is not controlled after application of the external fixator, it is important to rule out if the pelvic hematoma has freely ruptured into the peritoneal cavity, rapidly expanding, or hemorrhaging freely via an open wound. One should perform diagnostic peritoneal lavage to rule out intraperitoneal bleeding. An open supraumbilical technique is preferred. If free blood is aspirated or grossly bloody lavage fluid returned, exploratory laparotomy takes priority over the pelvic fracture. At surgery, unless direct operative control of pelvic fracture hemorrhage is mandated, evidence of significant ongoing pelvic hemorrhage is best treated by rapidly closing the abdomen and taking the patient from the operative room directly to angiography for localization and embolization of pelvic hemorrhage sites. When pelvic bleeding is demonstrated angiographically, successful embolization can be achieved in nearly all cases with long-term survival in excess of 80%.[12,13] Such results are far superior to the 10-15% survival associated with direct operative attempts at controlling pelvic fracture hemorrhage.[14] In general, angiography should be reserved for hemodynamically unstable pelvic fracture patients requiring more than four or six units of blood and in whom there is clinical evidence of ongoing hemorrhage. In reality, angiography will be indicated in only about 2% of all pelvic fractures.[12,13] Abdominal pelvic packing might be attempted to achieve at least transient control to angiography or, more often, to permit attention to other life-threatening injuries or underlying coagulopathy accepting a second look operation in 24-48 hours if the patient should survive. If angiography is not available, abdominal pelvic packing may be attempted and removed after forty hours when the general condition stabilizes. It is also important to monitor intra-abdominal pressure lest it may result in equivalent of an abdominal compartment syndrome.

If hemorrhage is not controlled with pelvic fixation, embolization, and blood and fluid replacement, mortality usually results.

Management of Associated Injuries

In polytrauma it is important that treatment algorithm are followed so that all members of the team have unified approach and treatment is given in a systemic fashion and one is less likely to miss severe associated injuries. Diagnostic workup for visceral injuries consist of clinical evaluation for signs of peritoneal irritation, per rectal examination, proctoscopy, sigmoidoscopy, X-ray of pelvis, abdomen, chest, ascending urethrogram, catheterization, retrograde cystogram and wash out films of bladder, IVU and DPL. Management of colon injuries is given in Protocol 1, rectal injuries in Protocol 2, and of bladder injuries in Protocol 3.

Open pelvic fractures need special mention. They carry a mortality of about 50%. They may be open outside or into a viscera, e.g. rectum, vagina or bladder. The clue comes from perineal lacerations or by rectal/vaginal examination—spicules from sacral/ramus fractures. Besides usual aggressive treatment if rectal injury is suspected a fecal divertion is essential-will require high placed end colostomy (Fig. 27.9).

Stabilization of Fracture Pelvis

Of late there is an increasing awareness of the requirement of restoring pelvic anatomy in order to achieve better functional results.

Tile has outlined treatment recommendations based on his classification (vide supra) type A fractures are stable and can be treated nonoperatively. For type B1 fractures (anteroposterior compression) he recommends external fixation or anterior plate fixation. Locking compression plate (LCP) offers better fixation than DCP. If laparotomy is required for other injuries, the application of a two hole plate is easier. One should not use internal fixation of the symphysis pubis if a suprapubic catheter is required for bladder disruption because of the risk of secondary

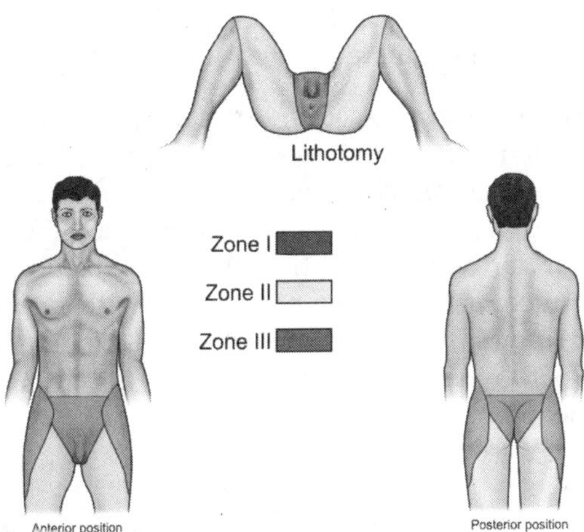

Fig. 27.9: Faringer's classification of wounds in different zones. Zone I injuries often require colostomy, zone II injuries are diverted selectively, with wounds into subcutaneous fat of anterior groin or medial thigh possibly requiring colostomy. Diversion is rarely required for zone III wounds *(For color version, see Plate 7)*

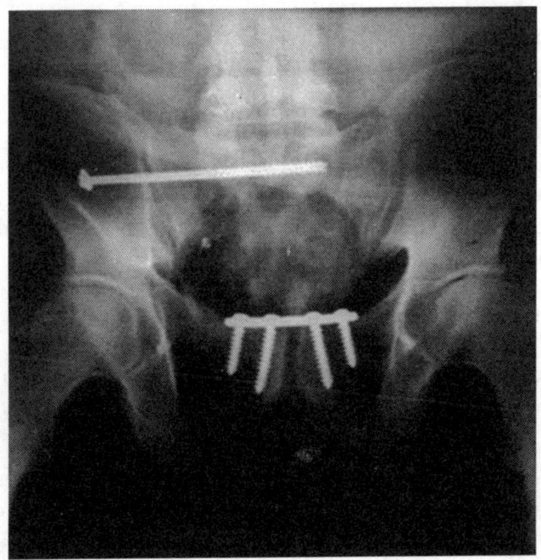

Fig. 27.10: Stabilization—anterior by plate and posterior by iliosacral rod

infection. For lateral compression injuries, usually bed rest is all that is required. If the lateral compression injury is unstable, however, both anterior and posterior stabilization are required. For type C fractures, the anterior ring can be fixed with either an external fixator or an anterior plate for symphysis pubis dislocations or midline fractures.

Posterior stabilization: SI joint instability can be addressed either by iliosacral screws or percutaneous anterior plates applied via ilioinguinal approach (Fig. 27.10). Transsacral instability is addressed by transsacral plate or sacral bars. For iliac wing fractures, standard open reduction and plate fixation techniques are used. Functional outcome of patients with unstable pelvic ring fractures stabilized with open reduction and internal fixation resulted in 62% returning to full work and 14% returned to job with modification.

REFERENCES

1. Johnston R. In Critical Decision in Trauma. (Eds.), Moore E, Eiseman S, Vanway III CW: St Louis, CV Mosby Co, 1984;238.
2. Melton LJ, Sampson JM, et al. Epidemiologic features of pelvic fractures. Clin Orthop 1981;155:43.
3. Siegel JH, Dalal SA, Burges AR, et al. Pattern of organ injuries and their implications for survival and death as a function of the direction and magnitude of impact forces in motor vehicle injuries. Presented at 33rd annual proceedings. AAAM, October2-4, 1989.
4. Watson-Jones R. Dislocation and fracture-dislocations of the pelvis. Br J Surg 1938;25:773-81.
5. Trunkey DD, Chapman MW, Lim RC Jr, et al. Management of pelvic fractures in blunt trauma injury. J Trauma 1974;14:912-23.
6. Pennal GF, Tile M, Waddell JP, et al. Pelvic disruption assessment and classification. Clin Orthop 1980;151:115-23.
7. Tile M. Pelvic ring fractures: Should they be fixed? J Bone Joint Surg 1988;70-B:1-12.
8. Bourdian GV, Jindal SL, Gilles RR, et al. Urinary ascites secondary to retroperitoneal fistula. Urol 1974;6:209.
9. Murr PC, et al. Abdominal trauma associated with pelvic fracture. J Trauma 1980;20:919.
10. Mwull KI, Sachatellow CR, Ernest CB. The deep perineal laceration, an injury frequently associated with open pelvic fractures, a need for aggressive surgical management. J Trauma 1977;17:685.
11. Poole GV, Ward EF, Mukkasa FF, et al. Pelvic fracture from major blunt trauma. Ann Surg 1991;213:532.
12. Mucha P Jr, Farnell MB. Analysis of pelvic fracture management. J Trauma 1984;24:379.
13. Mucha P Jr, Welch TJ. Haemorrhage in major pelvic fractures. Surg Clin North Am 1988;68:757.
14. Ravich MM. Hypogastric artery ligation in acute pelvic trauma. Surg 1964;56:601.

Chapter 28

Pediatric Trauma

M Arora

Traumatic injuries are the cause of more than half the deaths among children aged 1 to 14 years and are the second leading cause of emergency room visits after infections. The effects of trauma are different in children in comparison to adults. Blunt trauma accounts for more than 60% of childhood injuries. Head trauma is most common, but the most severely injured children have multisystem injuries. The smaller size of children results in the trauma forces affecting larger regions of the body. Multi-system injuries are thus more common in children. The internal organs of the child are more susceptible to injuries because of the limited amounts of protective muscle and subcutaneous tissue in the body. The increased flexibility and resilience of the pediatric skeleton and connective tissue allows external forces to be transmitted to deeper internal structures more readily than in adults. Hence in children, absence of external signs of injury does not rule out internal injuries. Careful investigation of pediatric trauma victims is advocated in all cases. In penetrating trauma increased numbers of organs are involved in children and surgical intervention becomes mandatory in a majority of cases. The most commonly injured organs are spleen and liver. In children even the response to injury differs from that of the adult, and specific patterns are seen with blunt injury; recognition of these patterns is essential for proper management.

EPIDEMIOLOGY

Several factors influence childhood injuries, including age, sex, behavior, and environment. Of these, age and sex are the most important factors affecting the patterns of injury. Male children younger than 18 years have higher injury and mortality rates, perhaps in part because of their more aggressive behavior and exposure to contact sports. In the infant and toddler age group, falls are a common cause of severe injury, whereas bicycle-related mishaps, with or without the interaction of motor vehicles, are the main culprits for injury of older children and adolescents. Use of helmets results in fewer head injuries and decreases the severity of them as well. Tragically, the home environment is the next most common scene of pediatric injury. Approximately 35% of significant injuries occur as the result of accidents in the very environment that should be the most sheltering and nurturing to children.

Most pediatric trauma occurs as a result of blunt trauma, with penetrating injury accounting for 10-20% of all pediatric trauma admissions at most centers. A rising incidence of pediatric penetrating trauma, particularly penetrating thoracic trauma, has occurred in recent years.

Developmental milestones correlate with mechanisms of childhood injuries. Head injuries, either alone or in association with multiple system injuries, are the most severe and cause the most deaths. Head injuries also account for most disability in children. All factors considered, clinicians must become aware of the anatomic and physiologic characteristics that make children unique.

Furthermore, traumatic injury in children dramatically affects the economy because of expenses for medical care and rehabilitation and costs related to the inability of the children to function independently in society. Therefore, injury prevention should be a priority for everyone.

SPECIFIC INJURIES

Central Nervous System Injuries

Pediatric head trauma is common and is the leading cause of death in injured children. Unlike adults who suffer focal injuries, children are more likely to have diffuse injury. As a result, they are prone to elevations in intracranial pressure. The goal in children with head injuries is to reduce intracranial pressure and maintain cerebral perfusion pressure.

Among children, the central nervous system (CNS) is the most commonly injured isolated system. Because CNS injury is the leading cause of death among injured children, it is the principal determinant of outcome. However, numerous observations have shown that patients from the pediatric population recover more frequently and more fully than similarly injured adults. Although this might be euphemistically ascribed to the "physiologic reserve" of the child, it suggests that injured children respond exceedingly well to preservation of cerebral oxygenation and perfusion. Therefore, management of the whole patient must focus on preservation of cerebral perfusion and elimination of potential detrimental effects of extracranial lesions to it.

In children aged 2 years or younger, physical abuse is the most common cause of serious head injury. Shaken baby syndrome (SBS) is characterized by retinal hemorrhage, subdural or subarachnoid hemorrhage, and little evidence of external trauma. In children aged 3 years and older, falls and motor vehicle, bicycle, and pedestrian accidents are responsible for most traumatic brain injuries.

Children tend to sustain injuries that produce diffuse edema rather than those that cause focal space-occupying lesions. For this reason, severely injured children who undergo early computed tomography (CT) scanning may have minimal radiologic evidence of parenchyma injury. Follow-up studies may reveal much worse injury. Magnetic resonance imaging (MRI) may reveal obscuring of the gray and white matter junction in the setting of cerebral edema. At this point, precise management makes the difference between disaster and success. Judicious fluid resuscitation, precise ventilatory care, and careful titration of cerebral perfusion pressure are the keys to success.

The Glasgow coma scale (GCS) score is the universal tool for the rapid assessment of the consciousness level of injured children. A modified verbal and motor version has been developed to aid in the evaluation of consciousness level in infants and young children. The GCS score and its modified version (with scores of 3-15) are based on children's best response in 3 areas: (1) motor activity, (2) verbal response, and (3) eye opening. Traumatic brain injury in children is classified as mild (GCS 13-15), moderate (GCS 9-12), or severe (GCS 3-8). Regardless of the GCS score, a head CT scan should be performed on any child with a history of trauma and loss of consciousness longer than 5 minutes or an altered level of consciousness.

Several factors predict mortality with head injury. A presenting GCS score of less than 8, unilateral dilated pupil, and transcranial missile injury are associated with mortality of almost 70-98%. Hypotension and hypoxia should be aggressively avoided and are known to produce secondary injury. This secondary injury, when present, is a substantial cause of morbidity, and aggressive protocols to prevent it should be in place.

Metabolic Demand

Metabolic studies of children with multiple injuries and severe CNS trauma suggest that total body metabolic demand is significantly elevated; therefore, controlling seizures and fever is of utmost importance because both significantly increase metabolic demands of the brain. Initiation of good nutritional support within hours of definitive stabilization to meet the needs of increased metabolism and oxygen consumption is important. Enteric feeding is preferred.

Mild Head Injury

A concussion is defined by the American Academy of Neurology as "trauma-induced alteration in mental status that may or may not involve loss of consciousness."

Children with a mild head injury (GCS 14-15) with a history of transient loss of consciousness or amnesia of the events and normal findings on a head CT scan can be discharged and observed at home after at least 6 hours of uneventful observation in the emergency department. Caretakers should be provided with specific discharge instructions. The discharge instructions should include neurological consultation if the child complains of constellation of headaches, memory loss, behavior disturbances, and impaired concentration. A prompt re-evaluation and possibly a repeat head CT/MRI scan are in order.

The post-concussive symptoms can last up to months after the injury but only rarely extend beyond 3 months. No specific treatment exists for these symptoms other than symptomatic support; however, with severe mood alteration, psychiatric treatment may be indicated.

Determining which pediatric patients with mild head injury need neuroimaging studies has been difficult. It has been reported that less than 5% of children with mild head injury have CT findings indicative of traumatic brain injury. The concern for limiting radiation exposure has led to scrutiny of this practice. A meta-analysis of 16 studies, including over 20,000 children with mild head injury, defined associated risk factors for traumatic brain injury. Skull fracture, focal neurologic signs, GCS less than 15, and loss of consciousness were all associated with traumatic brain injury. Headache and vomiting were not associated with traumatic brain injury with a presentation of mild head injury.

The very young child (<2 years) with mild head injury is perhaps the most difficult evaluation. The limitations of the neurologic examination often present a decision-making dilemma as to the appropriate imaging studies. The key point to remember in this evaluation is that a higher index of suspicion is required in a young child as compared with an older child because there is a higher incidence of skull fracture and traumatic brain injury in a child younger than 2 years after mild head injury. Up to 30% of children younger than 2 years with a skull fracture may have traumatic brain injury demonstrable on CT scan.

Severe Head Injury

The goal of initial resuscitation must be to limit or prevent secondary brain injury by maximizing cerebral perfusion and oxygen delivery while minimizing increased intracranial pressure (ICP). Hypoxia and hypotension should be aggressively treated. ICP monitoring is recommended in infants and children with a GCS score of 8 or less. Epidural hematoma occurs in about 2% of pediatric head trauma admissions. The characteristic lucid interval occurs in about 33%. A biconcave hyperdense lesion is seen on CT scan. Lesions associated with neurologic symptoms or mass effect should be evacuated. Intracranial hypertension can occur with open cranial sutures and does not alter this recommendation. Ventriculostomy catheters offer the benefit of allowing therapeutic cerebrospinal fluid (CSF) drainage.

An age dependent spectrum exists for cerebral perfusion pressure (CPP); in general, the CPP should be maintained above 40 mm Hg. CPP is the difference between mean arterial pressure (MAP) and ICP. ICP should be kept at less than 20 mm Hg. CPP is a predictor of outcome in pediatric severe head injury; however, whether this trend represents a marker of injury or a value that can alter the disease course is unclear. Current treatment of elevated ICP includes CSF drainage, sedation, neuromuscular blockade, mannitol, and hypertonic saline. Enthusiasm for hyperventilation therapy has waned with the finding of hypocapnic induced vasoconstriction further compromising cerebral blood flow. The only recommended role for hyperventilation is in the setting of acute herniation, to briefly assist, while definitive measures are being pursued. Another second tier therapy is hypothermia, which seems to be more efficacious in younger patients with traumatic brain injury.

Elevated ICP that is refractory to medical treatment may ultimately require decompressive craniectomy. The rationale for this treatment is founded on the Monro-Kellie doctrine, which allows for a stable intracranial volume via shifts in the amount of CSF, blood, or brain tissue. The Monro-Kellie doctrine defines ICP as a function of the relative composition of the 3 intracranial occupants: brain parenchyma, CSF, and blood. Decompressive craniectomy reduces the risk of death and unfavorable outcomes when maximal medical therapy fails to control ICP. Similar conclusions cannot be drawn from data on adults. Predictors of outcome after traumatic brain injury in the pediatric population have been noted to include initial GCS, pupillary reaction, and severity of findings on initial head CT scan.

Prospective data is limited in pediatric traumatic brain injury. One randomized trial of patients younger than 18 years examined 27 traumatic brain injuries. Findings supported improved outcome and less mortality with decompressive craniectomy in the pediatric population with refractory intracranial hypertension. Post-traumatic seizures may occur in up to 30%, and a lower GCS score portends a higher risk. There is insufficient data on prophylactic treatment in the pediatric population. When present, seizures should be treated to decrease metabolic demand and elevation of ICP that may extend an insult.

Adult literature supports the view that ICP management is more important than an absolute CPP threshold. The Lund concept–guided therapy has been validated in several clinical trails, in which this method of management improves outcomes and decreases mortality. It is designed as a treatment of vasogenic edema. This concept believes that systemic hypertension, in the setting of pathophysiology that may disrupt the blood-brain barrier and its autoregulation, increases intracapillary hydrostatic pressure, leading to accumulation of intracerebral water content. Thus, the emphasis is shifted to volume-targeted therapy, with judicious use of antihypertensive therapy to maintain normotension, in conjunction with aggressive maintenance of normovolemia.

The primary interventions used in the Lund concept–guided therapy are aggressive maintenance of normovolemia and reduction in ICP via manipulation of systemic arterial pressure. The Lund concept–guided therapy accepts a CPP of 40 mm Hg, in accordance with current pediatric guidelines. A recent review of the Lund concept–guided therapy toward children with severe traumatic brain injury by Whalstrom et al demonstrated favorable outcomes in 80% of patients and a survival rate of 93%. The treatment goals were as follows: ICP less than 20 mm Hg, CPP greater than 40 mm Hg, normovolemia, normotension, normoventilation, and sedation as needed. Albumin and packed red blood cell transfusion were used to promote colloid osmotic pressure and to ensure adequate cerebral oxygenation. Larger prospective trials are needed to validate this therapy.

Spinal Cord Injury

Although spinal cord injury is relatively uncommon in the pediatric population, cervical spine injury must be presumed until proven otherwise. The most common cause of spinal cord injury (SCI) in the pediatric population is motor vehicle collision, accounting for about 40%. The common cervical fracture usually involves the first 2 vertebrae. If it remains undetected, cervical fracture can result in devastating injuries. Other common spinal fractures among pediatric patients with trauma are compression fractures and flexion-distraction (Chance) fractures of the lumbar spine, usually from inappropriate use of a lap seat belt. Cervical spine injury is a rare event in children, but if it's unrecognized, it can lead to severe morbidity. Therefore, keep the child immobilized until the appropriate radiographs are evaluated.

Spinal cord injury without radiologic abnormality (SCIWORA) syndrome is a problem unique to the pediatric population. SCIWORA has been reported in 10-20% of children with SCI. The incompletely calcified vertebral column of the child may transiently deform and allow stretching of the cord or nerve roots with no residual anatomic evidence of injury. The hallmark of this syndrome is documented neurologic deficit that may have changed or resolved by the time the child has arrived in the emergency department. Immediate re-injury of the same area may produce permanent disability, so thorough neurosurgical evaluation is essential whenever reliable evidence of even a transient neurologic deficit is present.

MRI evaluation of SCIWORA is important in determining a prognosis but is not useful in determining stability of the spine. Radiologic evaluation should consider normal variants, such as C2-C3 pseudosubluxation occurring in 9% of children up to age 7 years. This is due to the elastic nature of the pediatric spine in that the ligaments and joint capsule can stretch without tearing. The pediatric spine hypermobility accounts for the SCIWORA syndrome being unique in the pediatric population.

Controversy exists regarding the use of methylprednisolone for children with SCI. They are not indicated for penetrating SCI.

Neck Injuries

There are three horizontal zones of the neck for classification of injury location. Zone 1 extends from the sternal notch to the cricoid cartilage. Zone 2 extends from the cricoid cartilage to the angle of the mandible. Zone 3 extends from the angle of the mandible to the skull base. Early airway control is paramount. Gross laryngotracheal injury, stridor, pulsatile bleeding, or expanding hematoma requires urgent operative treatment. In the absence of hemoptysis, hematemesis, dysphagia, subcutaneous emphysema, or the aforementioned urgent criteria, Zone 2 injury has been observed with success. Angiography, endoscopy, and bronchoscopy are useful for a complete examination. Missed esophageal injury can be greatly minimized by endoscopy, esophagram, and careful physical examination. Critical examination and the judicious use of ancillary studies is the cornerstone of successful result in neck injuries.

Oropharyngeal injury represents a complex array of injury, and most are due to falls in the pediatric population. The generous blood supply to this area usually leads to excellent healing but also can result in copious bleeding from wounds. Laceration of the lip or the tongue is usually treated with primary repair with non-absorbable sutures for the tongue and absorbable sutures for the lip. For optimal cosmesis, close attention should be given to approximation of the vermillion border of the lip. Recommendations vary for repair of a tongue laceration, but deformity from a significant, deep laceration should be prevented. Silk sutures are preferred for suturing tongue lacerations. Superficial facial laceration is treated with absorbable fine sutures and should be removed in 5-7 days to minimize scarring.

Suspected injury to the parotid region should be evaluated with close attention to facial nerve function and ductal laceration. General wound care principles with irrigation and removal of foreign debris will suffice for most wounds in this region.

Thoracic Injuries

A child can have significant injury to the chest cavity even when external signs are absent. If rib fractures are present, significant trauma has occurred. In addition to the life-threatening injuries as tension pneumothorax and pericardial tamponade, other serious injuries are likely, such as an open pneumothorax from a penetrating wound to the chest. If the thoracic wall wound is larger than 2/3 the diameter of the trachea, adequate ventilation cannot occur because air preferentially exits the wound, the path of least resistance. Close the wound temporarily with a flutter-type of dressing secured on three sides. When the child breathes in, the dressing is sucked in and occludes. When the child exhales, the air can exit and a tension pneumothorax is prevented. In addition, a massive hemothorax can occur and is usually the result of injury to the great vessels or heart. Evacuation of blood using a tube thoracostomy is a short-term measure; a significant portion of these children will require surgical intervention. If multiple ribs are fractured, a flail chest may occur and you see paradoxical respiratory motion. In addition to the external trauma seen in these children, there is usually significant pulmonary contusion that contributes to hypoxia. Supplemental oxygen, chest physiotherapy and adequate pain control are mandatory in the management of these children.

Thoracic injury is the second leading cause of death in pediatric trauma. Thoracic injury occurs in about 5% of children hospitalized for trauma. Blunt trauma, particularly from MVAs, is responsible for most thoracic injuries. Not surprisingly, isolated thoracic injuries seen commonly in adults are relatively uncommon in children. The pediatric thorax has a greater cartilage content and incomplete ossification of the ribs. Due to the pliability of the pediatric rib cage and mediastinal mobility, significant intrathoracic injury may exist in the absence of external signs of trauma. Pulmonary contusion and pneumothorax are frequently present without rib fractures. Pulmonary contusion, pneumothorax, and rib fractures are the most common injuries. Hemothorax and pneumothorax are the most common thoracic injuries from penetrating trauma.

Chest exploration is indicated for an immediate return of 20% of the patient's estimated blood volume or a continued output of 2 ml/kg/h. Intercostal artery bleeding is commonly found in this setting. Helical chest CT scan can identify these injuries and may identify unsuspected injuries in up to 15% of children with normal chest X-ray film results. Physical examination of the traumatized pediatric thorax is notoriously unreliable and requires careful assessment.

Unfortunately, because of the variety of criteria used to diagnose pulmonary contusion and concomitant aspiration of gastric content in pediatric trauma, any radiographic evidence of pulmonary parenchymal injury must be treated aggressively to ensure adequate oxygenation and ventilation. Assessment of adequate ventilation can be determined with arterial blood gas (ABG) analysis and pulse oximetry. Approximately 90% of blunt pediatric thoracic injuries can be managed conservatively or with tube thoracostomy. Severe pulmonary injury may require mechanical ventilation. Epidural catheter may be useful to provide adequate analgesia while avoiding excessive sedation.

Over half of rib fractures in children younger than 3 years may be due to child abuse. Pain control and aggressive pulmonary toilet are the mainstays of treatment of rib fractures. Fixation of flail segments is rarely required. With pulmonary contusion, progressive inflammation may lead to edema, atelectasis, and consolidation. Hypoxemia, hypercarbia, and tachypnea may result. Radiographic findings are variable in appearance and time course. The initial chest X-ray film result is abnormal in up to 70% of patients, but a normal chest X-ray film result does not exclude the diagnosis. Most respond to supportive treatment and heal in 7-10 days.

Parenchymal cavitation from blunt trauma may cause pneumatocele. They may become infected or expand requiring surgical intervention, while most resolve slowly. Pulmonary laceration can be a source of persistent bleeding and air leak. Tube thoracostomy allows small lacerations to seal spontaneously, while larger lacerations require surgical treatment. Tracheobronchial injury usually occurs near the carina and is thought to stem from anteroposterior compression of the pliable pediatric chest. Multiple findings may be present including pneumothorax, hemothorax, pneumomediastinum, subcutaneous emphysema, and hemorrhage. Persistent air leak is common. If the injury involves less than one-third of the diameter of the bronchus, nonoperative therapy may be suitable; otherwise, most require open repair.

Great vessel injury is rare. The diagnosis is suggested by a finding of widened mediastinum on plain film. Most thoracic aortic injury occurs via blunt mechanism (e.g. MVA, pedestrian, falls), in older children (mean age, 12 years), and at the ligamentum arteriosum (77-90%). This injury is highly morbid and requires rapid diagnosis and treatment. Preoperative blunt aortic injury management should include aggressive blood pressure control with beta blockade. Blunt cardiac injury is rare in children. Traumatic cardiac rupture is uniformly fatal. Traumatic cardiac contusion may result in arrhythmia, myocardial hypokinesis, and abnormal cardiac serum enzymes.

Traumatic diaphragmatic rupture occurs in about 1% of children with blunt chest trauma, with left-sided rupture being more common. Diagnosis is suggested with passage of a nasogastric tube noted to be in the chest on plain film. Laceration to the heart can be repaired with pledgeted 3-0 or 4-0 non-absorbable monofilament sutures. Respiratory embarrassment from herniation of viscera into the thorax is commonly found. Early diagnosis usually results in repair via abdominal approach. Esophageal perforation from blunt trauma is rare in children. Primary repair is indicated if the perforation is diagnosed early. Evaluation with contrast esophagram and esophagoscopy is recommended.

Traumatic Asphyxia

Traumatic asphyxia is a unique injury in pediatric trauma because of the compliance of the chest wall. This injury is commonly the result of blunt compressing thoracic trauma, with sudden airway obstruction and abrupt retrograde high pressure in the superior vena cava. Patients with traumatic asphyxia have a dramatic physical presentation characterized by cervical and facial petechial hemorrhages or cyanosis associated with vascular engorgement and subconjunctival hemorrhage. Despite its dramatic presentation, this injury has a good prognosis. CNS injuries, pulmonary contusions, and intra-abdominal injuries are common associated injuries.

Abdominal Injuries

Unstable vital signs after proper resuscitation and evaluation of the thoracic cavity can be a sign of significant intra-abdominal or pelvic injury. Assess stable patients for tenderness or distention of the abdomen. If you suspect any injury, the choice for evaluation is the CT. Anatomical differences in children make them more vulnerable to major abdominal injuries with very minor forces. In children, the abdomen begins at the level of the nipple. Children's small, pliable rib cages and undeveloped abdominal muscles provide little protection of major organs. Solid organs (spleen, liver, kidneys) are vulnerable to injury.

Abdominal Wall Bruising

Bruising of the abdominal wall after a motor vehicle collision is an important finding. This is usually the result of a lap seat belt or a restraint device. A seat belt syndrome has been described as the concurrent findings of abdominal wall bruising, intra-abdominal injury, and vertebral fracture. The finding of fluid in the abdomen on CT scan without associated solid organ injury should raise suspicion for bowel injury. The most common intra-abdominal injury associated with abdominal wall bruising is a hollow viscus. In the setting of abdominal wall bruising and unexplained fluid in the abdomen, serial abdominal examination and further investigation are indicated.

Vertebral fracture is also highly associated with abdominal wall bruising and may be present in up to 50% of patients.

Gastric Injuries

The great majority of abdominal injuries are secondary to blunt trauma, and blunt injuries to the stomach occur more frequently in children than in adults. The injury is usually a blowout or perforation of the greater curvature. Children who are struck by a vehicle or who fall across bicycle handlebars shortly after eating a meal are at greater risk. Consider injury to the stomach if the child has peritoneal signs and/or bloody nasogastric drainage. Abdominal X-ray films may show pneumoperitoneum.

Penetrating Duodenal Injuries

These injuries are relatively uncommon in children compared to adults. Most pediatric duodenal injuries, such as intramural duodenal hematoma, are from blunt trauma and are often associated with child abuse. Hyperextension injuries of the spine can also lead to duodenal injuries. The diagnosis of intramural duodenal hematoma may be suggested by a coiled-spring appearance on contrast imaging. Other culprits include falls or mishaps with bicycles or go-carts.

Small Intestinal Injury

The most common intra-abdominal organs injured in restrained children involved in MVAs are hollow viscus type. Several mechanisms have been proposed for this type of injury. Rapid deceleration may cause the lap belt to compress the intestines against the spine. An increase in intraluminal pressure may lead to rupture or tear. This is the most common mechanism of injury to the pediatric duodenum. Duodenal hematoma may result and cause obstruction. Luminal stricture may present several weeks after blunt intestinal injury as persistent nausea and bilious emesis. Mesenteric hematoma or rent is also possible.

The incidence of intestinal injury in children with blunt trauma is estimated to be 1-15%. In comparison, colon injury from blunt trauma is rare. The small intestinal injury in children occurs in the areas of fixation at the ligament of Treitz (most common site of the intestinal tract to be injured) or at the ileocecal valve. Such injury occurs in association with lap seat belt use or rapid deceleration. Up to 50% of children with lap seat belt injuries have associated retroperitoneal injuries. Associated injuries, such as flexion-distraction lumbar spine injury, may also occur. Penetrating intestinal injury presents unique diagnostic and therapeutic challenges. If the peritoneum has been violated by such an injury, exploratory laparotomy is recommended.

With blunt or penetrating abdominal trauma, a high index of suspicion should be maintained for small intestine injury, because a delay in diagnosis or an unrecognized injury can result in substantial morbidity. Fewer than 50% of children with blunt intestinal perforation have peritonitis on initial examination. Abdominal tenderness is a consistent finding. Pneumoperitoneum or contrast extralumination on imaging study should prompt exploration. Close observation and serial examinations should guide unclear findings.

Rectal Injuries

Except for the occasional straddle injury, child abuse or deviant sexual activity causes most isolated rectal injuries in children. Examine rectal injuries while the patient is under anesthesia because tissues are frequently painful. Examination under anesthesia also decreases the psychologic trauma of such an invasive examination. Rectal mucosal or superficial anal injuries usually resolve with conservative treatment, but full-thickness injuries or internal sphincteric injury may require surgical repair. If the injury involves full thickness of the rectal wall covering colostomy should always be an option to optimize surgical repair. If child abuse is a possibility, the appropriate agency should be informed.

Solid Organ Injury Management

Nonoperative management is considered the standard of care for most children with blunt solid organ injury who are clinically stable. This approach was pioneered in children and has led to a dramatic change in practice in adult patients regarding management of solid organ injury. The overall incidence of nonoperative management failure is 5%. The reasons for nonoperative management failure are shock, peritonitis, persistent hemorrhage, pancreatic injury, hollow viscus injury, and ruptured diaphragm. A significantly increased risk of failure is associated with bicycle-related mechanism of injury, isolated pancreatic injury, and isolated grade 5 injury. Multiple solid organ injuries were associated with a higher risk of failure as well.

There is importance of early vigilance in the care of the child with a solid organ injury. Those who will fail nonoperative management will likely do so early, within the first 12 hours. An important fact is that pancreatic injuries do not behave like other injured solid organs and are associated with a higher need for operative intervention. A key distinction between adult and pediatric nonoperative management of solid organ injury is that adults are more prone to late failure (e.g. >5 d), whereas 98% of pediatric failure is within 72 hours.

For isolated liver or spleen injury, current recommendations for length of stay and observation are per the American Pediatric Surgical Association (APSA). These recommendations are based on CT grade of injury. For grade 1 injury, no ICU stay, 2 total hospital days, and 3 weeks activity restriction. For grade 2 injury, no ICU stay, 3 total hospital days, and 4 weeks activity restriction. For grade 3 injury, no ICU stay, 4 total hospital days, and 5 weeks activity restriction. For grade 4 injury, 1 day of ICU stay, 5 total hospital days, and 6 weeks of activity restriction. These guidelines have been prospectively evaluated and demonstrate significant reduction in length of stay without adverse sequelae.

Splenic Injuries

Splenic injuries are relatively common in pediatric trauma. Successful conservative management of splenic injury was reported in 1968 by Upadhyaya et al. Because of the risk of overwhelming sepsis following splenectomy (OPSS), the current philosophy is to manage splenic injuries conservatively unless the spleen is hemodynamically compromised. OPSS occurs slightly more frequently after splenectomy in the treatment of hematologic disease compared with the lower incidence after traumatic splenectomy. Age younger than 5 years at the time of splenectomy also increases the risk.

A child's spleen stops bleeding spontaneously; therefore, most patients with splenic injuries respond to nonoperative management. Perform CT scanning, ultrasound, or isotope imaging to define the site and the extent of injury in every child with splenic injury. Conservative treatment can be used, provided the child is in a pediatric intensive care unit for at least 48 hours, with an experienced surgical team who are prepared to intervene if needed, and adequate anesthesia and transfusion services are immediately available. In adults, the presence of a splenic arterial blush is a risk factor for failure of nonoperative management. Contrast blush is rare in children; its presence does not predict nonoperative treatment failure. A role for splenic artery embolization in the management of pediatric splenic injury has yet to be clarified.

Hepatic Injury

Isolated hepatic injury, without disruption of the portal vein, hepatic vein, or suprarenal inferior vena cava, behaves clinically like a splenic injury. Most patients with these injuries respond to nonoperative management. The same criteria for selecting nonoperative or operative treatment for patients with splenic injury are now being selectively used for patients with documented hepatic injuries. The success rate for nonoperative management of blunt hepatic injury is about 85-90%. The exception, of course, is for children with a massive hepatic injury or with perihepatic vascular involvement who are not hemodynamically stable and transfusion requirements of greater than 25-40 ml/kg/d.

The definition of the degree of hepatic injury from CT scan evaluation provides important prognostic information regarding the potential for complications, such as hematobilia or delayed rupture, as well as an indication of the expected speed of recovery. Delayed bleeding after liver injury may occur in 1-3%, and mortality from this injury has been reported as high as 18%. Delayed bleeding has been reported from 3 days to 6 weeks after injury. Hemodynamic instability should prompt surgical treatment; however, a role for angiographic embolization may exist.

Combined hepatosplenic injury occurs in 2.9% of children having sustained blunt abdominal injury. Mortality rate for isolated splenic injury was the lowest at 0.7%, followed by isolated hepatic injury at 2.5%, and hepatosplenic injury was the highest at 8.6%. Most deaths (89%) occurred during the first 48 hours after injury. Hemorrhage was the most common cause of death for each group. Clearly, combined hepatosplenic injury portends a higher risk and requires vigilance.

Pancreatic Injury

Blunt trauma causes most pancreatic injuries. A frequently cited mechanism involves falling into bicycle handlebars.

CT scanning is a useful diagnostic modality in evaluating most pancreatic trauma. It is insufficient to evaluate pancreatic ductal injury. Operative exploration may be required to fully evaluate pancreatic injury. Endoscopic retrograde pancreatography (ERP) can reliably evaluate pancreatic duct injury. A few reports have described using this technique to provide definitive treatment of pediatric blunt injury associated pancreatic ductal injury with ERP and stent placement. In most cases, diagnosis of pancreatic injury is suggested by an elevated amylase level. However, the amylase level has been demonstrated to be neither sensitive nor specific in the evaluation of pancreatic trauma. In the setting of major pancreatic ductal injury, the serum amylase level is usually elevated significantly. With severe ductal injury or pancreatic transaction, distal pancreatectomy is indicated.

Timely diagnosis of major pancreatic injuries and prompt surgical treatment are essential to decrease mortality and morbidity rates in pediatric patients.

Renal Injury

Blunt abdominal trauma involves renal injury in 10-20% of cases. Renal trauma comprises 1.6% of total injuries, and 90% of these injuries are from a blunt mechanism of injury. The pediatric kidney is more susceptible to blunt injury due to the relative lack of perirenal fat and decreased protection from incompletely ossified ribs. Contusion is the most common renal injury encountered in children. Disruption of the ureteropelvic junction from transient axial torsion and parenchymal injury due to pre-existing renal abnormalities are the next most common renal injuries. These lesions are commonly associated with direct blows to the back or flank.

The concept of nonoperative management has been expanded to include renal injuries as well. Conservative management is standard for low-grade renal injury (grades I-III). A treatment strategy adopted by some level I trauma centers includes bed rest for 24 hours, serial hematocrit, heart rate monitoring, and frequent physical examinations.

Management of high-grade renal injury is more controversial (grades IV-V). Absolute indications for renal exploration are an expanding or pulsatile renal hematoma. Relative indications include urinary extravasation, nonviable tissue, arterial injury, and the need for complete staging. The presence or absence of hematuria and the amount thereof do not correlate with the severity of renal injury. A recent experience reported by Rogers et al demonstrated successful management of most grade IV injuries with a blunt mechanism. Management consisted of bed rest, catheter drainage, and documentation of the resolution of extravasation or urine leak via CT scan or ultrasound. A trial of ureteral stenting and catheter drainage should be used for urinary extravasation or renal fracture. All grade V injuries required operative management and only 30% achieved long-term renal salvage.

Vascular Injuries

Vascular injuries in children require early diagnosis and aggressive operative management to prevent serious sequelae. An injury to a major artery in a child's extremity can result in ischemia and growth retardation of that limb if not detected in a timely manner.

Most vascular injury is associated with orthopedic injuries, such as supracondylar fracture or long-bone fracture. The presence of hard signs mandates operative exploration and repair. These signs are pulsatile bleeding, expanding hematoma, absent pulses, cold limb, and bruit/thrill. If a vascular injury is thought to be present, objective studies (Doppler studies, arteriography) may be required. The most important differential diagnosis in pediatric vascular trauma is between thrombosis and spasm of the injured vessel. Spasm usually lasts less than 3 hours. When the pulses remain absent longer than 6 hours, thrombosis or transection of the vessel must be excluded. A delay in diagnosing vascular injury could lead to prolonged ischemia, compartment syndrome, and Volkmann contractures, with consequent long-term disability.

Penetrating Injuries

The lethality of penetrating injuries is about 3 times that of blunt injury. Several factors having prognostic value have been identified. An arrival systolic blood pressure of less than 90 mm Hg and an initial core temperature of less than 34°C correlate with mortality of penetrating trauma patients. Impalement injuries are uncommon, and the recommendation is to leave them in place until they can be removed in the operating room because of the potential for hemorrhage. All potential gunshot wounds should be marked with radiopaque clips to allow estimation of trajectory on imaging study. The current trend is in preference of the primary repair of colon injuries.

Orthopedic Injuries

Approximately 30-45% of children with trauma have multiple injuries and at least 1 skeletal fracture. Careful evaluation of every extremity is essential, and the possibility of deformity or associated fracture must be excluded. Splint fractured limbs effectively to prevent ongoing hemorrhage and to reduce occurrence of fat emboli syndrome. Carefully assess every limb for the presence of distal pulses. Adequate documentation of intact sensation is critical. Pediatric bone is relatively soft and prone to incomplete fracture, such as greenstick type. Inappropriate use of a seat belt in children can also result in associated lumbar spine fractures (Chance fractures) and hollow visceral injuries, primarily of the small bowel. The clinician must be aware of associated injuries when lap seat belts are involved.

Air Bag Injuries

Air bags can save lives and prevent injuries when seat belts and car seats are used correctly. Failure to adhere to safety regulations can result in childhood fatalities. The American Academy of Pediatrics has recommended that children aged 12 years and younger ride in the back seat. Most pediatric injuries are a result of proximity to air bag deployment and unused or improperly used seat belts. A deploying air bag can reach speeds of more than 240 km/h (150 mph), so it is not surprising that internal organ injuries have been reported. In children facing forward, injuries include abrasions and friction burns to the face, neck, chest, inner arms, and upper thighs. As the child moves closer, more severe head and neck injuries can occur, such as basilar skull fractures and/or SCIWORA. The safest place for a child is in the middle of the back seat, either in a safety seat or in a 3-point restraint.

Burns

Major burns contribute to a substantial percentage of the mortality in children. Airway management is important and elective intubation is considered if you find inhalation injury, facial burns, singed eyebrows or nasal hair, or carbonaceous sputum. Assess the percentage of the body surface area (BSA) burned but do not follow the "rule of 9's" in children; a chart can be useful for this determination. Provide volume resuscitation initially as you would in all trauma patients but after you have assessed the area of burn, the fluid replacement recommended is lactated Ringer's at 3–4 ml/kg/% BSA in addition to maintenance fluids. Infuse this volume over the first 24 hours, with half going in during the initial eight hours. After all the clothing is removed, clean the burns with sterile saline and apply a moist non-occlusive dressing. Transfer children to a burn center if any of the following are present: partial or full thickness burns over 10% of the BSA; full thickness burns over 5% of the BSA; burns to the face, hands, feet, genitalia, perineum or major joints; circumferential burns; electrical or chemical burns; burns associated with inhalation injury.

Child Abuse: Possibility of Abuse

Whenever you treat children with traumatic injuries, you must be attuned to the possibility of abuse. Many types of injury can be the result of an abusive family member or friend. Clues to abuse include a history that is not consistent with the injury, a delay in seeking treatment, injuries in different phases of healing and multiple healed fractures on radiographs. Because your goal is to ensure the safety and well being of the children you treat, thoroughly investigate any suspicious circumstances and, if needed, report your findings to the appropriate authorities.

Child abuse includes physical abuse, sexual abuse, emotional abuse, and child neglect. Child abuse involves children of all ages and crosses all socioeconomic boundaries, although poverty, a young single parent, and substance abuse contribute to the risk factors. Most abused children are younger than 3 years, with one-third being younger than 6 months.

Because signs and symptoms of abuse can be subtle, maintain a high level of clinical awareness when evaluating these children. The history and mechanism of alleged trauma must be consistent. Infants and children younger than 2 years are more prone to present with closed-head trauma as a result of SBS. Older children, as they begin to explore their surroundings, are more likely to sustain physical abuse as a form of discipline, so abdominal trauma, skeletal trauma, and cutaneous injuries are more commonly observed. Prepubescent children and adolescents often experience sexual abuse and are less likely to report such assaults. Certain characteristic findings may suggest child abuse.

Fundoscopic examination may reveal retinal hemorrhages suggesting SBS. Radiographic skeletal survey may demonstrate multiple fractures in various stages of healing.

ACUTE CARE

Prehospital Care

Emergency medical team must be trained in rapid pediatric cardiorespiratory assessment, prompt establishment of effective ventilation (airway), oxygenation (breathing), and perfusion (circulation), as well as in stabilization and transport of injured or ill children to the treatment facility. The medical team is the first medical contact (first responder) that children have following an injury. No objective studies compare the "scoop-and-run" philosophy to the "stay-and-play" philosophy in children, but resuscitation should be tailored to each child and should begin in the field. Dedicate time in the field to securing the airway. Do not extend the time with multiple attempts to establish intravenous access. If direct transport to a designated trauma facility is not possible because of great distance or a child's instability, take the child to the nearest emergency department for stabilization.

Initial Assessment and Resuscitation

The primary survey or initial phase of resuscitation should address life-threatening injuries that compromise oxygenation and circulation. Make evaluation of the child's ABCs, disability, and exposure the priority of this initial phase. Airway control is the first priority.

Airway for Normal Breathing

Unlike in adults, the cause of childhood cardiac arrest is an initial respiratory arrest. A child's airway is anatomically different from an adult's. A child has a shorter neck, smaller and anterior larynx, floppy epiglottis, short trachea, and large tongue. If oral intubation is indicated, use the jaw-thrust maneuver to improve airway patency. All pediatric trauma patients must be assumed to have cervical spine injury until proven otherwise. Thus, if oral intubation is indicated, in-line cervical spine immobilization must be performed. Nasotracheal intubation is not recommended due to the small nasal passages in young children.

Estimate the size of the endotracheal tube by the child's fifth digit or by the formula (age + 16)/4. The subglottic trachea is the narrowest portion of the pediatric airway and provides a "physiologic cuff", so use uncuffed endotracheal tubes in children younger than 8 years in order to minimize tracheal trauma. Use a rapid-sequence intubation technique to facilitate successful intubation. If oral intubation is contraindicated in patients with severe maxillofacial or laryngotracheal trauma, then perform needle cricothyrotomy. Surgical cricothyroidotomy is rarely indicated in infants or small children because of the high association with secondary subglottic stenosis.

Infants and small children have proportionately larger heads than adults, and when a child is lying supine, flexion of the neck can occur to the point of airway obstruction. By placing small children in the "sniffing position", midface slightly anterior and superior, this problem can be prevented. Also, because a child's tongue is proportionately larger relative to the mouth than in an adult and may cause obstruction, the chin is lifted to move the tongue forward. Infants are obligate nose breathers, so take special attention to suction the nasal passages free from debris.

Depending on the status of the child, you may use various measures to maintain a patent airway. In a spontaneously breathing and crying child, you can use an oral airway to keep the tongue from occluding the posterior pharynx. Insert the appropriate size airway while maintaining C-spine control. By adding a mask, you can give additional oxygen to a child with a patent airway. For optimal results, be sure you have a tight seal.

For children who cannot maintain an airway, you must perform endotracheal intubation. You may also decide to intubate at-risk children before they are transported.

Breathing

After you have a secure airway in the traumatized child, adequate oxygenation and ventilation should be assured. Auscultate to assess for equal breath sounds. In small infants, breath sounds may be transmitted from the contralateral side so an early chest radiograph is important. In addition to listening for equal breath sounds, observe the child for grunting, nasal flaring and the use of accessory muscles; all are signs of impending respiratory distress. Monitor the respiratory rate; tachypnea is based on the normal respiratory rate for the child's age.

If respiration is inadequate, provide ventilatory assistance. Infants and small children are primarily diaphragmatic breathers; their ribs lack the rigidity and configuration present in adults. As a result, any compromise of diaphragmatic excursion significantly limits the child's ability to ventilate. Direct injury to the diaphragm, disruption and herniation of intra-abdominal contents, or gastric distention (aerophagia) can severely compromise the infant or small child's ability to breathe. The mediastinum of a child is very mobile; therefore, mediastinal structures can shift into the contralateral hemithorax as a result of a simple pneumothorax, hemothorax, or tension pneumothorax. The clinician must recognize these emergencies and intervene as needed.

In these very early moments of the child's care, one should be alert for two life-threatening thoracic injuries—tension pneumothorax and pericardial tamponade.

Tension pneumothorax: Tension pneumothorax can occur in the absence of external signs of thoracic trauma because children have a very compliant chest wall. Also, a simple pneumothorax can progress to a tension pneumothorax after the child is intubated and on positive-pressure ventilation. Signs of tension pneumothorax include absent breath sounds on the affected side, hypotension, tracheal deviation, jugular venous distention and possible electromechanical dissociation. If a tension pneumothorax is diagnosed, the child needs an immediate needle thoracostomy. You do this by inserting a venflon high and anterior on the chest wall so that the air may be released. This is attached to a IV tubing, the remote of which is inserted into a bottle of saline. After the child is stabilized, the definitive intercostal tube drain is inserted.

Pericardial tamponade: Pericardial tamponade is another problem that one must address immediately. Signs of tamponade include muffled heart tones, hypotension, jugular venous distention and possible electromechanical dissociation. This condition calls for an immediate pericardiocentesis. To do this, insert a needle attached to a syringe, into the subxiphoid space and direct the needle toward the left shoulder at a 15° to 30° downward angle. The needle is advanced while withdrawing on it until there is blood return. If blood or air is found in the pericardial space, connect the syringe to a stopcock for repeated aspiration. At the same time, prepare for an emergency thoracotomy or sternotomy.

Assess Child's Hemodynamic Status and Circulation

With the airway open and the child's breathing assured, the next step is to assess the child's hemodynamic status, control hemorrhage and make sure you have intravenous access.

Control Hemorrhage

To control ongoing hemorrhage, identify the external sites and use direct pressure and elevation techniques. Occasionally pneumatic splints can be used to assist in controlling bleeding, although the pneumatic antishock garment is no longer routinely used. If it has been placed on the child at another emergency facility, slowly decompress one compartment at a time to avoid severe shock due to large blood-volume shifts.

Assess for Shock

Recognizing hypovolemic shock in pediatric trauma patients is essential to ensure a positive outcome. Shock is a state of insufficient delivery of oxygen to the cells. The most common form of shock in a child who has sustained trauma is hemorrhagic shock from excessive blood loss. Acidosis occurs due to the accumulation of lactic acid, a byproduct of anaerobic metabolism. The child's respiratory rate increases to correct the pH. Tachycardia also occurs, although this is not a specific sign. Tachycardia is usually the earliest measurable response to hypovolemia. Heart contractility increases in the older child but is not a mechanism readily available to the infant and small child. In addition, an increase in vasomotor tone shunts the blood to the essential organs. This results in decreased capillary refill. To check capillary refill, compress the nail bed or hypothenar eminence and watch for immediate blanching. The time to return to normal color is the capillary refill time. Normally this is less than two seconds; a longer time indicates decreased perfusion. Late signs of hemorrhagic shock include hypotension and initial agitation and then decreased mental status and oliguria. Obvious signs of shock, such as hypotension or a decrease in urinary output, may not occur until more than 30% of blood volume has been lost.

Children are known to have an amazing cardiovascular reserve, so the initial normal vital signs should not impart any sense of security with regard to the status of the child's circulating volume.

Normal Vital Signs

	Pulse (beats/min)	*Systolic blood pressure (mm Hg)*	*Respiration (breaths/min)*
Newborn	95-145	60-90	30-60
Infant	125-170	75-100	30-60
Toddler	100-160	80-110	24-40
Preschool	70-110	80-110	22-34
School age	70-110	85-120	18-30
Adolescent	55-100	95-120	12-16

Vascular Access

Make vascular access the next priority once adequate ABCs are established. If possible, place two percutaneous intravenous catheters in the upper extremities. If peripheral venous access cannot be obtained after 3 attempts or in less than 90 seconds, establish intraosseous access in children younger than 6 years. You can use a bone marrow aspiration needle or a commercially available kit. The tibia is the most accessible site. Insert the needle with a screwing motion one to two centimeters below the tibial tuberosity until resistance gives way, and aspirate the marrow to confirm placement. In addition to replacing fluids with this site, you can use it for drawing laboratory samples for testing and for giving medications.

A saphenous vein cut down and cannulation of central veins is other option, but these techniques should be reserved for stable patients and skilled personnel. For central access one can use the subclavian or femoral veins. Femoral catheterization is easy to learn and has few complications in the acute period. To prevent infectious complications, replace all of the emergently placed access devices with more permanent access after the child is stabilized.

Fluid Resuscitation

Initial fluid resuscitation should consist of warm isotonic crystalloid solution (Ringer lactate or isotonic sodium chloride solution) at a bolus of 20 ml/kg. The goals of the initial resuscitation should be to achieve hemodynamic normality and to restore adequate tissue perfusion as soon as possible. The bolus can be repeated twice if complete response is not obtained initially. Children with evidence of hemorrhagic shock who fail to response to fluid resuscitation should also receive blood (10 ml/kg) and are evaluated by a pediatric surgeon for possible operative intervention.

Estimation of blood loss and normal blood volume may guide component replacement. In general, younger patients have a higher fraction of their body weight as blood volume. Obese patients tend to have a lower fraction. To estimate blood volume, multiply 70 by the patient's weight in kilograms. For example, a 30 kg child would estimate 2100 ml of blood volume. Estimation of volume required to replace loss multiplies the estimated blood volume by the fractional change in hematocrit. For example, a 30 kg child with a hematocrit of 0.26, whose normal hematocrit is 0.36, would have a fractional change in hematocrit of 0.28 ([0.36-0.26]/0.36) and an estimated blood loss of 588 ml (0.28 × 2100).

Avoid accidental hypothermia during the initial phase of resuscitation. Hypothermia results in vasoconstriction, low-flow state, acidosis, and consumptive coagulopathy. To prevent hypothermia, use warm intravenous fluids. Once the patient is exposed, cover the patient with a warm blanket. Connective air re-warmers (Bear Hugger) and warmed, humidified ventilation can help maintain core body temperature if hypothermia is detected (<35°C/95°F). Peritoneal lavage with warm saline may assist with hypothermia refractory to prior measures.

Once the primary survey has been completed, address the issue of pain control. Manage pain on a case-by-case basis. Pain relief can be provided with morphine (0.1 mg/kg) or a combination of fentanyl (1 mcg/kg) and midazolam (0.5-0.1 mg/kg).

Definitive treatment can be accomplished safely once hypoxia, tachycardia, hypotension, and hypothermia have been managed. The secondary survey involves a more detailed systemic evaluation and initiation of diagnostic studies.

Full exposure is necessary for a complete survey. To avoid missing any injuries, all the clothes are removed and the child is exposed fully so that a complete head-to-toe examination can be done. Roll the child to look at the back, and also do a rectal exam to assess tone and bleeding. Insert a nasogastric tube to prevent gastric dilatation or aspiration from vomiting. Place a urinary catheter to monitor urine output and to check for the presence of blood. If a boy has blood in the scrotum or at the urethral meatus, or if there is a high-riding prostate, do a retrograde urethrogram before catheter insertion.

DIAGNOSTIC MODALITIES

As with adults, radiographic evaluation of the cervical spine, chest, and pelvis has become an integral part of assessment of injured children. Radiographic evaluation of the pediatric cervical spine can be challenging because of normal anatomical variants and should be performed by experienced personnel. Once the initial trauma X-ray films (cervical spine series, anteroposterior chest and pelvis series) have been cleared, perform further imaging studies (CT scans of head, chest, abdomen, and pelvis) on a case-by-case basis, depending on the mechanism of injury.

Assessment of Blunt Abdominal Trauma in Children

Blunt trauma is responsible for most intra-abdominal injuries. Injuries of solid organs predominate, particularly injuries of the spleen, followed by the liver and kidney. However, the mortality rate for children from severe blunt trauma is higher than the rate from penetrating injuries because of concurrent CNS, chest, and skeletal injuries. Fortunately, nonoperative management has a 90% success rate and has become the standard of care. In children who are hemodynamically stable with possible thoracoabdominal injury, CT scan is the preferred imaging technique.

The most commonly used indications for an abdominal CT scan are abdominal bruising (seat belt sign) and gross hematuria. Establishing a diagnosis of hollow viscus injury with CT scan is extremely challenging. Common findings when a bowel perforation has occurred or is severely contused are thickening of the bowel wall and collection of free fluid. Focal points of free air, mesenteric thickening or stranding, bowel dilatation, and focal hematoma are also suggestive of hollow viscus injury when encountered on an abdominal CT scan. At least 30% of children with hollow viscus injury will have no evidence of such on CT scan, thereby emphasizing the need for clinical vigilance.

Diagnostic peritoneal lavage (DPL) has a limited role in the assessment of intra-abdominal injury. Children are more likely to have solid organ injury without hemoperitoneum; therefore, a CT scan is preferable. DPL is indicated for children with coexisting injuries (head or orthopedic injuries) requiring immediate surgical intervention and with no time for CT scanning.

FAST is slowly gaining acceptance as a reliable method to evaluate patients with trauma, particularly individuals who are hemodynamically unstable. FAST has several advantages over CT scan and DPL. FAST is portable and easy to use, and it can be performed in minutes. It is noninvasive, fairly accurate in identifying fluid in the peritoneal cavity or pericardial sac, and costs less than CT scan. A review of relevant pediatric literature performed by Murphy demonstrated the sensitivity of FAST examination to be 30-87.5% and the specificity to be 42-100%. Adult series have reported a higher sensitivity with FAST examination for hemoperitoneum. As noted in a recent review, a FAST examination can miss significant spleen or liver injury. Up to 40% of low-grade liver and spleen injury and 11% of high-grade liver and spleen injury will be missed based on a negative FAST examination.

A role for laparoscopy, as both diagnostic and potentially therapeutic, has been suggested for the evaluation of blunt and penetrating abdominal injuries in hemodynamically stable patients. Proposed benefits include avoiding morbidity of a negative laparotomy, improved diagnostic accuracy, and shorter ICU and hospital length of stays. With local wound exploration demonstrating penetration of anterior abdominal fascia, a laparoscopic survey may be useful. Indications for laparoscopic evaluation in patients with blunt abdominal trauma include suspicious examination findings, such as abdominal wall contusions, peritonitis, and a declining hematocrit. The child with blunt abdominal trauma and free peritoneal fluid but no radiographic solid organ injury presents the greatest dilemma. Delayed diagnosis of a bowel injury in this setting would be a substantial cause of morbidity.

BATTERED BABY

The term 'battered baby syndrome' is defined a clinical condition, usually in children under 3 years of age, who have suffered non-accidental injury, on one or more occasions, by an adult in a position of trust, generally a parent, guardian or a foster parent. The injuries may be minimal or severe, sometimes even fatal and there may be associated deprivation of care and nutrition. It is very common to find a discrepancy between the history and the clinical findings. The neglect and lack of care in these children may result in complications and deformities.

SHAKEN BABY SYNDROME

Shaken baby syndrome (SBS) is a violent act of abuse that can cause myriad neurologic, cognitive, and other functional deficits. In the most serious cases, death can result. Health care practitioners, child care providers, and parents must be educated on the signs of SBS. Cases should be thoroughly reviewed and prevention strategies developed to prevent future incidents.

Retinal hemorrhages are the most common fundus finding in the shaken baby syndrome. They vary in type and location; no particular type is pathognomonic for the condition. Retinal hemorrhages are not needed to make a diagnosis of shaken baby syndrome. However, in a child under age 3 years, the presence of extensive bilateral retinal hemorrhages raises a very strong possibility of abuse, which must be investigated. The other possible causes for hemorrhages in this age child can be investigated and eliminated. The diagnosis of abuse should be made by someone particularly trained in this area, who can put together the entire picture of inadequate or changing history, fractures of various ages, particularly rib fractures, subdural hematoma of the brain, and retinal hemorrhages. Photographs of retinal hemorrhages are very helpful to child advocacy experts who take these cases to court.

Shaken baby syndrome should be suspected in all children younger than one year of age who present with drowsiness, external trauma to the head or fracture of the clavaria. A combination of clinical findings in infants with intracranial and intraocular hemorrhage in the absence of coma, seizures or apnea should arouse the suspicion of SBS. These shaking injuries were thought to be caused by the easily torn bridging veins of infants head. The infants head and blood vessels are particularly vulnerable to shaking and whiplash because of the relatively large head and weak neck muscles of the child, the abundance of unmyelinated brain tissue which permits excessive stretching of the brain and vessels, and the increased pliability of the skull as compared to the rigidly fixed internal soft tissue structures such as falx cerebri.

In contrast to the "Battered baby syndrome" all the findings in whiplash shaken baby syndromes of infants are subtle and demand awareness, an index of suspicion and a fundus examination. Intraocular hemorrhages can range from minimal to severe. Therefore in a child under 3 years of age, the presence of extensive bilateral retinal hemorrhages raises a very strong possibility of SBS, which must be investigated. Ophthalmic examination of children with suspected SBS is important for prognostic as well as diagnostic purposes. Diffuse fundic bleeds, vitreous hemorrhage or large subhyaloid hemorrhages are usually associated with worse visual outcome. Nonreactive pupils and midline shifts of the brain structure correlates highly with mortality and more severe neurologic injury. Many are fatal. Of the survivors, up to 60% may have neurological sequalae which include seziures, cerebral palsy and blindness. There is a spectrum of the consequences of SBS and less severe cases may not be brought to the attention of medical professionals. A victim of sublethal shaking may have a history of poor feeding, vomiting, lethargy and or irritability occurring for days or week. Signs of SBS may vary from mild and nonspecific to severe and immediately identifiable clinically as head trauma. In the most severe cases which usually result in death or severe neurologic consequences the child usually becomes immediately unconscious and suffers rapidly escalating life-threatening CNS dysfunction.

SUMMARY

Caring for pediatric patients with trauma is a complex and integrated process that requires knowledge of the special considerations of pediatric trauma patients and understanding of the pathophysiology and special requirements of the pediatric population. Providing this care is an exercise in psychomotor skill, surgical judgment, and intellectual reasoning. Approach the treatment of the injured child with a rational and meticulous plan of action that not only leads to expeditious diagnosis and therapeutic intervention but also provides efficient and effective care for the patient.

The pediatric trauma patient is evaluated following the same general principles used for managing an adult trauma patient with the exceptions outlined in this article. The goal is to stabilize injured children by thoroughly assessing them for injuries, appropriately treating these injuries and transferring them to a tertiary care center when appropriate. In addition, education of parents, teachers and children about injury prevention should be a priority because of its value in saving countless lives and money.

BIBLIOGRAPHY

1. Ball JW, Liao E, Kavanaugh D, Turgel C. The emergency medical services for children program: accomplishments and contributions. Clin Pediatr Emerg Med 2006;7(1):6-14.
2. Densmore JC, Lim HJ, Oldham KT, Guice KS. Outcomes and delivery of care in pediatric injury. J Pediatr Surg 2006;41(1):92-8.
3. Jewett EA, Anderson MR, Gilchrist GS. The pediatric subspecialty workforce: public policy and forces for change. Pediatr 2005;116 (5):1192-1202.
4. Kissoon N, Dreyer J, Walia M. Paediatric trauma: Differences in pathology, injury pattern and treatment copared with adult trauma. Can Med Assoc J 1990;142:27-34.
5. MacKenzie EJ, Rivara FP, Jurkovich GJ, et al. A national evaluation of the effect of trauma-center care on mortality. N Engl J Med. 2006;354 (4):366-78.
6. Pressley JC, Barlow B, Durkin M, Jacko SA, Dominguez DR, Johnson L. A national program for injury prevention in children and adolescents: the injury free coalition for kids. J Urban Health 2005;82 (3):389-402.
7. Pyles LA, Knapp JF. American Academy of Pediatrics, Committee on Pediatric Emergency Medicine. Role of pediatricians in advocating life support training courses for parents and the public. Pediatr 2004;114(6):e761.
8. Walker PJ, Cass DT. Paediatric trauma: Urban epidemiology and an analysis of methods for assessing the severity of trauma in 598 injured children. Aust N Zealand J Surg 1987;57:715-22.
9. Yamamoto LG. American Academy of Pediatrics, Committee on Pediatric Emergency Medicine. Access to optimal emergency care for children. Pediatr 2007;119(1):161-4.

Index

Page numbers followed by *f* refer to figure and *t* refer to table

A

D

E

I

J

K

L

M

N

O

P

Q

R

S